READY RECKONER IN
COMMUNITY
MEDICINE

READY RECKONER IN
COMMUNITY MEDICINE

Dr. MANGALA S.

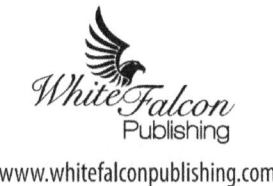

WhiteFalcon
Publishing

www.whitefalconpublishing.com

Ready Reckoner in Community Medicine
Dr. Mangala S.

www.whitefalconpublishing.com

CONTENTS

PART 2

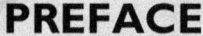

PREFACE

Community Medicine is a vast subject and the book "Ready Reckoner in Community Medicine" has been written keeping in mind the medical, dental, nursing and paramedical undergraduate and postgraduate students. I am sure this book will be of immense help to all the students, especially prior to their examinations.

I, wholeheartedly, thank the Chairperson, Mrs DA Kalpaja, of Vydehi Institute of Medical Sciences and Research Centre for her constant encouragement and invaluable help in my academic career.

I am grateful to all my colleagues in the Department of Community Medicine for their continued support in all my endeavours.

I am also thankful to my family and all my friends for inspiring me to write this book.

Dr Mangala Subramanian

PART 1

PART I

CHAPTER 1

HEALTH & DISEASE

Preventive Medicine

The science and art of preventing disease, prolonging life and promoting health and efficiency through organized community effort.

Social medicine

The study of man as a social being in his total environment and the role of social factors in disease etiology (eg. Socio-economic status, lifestyle, habits, interpersonal relationships).

Community Medicine

This deals with populations and comprises of doctors who measure the needs of the population, both sick and well, plan and administer services to meet those needs and engage in research and teaching in the field.

Health for All

The 30th World Health Assembly held in 1977 resolved that the main social target of governments and WHO in the coming decades should be the attainment by all citizens of the world, by the year 2000, a level of health that will permit them to lead a socially and economically productive life – HFA 2000.

Primary Health Care

It is the key to achieve HFA 2000; is essential health care made universally accessible to individuals and acceptable to them through their full participation and at a cost the community and country can afford.

CONCEPTS OF HEALTH AND DISEASE

Health

A state of complete physical, mental and social well-being and not merely the absence of disease or infirmity and the ability to lead a socially and economically productive life.

Dimensions of Health

1. **Physical Dimension:**
    state of perfect functioning of the body wherein every cell and organ functions at optimum capacity.
2. **Mental Dimension:**
    The ability to deal with experiences of life with flexibility and a sense of purpose.
    Psychosomatic diseases eg. Hypertension, Peptic Ulcer, Bronchial Asthma.
    Major mental diseases eg. Depression, Schizophrenia
3. **Social Dimension:**
    Man and his inter-relationship with other members of the society.
4. **Spiritual Dimension:**
    The role of God in health. Studies have shown that those who believe in prayers and God, heal faster and their duration of stay in the hospital also decreases
5. **Emotional Dimension:**
    It relates to feelings of joy, happiness, worry, grief, fear and anger.
6. **Vocational Dimension:**
    Work can promote health if it is fully adapted to human goals, capacities and limitations and leads to satisfaction and increased self-esteem
7. **Others:**
    Philosophical, Socio-economic, Cultural, Environmental, Educational, Nutritional, Curative and Preventive

Physical Quality of Life Index (PQLI)

indicator of quality of life.
Comprises of three indicators:
  1. Infant mortality
  2. Life expectancy at age one
  3. Literacy

For each component, the individual countries' performance is placed on a scale of 0-100 (0 represents the worst performance and 100 represents the best performance). Averaging these 3 indicators, the composite index is calculated.

GNP is not considered in PQLI, showing that money is not everything.

Middle East countries have a high per capita income but less PQLI than Sri Lanka and the state of Kerala in India.

The ultimate objective is to attain a PQLI of 100.

Human Development Index (HDI)

Comprises of three indicators
1. Longevity (Life expectancy at birth)
2. Knowledge (Adult literacy rate and mean years of schooling)
3. Income (Real GDP per capita in US $)

HDI is a more comprehensive measure than per capita income.
HDI values range between $0 - 1$.

For the indicators maximum and minimum values have been established.

- Life expectancy at birth: 25 years and 85 years
- Adult literacy rate: 0% and 100%
- Combined gross enrollment ratio: 0% and 100%
- Real GDP per capita: $100 and $40,000

Individual Indices can be calculated by the formula:

$$\text{Index} = \frac{(\text{Actual } X_1 \text{ Value}) - (\text{Minimum } X_1 \text{ value})}{(\text{Maximum } X_1 \text{ value}) - (\text{Minimum } X_1 \text{ value})}$$

Eg. India:

$$\text{Life Expectancy Index} = \frac{68.3 - 20}{83.2 - 20} = 0.764$$

$$\text{Mean years of Schooling Index} = \frac{6.3-0}{13.2-0} = 0.477$$

$$\text{Expected years of Schooling Index} = \frac{11.7-0}{20.6-0} = 0.568$$

$$\text{Education Index} = \frac{\sqrt{0.477 \times 0.568} - 0}{0.951 - 0} = 0.547$$

$$\text{Income Index} = \frac{5663 - 163}{108{,}211 - 163} = 0.546$$

$$\text{HDI} = \sqrt[3]{0.764 \times 0.547 \times 0.546} = 0.611$$

Health and Development

Health and development are interlinked. Economic development alone cannot solve the problems of poverty, hunger, malnutrition and disease. Non-economic issues namely education, employment, housing, equity, freedom and dignity, human welfare are equally important in development strategies.

Eg. Sri Lanka, Costa Rica and Kerala (India) have shown that health forms a part of development.

Kerala State

Through strong political commitment to equitable socio-economic development, high levels of health can be achieved with modest levels of income. Literacy, especially female literacy has played a key role in improving health by improving utilization of health services.

Improved transport network and promotion of land reforms has revealed that good health at a low cost is attainable by poor countries but it requires major political and social commitments.

Health Development

The process of continuous progressive improvement of the health status of a population.

Health Indicators

Health is multi-dimensional therefore measurement is also multi-dimensional.

1. Mortality indicators
2. Morbidity indicators
3. Disability rates

4. Nutritional status indicators

5. Health care delivery indicators

6. Utilizations rates

7. Indicators of social and mental health

8. Environmental indicators

9. Socio-economic indicators

10. Health policy indicators

11. Quality of life indicators

12. Other indicators

I. *Mortality Indicators*

(a) Crude Death Rate – No. of deaths per 1000 population per year in a given community

$$\frac{\text{No. of deaths}}{\text{Mid-Year Population}} \times 1000$$

(b) Life Expectancy – Average No. of years that will be lived by those born alive into a population, if current age specific mortality rates persist. Males 67; Females 69.

(c) Infant Mortality rate – ratio of deaths under 1 year of age in a given year to total No. of live births in the same year expressed as the rate per 1000 live births (34/1000 live births).

(d) Child Mortality rate – No. of deaths of children within the age of 1-4 years in a given year, per 1000 children of 1–4 years.

$$\frac{\text{No. of deaths of 1-4 years during a year}}{\text{Total children of 1-4 years in the middle of the year}} \times 1000$$

(e) Under 5 Mortality rate – Annual No. of deaths of children under 5 years expressed as rate per 1000 live births

$$\frac{\text{No. of deaths of children} <5 \text{ years during a year}}{\text{No. of live births in the same area and year}} \times 1000$$

(f)   Maternal Mortality Ratio (MMR)

$$\frac{\text{Total No. of female deaths due to complications of pregnancy, child birth or within 42 days of delivery from puerperal causes in an area during a given year}}{\text{Total No. of births in the same area and year}} \times 100,000$$

(g)   Disease specific mortality
      Eg. TB.

$$\text{Specific death rate due to TB} = \frac{\text{No. of deaths due to TB during the calendar year}}{\text{Mid-year population}} \times 1000$$

(h)   Proportional Mortality Rate – proportion of all deaths currently attributed to it eg. coronary heart disease causes 25 – 30% of all deaths in western countries.

2.   *Morbidity indicators*

(a)   Incidence and Prevalence
(b)   Notification Rates
(c)   Attendance Rates at OPDs and Health Centres
(d)   Admission, Re-admission, Discharge Rates
(e)   Duration of stay in hospital
(f)   Spells of sickness or Absence from work or school

3.   *Disability rates*

(a)   Event type indicators
      i.   No. of days of restricted activity
      ii. Bed disability days
      iii. Work loss days or school loss days within a specified period
(b)   Person type indicators
      i.   Limitation of mobility: Eg. Confined to bed, confined to house, special aid in getting around inside or outside the house.
      ii. Limitation of activity: Eg. Limitation in performing ADL (Activities of Daily Living) such as eating, washing, dressing, going to toilet, moving about
      iii. Limitation of major activity: Ability to work, ability to do house work

Sullivan's Index: Expectation of a life free of disability is calculated by subtracting duration of bed disability and inability to perform major activities from the life expectancy probable, according to cross sectional data from population surveys.

Eg. In USA the expectation of life is 70.2 and the Sullivan's Index is 64.9

HALE – Health Adjusted Life Expectancy:

The equivalent number of years in full health that a newborn can expect to live based on the current rates of ill health and mortality.

DALY – Disability Adjusted Life Year:

It measures the burden of disease in a defined population and the effectiveness of interventions.

DALYs expresses the years of life lost to premature death and the years lived with disability.

4. Nutritional status indicators

  (a) Prevalence of low birth weight
  (b) Anthropometric measurements of pre-school children
  (c) Heights, weights of children at school entry

5. Health care delivery indicators

  (a) Doctor - Population ratio
  (b) Doctor - Nurse ratio
  (c) Population - Bed ratio
  (d) Population per Health Centre/Sub-centre
  (e) Population per traditional birth attendant

6. Utilization rates

The proportion of people in need of service and who actually receive it in a given period, usually a year. Eg. Proportion of infants fully immunized against 6 EPI diseases, proportion of pregnant women who receive ante-natal care or have deliveries by trained birth attendants, the percentage of population using various methods of family planning, Bed Occupancy Rate, Average length of stay and the Bed Turn-over Ratio.

7. Indicators of Social and Mental Health

Indirect measures – Suicide, homicide, family violence, battered baby syndrome, battered wife syndrome, road traffic accidents, juvenile delinquency, alcohol abuse, smoking, drug abuse, consumption of tranquilizers, obesity

8. Environmental indicators

Proportion of population having access to safe water and sanitation
Indicators of air and water pollution, radiation, solid waste, noise, exposure to toxic substances in food or drinks

9. Socio economic indicators

Rate of population increase, per capita GNP, level of unemployment, dependency ratio, literacy especially female literacy rates, family size, housing: No. of persons per room, per capita calorie availability

10. Health Policy indicators

Proportion of GNP spent on health services, proportion of GNP spent on health-related activities (water, sanitation, housing, community development, nutrition), proportion of total health resources spent on primary health care.

11. Indicators of quality of life

PQLI – Physical Quality of Life Index (Infant mortality, Life Expectancy at age 1 and Literacy)

12. Other indicators

(a) Social indicators – Population, family formation, learning & educational services, earning activities, distribution of income, social security, welfare services, health services and nutrition, housing, environment, leisure, culture
(b) Basic needs indicators – Calorie consumption, access to water, life expectancy, deaths due to disease, illiteracy, doctors and nurses per population, rooms per person, GNP per capita.
(c) HFA indicators

Indicators for monitoring progress towards Health For All (HFA):

1. Health Policy Indicators:
   • Political commitment to HFA
   • Resource allocation
   • Health services – equity of distribution
   • Community involvement
   • Organizational framework and managerial process

2. Social & Economic Indicators
   • Rate of population increase
   • GNP or GDP

- Income distribution
- Work conditions
- Literacy rate
- Housing
- Food availability

3. Indicators for provision of Health Care
   - Availability
   - Accessibility
   - Utilization
   - Quality of care

4. Health Status Indicators
   - Low birth weight percentage
   - Nutritional status and psycho-social development
   - Life expectancy of children at birth
   - IMR
   - Child mortality rate (1-4 years)
   - Maternal mortality ratio
   - Disease specific mortality rate
   - Morbidity – Incidence; prevalence
   - Disability prevalence

(d) Millennium Development Goal Indicators
   Health related millennium development goals and indicators

Goal 1. Eradicate extreme poverty and hunger
   Indicator 1. Prevention of underweight children under 5 years of age
            2. Proportion of population below minimum level of dietary energy consumption

Goal 2. Reduce child mortality
   Indicator 1. Mortality rate of children under 5 years of age
            2. Infant mortality rate
            3. Proportion of 1 year old children immunized against measles

Goal 3. Improve Maternal Health
   Indicator 1. Maternal mortality ratio
            2. Proportion of births attended by skilled health personnel

Goal 4. Combat HIV/AIDS, malaria & other diseases
   Indicator 1. HIV prevention among young people 15-24 years
            2. Condom use rate
            3. Number of children orphaned by HIV/AIDS

    4. Prevalence and death rates associated with malaria

    5. Proportion of population in malaria risk areas using effective malaria prevention and treatment measures

    6. Prevention and death rates associated with TB

    7. Proportion of TB cases detected and cured under DOTS

Goal 5. Ensure environmental sustainability

    Indicator 1. Proportion of population using solid fuel

    2. Proportion of population with sustainable access to improved water sources, urban and rural

    3. Proportion of urban population with access to improved sanitation

Goal 8. Develop a global partnership for development

    Indicator 1. Proportion of population with access to affordable essential drugs on a sustainable basis.

(e)   Sustainable Development Goals (SDGs)

    In Sept 2015, the UN General Assembly adopted the new development agenda: Transforming our world - the 2030 agenda for sustainable development comprising 17 goals.

    Goal 1 - No Poverty

    Goal 2 - Zero Hunger

    Goal 3 - Good Health & Well-being - Ensure healthy lives and promote the well-being of all at all ages

    Goal 4 - Quality Education

    Goal 5 - Gender Equality

    Goal 6 - Clean Water & Sanitation

    Goal 7 - Affordable & Clean Energy

    Goal 8 - Decent Work & Economic Growth

    Goal 9 – Industry, Innovation, Infrastructure

    Goal 10 - Reduced Inequalities

    Goal 11 - Sustainable Cities & Communities

    Goal 12 - Responsible Consumption & Production

    Goal 13 - Climate Action

    Goal 14 - Life Below Water

    Goal 15 - Life on Land

    Goal 16 - Peace, Justice & Strong Institutions

    Goal 17 - Global Partnership

SDG 3: Health has 13 Targets and 26 Indicators

Goal & Targets (By 2030)	Indicators
3.1: Reduce Global MMR <70/100,000 LB	3.1.1: MMR 3.1.2: Proportion of births attended by skilled health personnel
3.2: End preventable deaths of newborns & children < 5 years Neonatal mortality < 12/1000 LB Mortality under 5 years < 25/1000 LB	3.2.1: Neonatal mortality rate 3.2.2: Mortality rate under 5 years
3.3: End epidemics of AIDS, TB, Malaria, neglected tropical diseases, combat hepatitis, water borne diseases & other communicable diseases	3.3.1: No. of new HIV/1000 uninfected population 3.3.2: TB incidence/1000 persons/year 3.3.3: Malaria incidence/1000 persons/year 3.3.4: Hepatitis incidence/100,000 population/ year Hepatitis B vaccination coverage of 3 doses 3.3.5: No. of people requiring interventions against neglected tropical diseases
3.4: Reduce by one third premature mortality from NCDs through prevention treatment promote mental health and well-being	3.4.1: Mortality of Cardiovascular disease, Cancer, Diabetes or Chronic Respiratory diseases 3.4.2: Suicide mortality rate
3.5: Strengthen the prevention & treatment of substance abuse including narcotic drug abuse & harmful use of alcohol	3.5.1: Coverage & treatment interventions for substance use disorders Harmful use of alcohol
3.6: Halve the No. of global deaths & injuries from RTA	3.6.1: No. of road traffic fatal injury deaths within 30 days/100,000 population
3.7: Ensure universal access to sexual & reproductive health care services including FP information & education introduction of reproductive health into national strategies & programmes	3.7.1: Percentage of women of reproductive age (15-49 years) whose need for FP is satisfied with modern methods 3.7.2: Adolescent birth rate (10-14; 15-19 years) per 1000 women in that age group
3.8: Achieve Universal Health Coverage including Financial Risk Protection, access to quality essential health care services, access to safe effective quality affordable essential medicines & vaccines	3.8.1: Coverage of tracer interventions eg. child fully immunized, ART, TB treatment, Hypertension treatment, Skilled birth attendant at birth 3.8.2: Proportion of population protected against catastrophic out of pocket health expenditure

3.9: Substantially reduce the No. of deaths & illnesses from hazardous chemicals, air, water and soil pollution & contamination	3.9.1: Mortality rate due to household & ambient air pollution/lakh population Mortality rate due to hazardous chemicals, water and soil pollution and contamination
3.10: Strengthen the implementation of WHO Framework Convention on Tobacco control in all countries	3.10.1: Age standardised prevalence of current Tobacco use among persons 15 years and older
3.11: Support Research & Development of vaccines & medicines for communicable & non-communicable diseases	3.11.1: Proportion of population with access to affordable medicines & vaccines 3.11.2: Total net official development & assistance to medical research & basic health sectors
3.12: Substantially increase health financing & recruitment, development, training and retention of health workforce in developing & least developed countries and small island developing states	3.12.1: Health worker density & distribution per 10,000 population
3.13: Strengthen the capacity of all countries for early warning, risk reduction & management of national & global health risks	3.13.1: Percentage of attributes of 13 core capacities that have been attained at a specific point in time

*LB is Live Births

Levels of Health Care

Health services are organized at 3 levels:

1. **Primary Health Care**:
   It is the first level of contact for the individual with the health system.
   Essential health care is provided at the Primary Health Centers and Sub-centres
   Common health problems are managed here.

2. **Secondary Health Care:**
   The first is the referral level
   More complex problems are managed, mainly curative services at the District Hospitals and Community Health Centers

3. **Tertiary Health Care**
   Super-specialist care is provided at Regional and central level institutions and medical college hospitals.

Health Team

Definition:
A group of persons who share common health goals and objectives determined by community needs and towards the achievement of which each member contributes in accordance with his competency and skills, respecting the functions of others.

Types:
Hospital team,
Community health work team

Members:
Doctors, nurses, social workers, health assistants, female health workers, male health workers, trained dais, village health guides

Leader:
The Team must have a leader who will plan, monitor and evaluate the health services.

Services:
Depending on community needs
HFA - Referred later
Primary Health Care - Referred later

Spectrum of Health

Health and disease lie along a continuum where death is the lowest and WHO's positive health is the highest

> Positive health
> Better health
> Freedom from sickness
> Unrecognized sickness
> Mild sickness
> Severe sickness
> Death

Determinants of Health

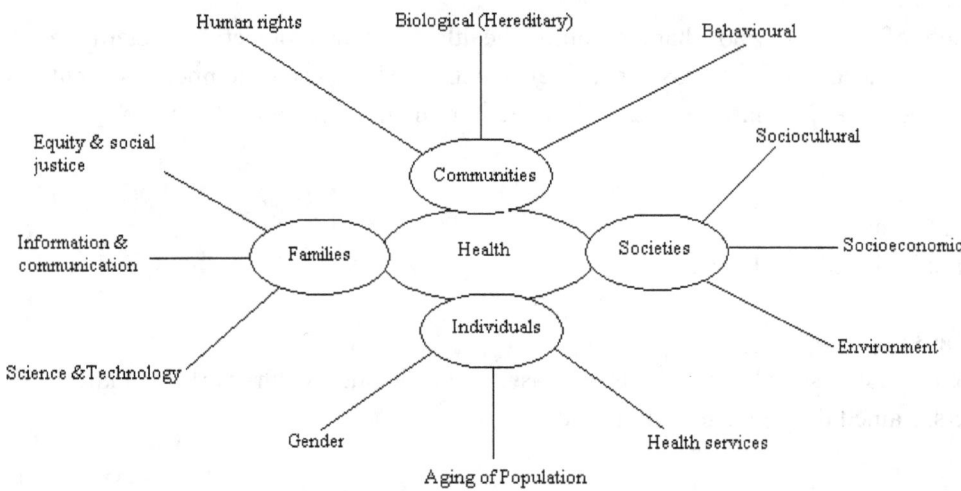

1. ***Biological determinants (Heredity)***
    Genetic constitution determines diseases e.g. Chromosomal Anomalies, Mental Retardation, Errors of Metabolism, Diabetes.
    Prevention is by Genetic Screening and Gene Therapy.

2. ***Behavioural determinants***
    Lifestyle – The way people live e.g. smoking, drinking, drugs, diseases e.g. Coronary Heart Disease, Hypertension, Obesity, Lung Ca, illnesses associated with lack of sanitation, poor nutrition, poor personal hygiene, customs, cultural patterns.

3. ***Environmental determinants***
    - Hippocrates related disease to environment e.g. Cimate, water, air
    - Internal environment - Harmonious functioning of every tissue, organ, organ system
    - External environment - External to the human host – Physical, Biological, or macro environment, Psycho-social.
    - Microenvironment – The individual's way of living and lifestyle e.g. Eating habits, personal habits (smoking, drinking, drugs)
    - Occupational environment – The environment at work
    - Socio-economic environment – Education, occupation, income, social group for interaction.
    - Moral environment

4. ***Socio economic conditions***
    - Socio economic development e.g. Per capita GNP, education, occupation, nutrition, housing, political system

- Economic progress leads to increased purchasing capacity, standard of living, quality of life, small family norms, pattern of diseases, health seeking behaviour
- Illiteracy associated with poverty, malnutrition, ill health, high infant and child mortality rates Education compensates the effect of poverty eg. Kerala state's female literacy rate is 95.2% compared to 70.3% for All India.
- Occupation – Employment promotes health because it gives income and status
- Political system – Resource allocation for health, WHO expects 5% of GNP for health whereas India spends 3% on health.

5. *Socio-cultural determinants*
   From birth to death socio-cultural factors can be seen eg. Infant and child feeding, nutrition, exercise, diet patterns, customs, habits such as open defaecation, urination, spitting everywhere

6. *Health services*
   Family welfare services – Mother and child immunization, provision of safe water, sanitation
   Primary health care - Equitably distributed, accessible at a cost the community and country can afford.

7. *Aging of population*
   8% of population in India > 60 years face Geriatric problems.

8. *Gender determinants*
   Lesser child – female child
   Women - Nutrition, reproductive health, violence, lifestyle related conditions, occupational environment

9. *Science & Technology*
   Food production, green revolution, white revolution, better treatment facilities.

10. *Information & communication*
    Easy access to information on the Internet

11. *Equity & Social Justice*
    Health care for all irrespective of paying capacity

12. *Human Rights*
    Everyone has the right to a standard of living adequate for the health and well-being of himself/herself and family.

Responsibility for Health

Individual Responsibility	Community Responsibility	State Responsibility	International Responsibility
Individuals should take responsibility for their health. Self-care: Diet, exercise, weight, sleep, smoking, alcohol, drugs, personal hygiene, yearly screening above 30 years, immunization, disease prevention measures, report early when sick and accept treatment, family planning, recording own BP, sugar	Primary health care, community participation, health care of the people by the people for the people. Community can: (i) Provide facilities, manpower, logistic support, funds. (ii) Be actively involved in planning, management & evaluation. (iii) Use the health services	Health is a state responsibility. The state shall regard raising the level of nutrition, standard of living and improvement of public health - Primary health care approach.	WHO helps nations to strengthen their health system to combat diseases eg. Eradication of small pox, health for all, campaign against smoking, AIDS

Comparison of Kerala and All-India Health Statistics (2018):

Current Status	Kerala	All-India
Death Rate/1000 population	6.9	7.3
Rural Birth Rate	13.8	21.6
Infant Mortality Rate	6.0	32
U5MR	10	36
Maternal Mortality Ratio	43	113
Annual Growth Rate	0.71	1.38
Life expectancy at birth Male Female	73.2 77.6	67.3 69.1
Literacy Rate (%)	96.2	77.7
Female Literacy Rate (%)	95.2	70.3
Mean age at marriage	23.2	22.3
Per capita income	204,105	126,521

Concept of Disease

Definition:

Disease – dis-ease, without ease; deviation from complete physical and mental well-being.

Concept of Causation

Germ Theory of Disease

Disease agent→Man→Disease

There is one to one relationship between causal agent and disease. A single agent causing disease is rare.

Epidemiological Triad

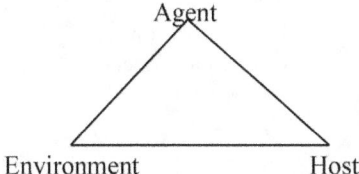

Agent Factors	Host factors	Environmental factors
1. Biological agents: Virus, bacteria, fungi, protozoa, rickettsiae 2. Nutrient agents: Proteins, fats, carbohydrates, vitamins, minerals, water. Malnutrition causes PEM, anemia, Vit A deficiency, Goitre, obesity 3. Physical agents: Heat, cold, humidity, pressure, radiation, electricity, sound 4. Chemical agents: Endogenous - Bilirubin, urea, ketones, uric acid, calcium carbonate. Exogenous – Allergens, fumes, dust, insecticides, gases 5. Mechanical agents: Friction may lead to sprains, dislocation, death 6. Absence, insufficiency, excess of a factor Chromosomal - Mongolism, congenital heart disease, nutrient factors. 7. Social agents: Poverty, smoking, drug abuse	1. Demographic characteristics: Age, sex, ethnicity 2. Biological characteristics: Genetic factors, biochemical levels of blood e.g. cholesterol, blood groups, immunological factors, physiologic functions - BP, PEFR 3. Social & economic characteristics: Socio-economic status, education, occupation, housing, marital status. 4. Lifestyle factors: Smoking, alcohol, drugs, nutrition, physical exercise	1. Physical environment: Air, water, soil, housing, climate, heat, cold, light, noise, radiation 2. Biological environment: Virus, bacteria, fungi, vectors, rodents. 3. Psycho-social environment: Man and interaction with his social group Social factors: Poverty, urbanization, migration, exposure to stress

Interaction of Agent - Host - Environment

Web of Causation for Myocardial Infarction

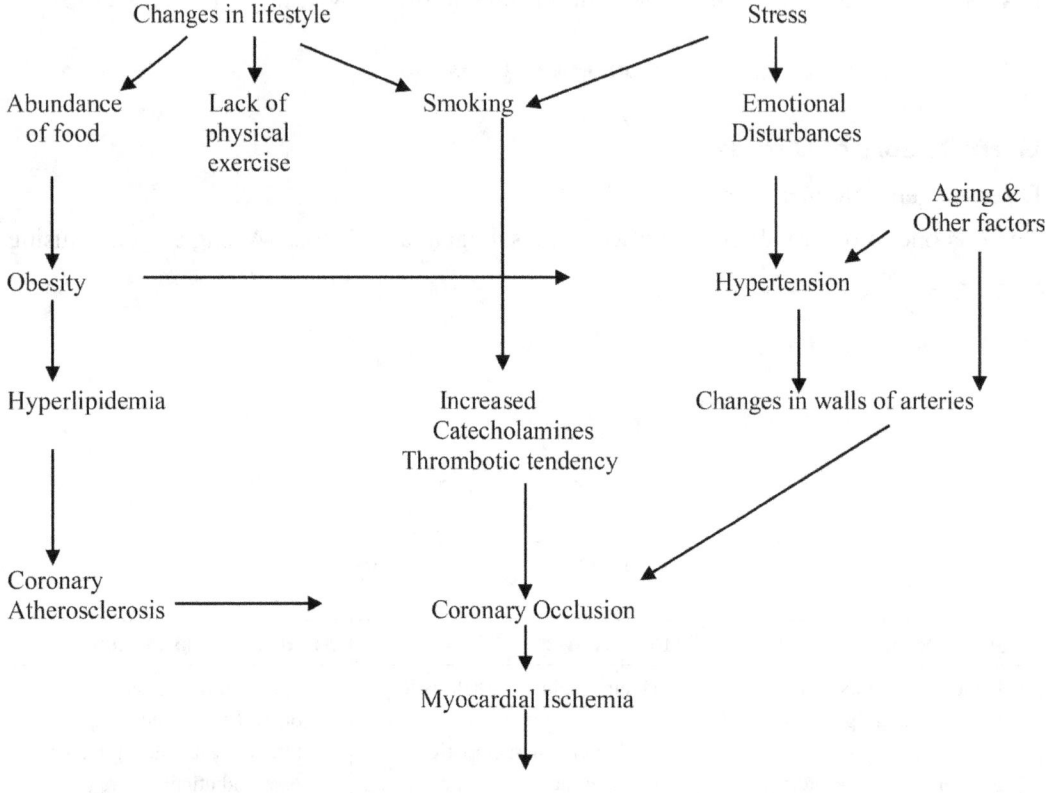

Myocardial Infarction

Web of causation considers all predisposing factors and their complex inter-relationships with one another. It depicts a variety of possible interventions that could be implemented to reduce the disease, for e.g. Myocardial Infraction.

It does not mean that all causes have to be removed to prevent the disease. Sometimes only one significant factor needs to be removed. E.g. If smoking is removed it can control the disease.

Natural History of Disease

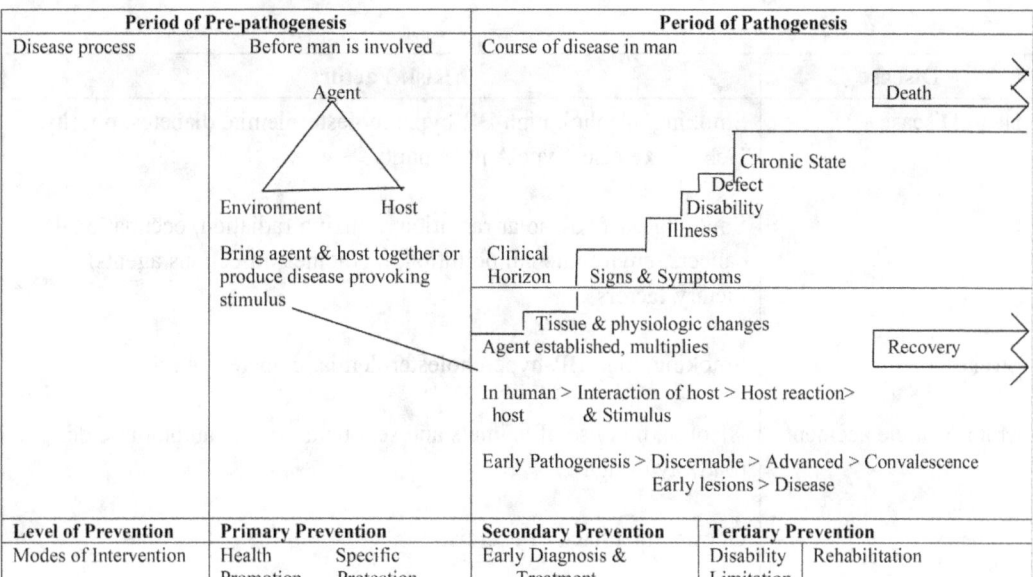

Period of Pre-pathogenesis		Period of Pathogenesis
Disease process	Before man is involved	Course of disease in man

Definition

The natural history of a disease is the way in which it evolves over time from the earliest pre-pathogenesis phase to termination which could be recovery, disability or death in the absence of treatment or prevention.

Each disease has its own natural history.

Method of Study

The best is by Cohort Study but it is costly and there is also a problem of attrition. Therefore, Cross Sectional or Case Control Studies are used.

Pre-pathogenesis phase	Pathogenesis Phase
The period prior to onset of disease in man - "Man in the midst of disease"	It begins with the entry of disease agent in the susceptible host where the → Disease agent multiplies→ Tissue & Physiological changes occur→
Epidemiological Triad – The results of interaction between the agent, host & environment	Incubation period, early & late pathogenesis→ recovery, disability or death This phase may be modified by intervention e.g. immunization, chemotherapy

Risk Factors

Disease	Risk Factors
Heart Disease	Smoking, alcohol, high BP, hypercholesterolemia, diabetes, obesity, lack of exercise, Type A personality
Cancer	Smoking, alcohol, solar radiation, ionizing radiation, occupational cancers, environmental pollution, medicines, infectious agents, dietary factors
Stroke	Smoking, high BP, hypercholesterolemia, diabetes, obesity
Motor vehicle accident	Alcohol, non-use of helmets and seat belts, speed, automobile design, roadway design
Diabetes	Obesity, diet, lack of exercise
Cirrhosis of Liver	Alcohol

Definition

An exposure which is significantly associated with the development of a disease.

The Risk factor may be:
  (i)   Truly causative e.g. Smoking for Lung Cancer
  (ii) Contributory to the undesired outcome e.g. Lack of physical exercise for Coronary Heart Disease
  (iii) Predictive only in statistical sense e.g. Illiteracy for Perinatal Mortality.

Some Risk factors are modifiable (smoking, high BP, hypercholesterolemia, diabetes, obesity) while others are not modifiable (age, sex, race, family history)

Risk factors may characterize the:
  Individual – Age, sex, smoking, hypertension
  Family – Education, occupation, income
  Community – Malaria, TB, poor sanitation

Methods to Identify Risk factors
Epidemiological studies – Case Control and Cohort Studies

Prevention and Control of Risk factors
Primordial and primary prevention is important e.g. Health Education during the school Health Programme

Iceberg of Disease

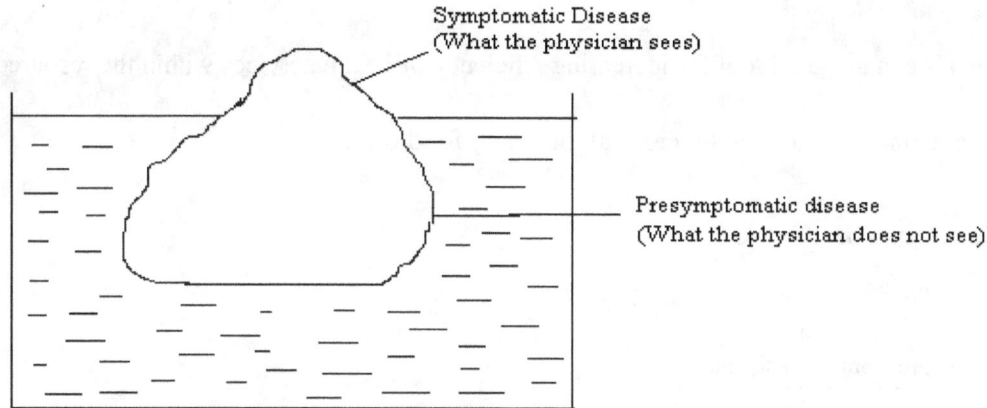

- Disease in a community can be compared with an iceberg.
- The floating tip represents what the physician sees – Clinical Cases
- The major, submerged portion represents the hidden mass of the disease - Latent, inapparent, pre-symptomatic, undiagnosed cases, carriers in the community
- E.g. Malnutrition, polio, hypertension, diabetes mellitus, anemia, mental illness
- The hidden part is undiagnosed. It is the reservoir of disease and its detection and control is a challenge to modern techniques in preventive medicine.

Risk Groups

(a) Biological Situation

Age group – Infants, toddlers, elderly
Sex – Females in reproductive age
Physiological state – Pregnancy, cholesterol level, high BP
Genetic factors – Family history of genetic disorders

(b) Physical Situation

Rural, urban slums
Living conditions, over-crowding
Environment – Water supply, proximity to industries

(c) Socio-cultural & cultural situation

Social class
Ethnic and cultural group
Family disruption, education, housing
Customs, habits, behaviour (smoking, overeating, lack of exercise, drug addiction)
Lifestyles & attitudes
Access to health services

Identification of Risk Groups e.g. At risk mothers, at risk infants, at risk families, chronically ill, handicapped and elderly in the population are known as risk approach.

This is a managerial tool for increasing efficiency of health services within the resources.

It is summed up as something for all but more for those in need

Spectrum of disease

Positive health
Better health
Freedom from sickness

Unrecognized sickness
Mild sickness
Severe sickness
Death

The Spectrum of disease varies from sub-clinical infections to fatal illnesses.
The different clinical manifestations are reflections of the individuals' different states of immunity. e.g. Leprosy
It can be modified by interventions – early diagnosis and treatment

Concepts of Control

Disease Control	Disease Elimination	Disease Eradication
Definition: The disease agent is permitted to persist in the community at a level where it ceases to be a public health problem e.g. Malaria control Activities aimed at reducing the incidence of disease, duration of disease, effects of infection both physical and psycho-social complications and financial burden to community Controlled activities may incorporate primary prevention, secondary prevention or both	Definition: An intermediate goal between control and eradication. Interruption of the transmission of disease e.g. Measles, polio, diphtheria	Definition: To tear out by the roots Termination of all transmission of infection by extermination of infectious agent e.g. Smallpox

Concepts of Prevention

Levels of Prevention	Modes of Intervention
Primordial Prevention: Prevention of emergence or development of risk factors in countries or population groups in which they have not yet appeared	Individual & Mass Health Education: E.g. During school health programmes to promote healthy lifestyle through diet, physical exercise, not picking up habits like smoking, alcohol, drugs

Primary Prevention:
Action taken prior to the onset of disease which removes the possibility of the disease ever occurring
 	
Each individual should take responsibility for his health, his family's health & community health.
 	
Strategies:
(i) Population strategy
  E.g. North Karelia project to decrease coronary heart disease through health education
(ii) High Risk strategy
  E.g. Oslo diet/smoking intervention study
	(a) Health Promotion:
	  (i) Health education -
	    A cost-effective intervention for diseases prevalent in the region & measures to control & prevent them
	  (ii) Environmental Modification -
	    Provision of safe water, sanitary latrines, improvement of housing, control of insects & rodents, prevention of air pollution, solid waste management.
	    Mawlynnong, the cleanest village in India and Asia
	  (iii) Nutritional Interventions -
	    Food supplementation programmes to improve nutrition of vulnerable groups, child feeding programmes, nutrition education, food fortification.
	  (iv) Lifestyle & Behavioural Changes - Health education to promote healthy lifestyle, diet, physical exercise, prevent smoking, alcohol, drugs.
	  (v) Family Life Education
	    Educating the population & importance of family planning.

Secondary Prevention: Action which halts the progress of a disease at its incipient stage & prevents complications	(b) Specific Protection: Immunization, Nutritional supplement, Chemoprophylaxis e.g. malaria, Immuno-prophylaxis, protective device in industry, protective device for traffic accident e.g. Helmets, safety belts, protection from carcinogens, protection from allergens Early Diagnosis & Treatment: E.g. Diabetes mellitus, hypertension, Ca cervix, Ca breast, TB, leprosy, malaria Screening for diabetes, hypertension, cancer

Tertiary Prevention: Intervention in late pathogenesis phase - All measures are taken to reduce impairments & disabilities, minimize suffering caused by existing departure from good health & promote patients' adjustment to irremediable conditions	(a) Disability Limitation: Impairment - Any loss or abnormality of psychological, physiological or anatomical structure or function e.g. Mental retardation, defective vision, loss of foot Disability – Lack of ability to perform an activity in the manner or within the range considered normal for a human being Handicap – A disadvantage for an individual resulting from an impairment or disability that limits the fulfillment of a role that is normal e.g. Disease – Impairment – disability –Handicap Accident – loss of foot – cannot walk – unemployment (b) Rehabilitation: Combined & coordinated use of medical, social, educational & vocational measures for training & re-training the individual to the highest possible level of functional ability Medical Rehabilitation – Restoration of function e.g. Reconstructive surgery of hand after accident or leprosy Social rehabilitation – Restoration of family & social relationship Economic rehabilitation – Financial assistance to recover from handicap e.g. Loan under self- employment scheme Vocational rehabilitation – Restoration of earning capacity Psychological rehabilitation – Restoration of personal dignity & confidence

Functions of a Physician

Definition:

A Physician is a person who has been regularly admitted to a duly recognized medical school in the country, having successfully completed the prescribed courses in medicine and has acquired the requisite qualification to be legally licensed to practice medicine (comprising prevention, diagnosis, treatment and rehabilitation) using independent judgement to promote community & individual health.

Functions:
(i) Care of an individual:
    To diagnose and treat individuals regarding their illness, nutritional problems and emergency care
(ii) Care of the community:
    A Physician is the leader of the health team and renders primary health care to the community
(iii) A teacher:
    "Doctor" means to teach
    A Physician has a major responsibility as a teacher and health educator

Community Diagnosis

Definition:
The pattern of disease in a community and factors influencing them.
Based on collection of data pertaining to: Age, sex, socio-economic status, vital statistics e.g. birth rate, death rate, incidence and prevalence of important diseases in the area.
Mainly assesses the health needs and health problems of the community.
These needs should be investigated and listed according to priority for community treatment.

Community Treatment

Based on community diagnosis, community treatment is undertaken to meet the health needs.

Community health interventions:
E.g. Improvement of water supply, immunization, health education, control of specific diseases, health legislation

Characteristics of community action:
(i) It must effectively utilize the available resources
(ii) There should be intersectoral coordination
(iii) There should be community participation in planning, monitoring, evaluation of the programmes

CHAPTER 2

NUTRITION

Assessment of Nutritional Status

Nutritional assessment can be done by 1) Direct and 2) Indirect methods

Direct	Indirect
Clinical Examination	Morbidity Data
Nutritional Anthropometry	Mortality Data
Biochemical Tests	Food Consumption Data
Biophysical Tests	Food Production Data
	Ecological Studies

Clinical Examination

For Anemia:	Palor of Conjunctivae, Tongue, Skin
Vit A Deficiency:	Bitot's Spots, Conjuctival Xerosis, Corneal Xerosis, Keratomalacia
Iodine Deficiency:	Enlargement of Thyroid, Cretin
PEM:	
Kwashiorkor:	Decreased weight, Pitting Edema, skin and hair changes, loss of appetite, Diarrhoea
Marsmaus:	Decreased weight, muscle wasting, fat wasting, irritability, good appetite

Nutritional Anthropometry

Weight: (IAP Classification: N 80–100%, Gr I 70 – 80%, Gr II 60 – 70%, Gr III 50 – 60%, Gr IV <50% malnutrition)

Height: Growth charts should be maintained for children under 5 years

MAC: N = >13.5 cm, Mild to moderate PEM = 12.5–13.5 cm, Severe PEM = < 12.5 cm.

Skinfold thickness: To measure subcutaneous fat

Head Circumference (HC) & Chest Circumference (CC): At birth HC > CC whereas at 9 months CC > HC in Western Children but for Indian children at 2 yrs CC overtakes HC

Laboratory & Biochemical Tests

Hb %

Stools for Parasites

Urine for Albumin, Sugar

Biochemical tests

Eg. Se Retinol, Se Iron, Urinary Iodine, Enzyme measurement

These tests are expensive and time consuming but may be done on sub-sample of the population

Biophysical Tests

These are not widely used for community surveys

Eg. Radiological examination for Rickets, Osteomalacia, Fluorosis, Dark Adaptation for Vit A deficiency

Functional Indicators

These are emerging as important diagnostic tools.

Eg. Structural Integrity	–	Erythrocyte Fragility, Capillary Fragility
Host Defense	–	Leukocyte Chemotaxis, Leucocyte Bactericidal Capacity, Delayed Cutaneous Hypersensitivity
Reproduction	–	Sperm Count
Nerve Function	–	Nerve Conduction, Dark Adaptation, EEG
Work Capacity	–	Heart Rate

Assessment of Dietary Intake

Food consumption surveys comprise of:

   i.   Weighment of Raw Foods
        Weighment of Cooked Foods
        Duration 1-21 days, commonly 7 days is one dietary cycle
  ii.   Weighment of Cooked Foods
        Foods analysed after being cooked

iii. Oral Questionnaire Method

24–48 hour Recall Method, most commonly used

The data is collected, analysed and interpreted in terms of cereals, pulses, vegetables, fruits, milk, meat, fish, eggs and the mean nutrients are calculated.

Vital Statistics

Morbidity Data – PEM Status, Diarrhoeal Disease, Measles, Beri-beri, Rickets, Anemia, Night Blindness, Low Birth Weight, Goitre

Mortality Data – IMR, 1- 4 year Mortality

Assessment of Ecological Factors

(a) Food Production Data

At National level – Total food consumed divided by total population.

Average national consumption per reference consumption unit can be obtained.

(b) Socio Economic Factors

Factors such as Family size, occupation, income, education, customs, cultural patterns influence food consumption patterns

(c) Health Educational Services

Primary health care, feeding, immunization programmes also play a part

(d) Conditioning Influences

Parasitic, Bacterial, Viral infections precipitate malnutrition

Nutritional Surveillance

Definition:

Keeping watch over nutrition to make decisions that will lead to improvement of Nutrition in the population.

Objectives

1. Planning for Health and Development

2. Programme Management and Evaluation

3. Give timely warning and intervention to prevent short-term food consumption crisis

1. To give timely warning and intervention to prevent short term food consumption crisis

Factor	Growth Monitoring	Nutritional surveillance
Strategy	Preservation of normal growth	Detection of undernutrition
Approach	Educational – Motivational	Diagnostic Interventional
Enrolment	all infants	Representative sample
Age	start before 6months	Representative ages
Number	Small groups – 10 to 20	Any size – 50 to 100
Weigher/Recorder	Mothers guided by worker	Trained workers
Weight Card	Simple, emphasis growth	Precise, nutritional status
Nutritional emphasis	Maintaining good nutrition	Detect malnutrition
Response	Early home intervention based on local knowledge	Nutritional rehabilitation with supplements
Response time	Brief, resumption of N growth	Long, regain of good nutrition in community
Interventions	Primary health care, vaccinations, Vit A, oral rehydration therapy, deworming, chloroquinine, contraceptives	food supplements food subsidy
Referral	Health system for checking & brief food supplements	Malnutrition rehabilitation in special centre

Nutritional Status Indicators

Phenomenon	Indicator
Maternal Nutrition	Birth Weight
Infants & Pre-school Child Nutrition	Proportion on weaning foods by age in months Mortality rates in children aged 1-4 years If age known: Height for age Weight for age If age unknown: Weight for height Arm Circumference Clinical Signs of Syndromes
School Child Nutrition	Height for age Weight for height at 7 years or school admission Clinical Signs

Food Surveillance

Definition

All conditions and measures necessary during production, processing, storage, distribution and preparation to make food safe for human consumption

1. **Food Hygiene**
   Production, handling, distribution and serving all food in a hygienic manner to prevent food poisoning and food borne diseases.
2. **Milk Hygiene**
   This includes:
   Clean and safe milk
   The cow – Clean animal, cow shed sanitation to be maintained, clean milk vessels, milk handlers to be free of disease, handwashing mandatory, milk cooled immediately to <10°C.
   Pasteurization
   (a) Holder Method (Vat) – Milk kept at 66°C for 30 mins and quickly cooled to 5°C
   (b) HTST Method – High Temperature Short Time Method
   Milk rapidly heated to 72°C, held for 15 secs, rapidly cooled to 4°C.
   (c) UHT Method – Ultra-High Temperature method
   Milk rapidly heated in 2 stages to 125°C (2nd stage) under pressure, kept for few seconds then rapidly cooled and bottled.
   Pasteurized milk is tested by:
   (a) Phosphatase Test
   (b) Standard Plate Count
   (c) Coliform Count
   Milk borne diseases:
   • Tuberculosis
   • Brucellosis
   • Streptococcal Infections
   • Staphylococcal Enterotoxin Poisoning
   • Salmonellosis
   • Q Fever
   • Anthrax
3. **Meat Hygiene**
   Necessary for preventing following diseases:
   (a) Tapeworm Infestations – Tinea Solium, T Saginata, Trichinella Spiralis, Fasciola Hepatica
   (b) Bacterial Infections – Anthrax, Actinomyosis, Food Poisoning, Tuberculosis
   Meat Inspection

Veterinary staff to inspect animals for slaughter, antemortem and postmortem
Good meat should be neither pale pink nor deep purple, firm and elastic, have agreeable odour, should not be slimy

Slaughter Houses

Hygiene is important

Location – Away from residential areas

Structure – Floor, walls to be impervious, easy to clean

Disposal of wastes – Blood, offal to be separately collected and not discharged into public sewers

Water supply – Adequate

Examination of animals – Antemortem, postmortem examinations

Storage of meat – In fly proof, rat proof rooms at < 50°C

Transportation of meat – In fly proof, covered vans

4. **Fish Hygiene**

Important to prevent D Latum Infection, Vibrio Parahaemolyticus, Salmonella SPP, Cl Botulinum

Signs of fresh fish – Stiff or rigor mortis, gills bright red, eyes clear

Tinned fish - Tin must be new, clean with no rusting; No evidence of tampering of seal, contents should not be blown out

5. **Egg Hygiene**

Proper egg preservation

Eggs may become contaminated by faecal matter of hens

Salmonella can penetrate the cracked shell

6. **Fruits and Vegetable Hygiene**

They are important source of Pathogenic Organisms, Protozoans, Helminths

Vegetables and fruits eaten raw should be washed thoroughly eg Salads

7. **Sanitation of Eating Places**

Model Public Health Act

Location – Should not be near filth, open drains or manure pits

Floors – Higher than adjoining land, impervious, easy to keep clean

Rooms – Accommodation for maximum 10 persons and not <100 sq ft

Walls – Impervious, easily washable

Lighting – Adequate

Ventilation – Good circulation of air

Kitchen – Floor space minimum 60 sq ft

Windows – 25% of floor space

Doors & windows – Rat proof, Fly proof with Ventilators & Smoke Pipes

Separate room for storage of cooked food

Storage of uncooked food – Rat proof, Vermin proof room

Furniture – Strong, easy to keep clean

Disposal of Refuse – Collected in covered dustbins and disposed off twice a day

Water Supply – Adequate and safe

Washing Facilities – To be provided, Hot water provision

Food Handlers

To prevent infections eg. Diarrhoea, Dysenteries, Typhoid, Enteroviruses, Viral Hepatitis, Protozoal Cysts, Eggs of Helminths (Parasitic Worms), Streptococcal, Staphylococcal Infections, Salmonellosis

(a) Complete Medical Examination of Food Handlers
(b) Persons with wounds, boils, otitis media, skin infections should not be permitted to handle food
(c) Personal Hygiene
(d) Health education on food hygiene – handling, storing food
(e) Handwashing
(f) Hair – Head coverings (caps)
(g) Overalls – Clean white overalls
(h) Habits – Coughing, sneezing, licking fingers, scratching hair, smoking to be avoided

Protein Energy Malnutrition (PEM)

Definition

PEM is a group of pathological conditions of varying degrees of severity arising from lack of proteins and calories and extremes of condition manifested as Kwashiorkor or Marasmus.

Kwashiorkor is a Ghana word meaning condition in an older child who has been weaned from the breast when a younger sibling comes. In India, Undernutrition - 36%; Stunted 38%; Wasted 21%; Kwashiorkor/Marasmus <1% in children under 5 years.

Classification

IAP Classification:

Gr I: 71-80% of reference weight for age {50th percentile (median) weight of Harvard standards}

Gr II: 61-70%

Gr III: 51-60%

Gr IV: 50% or less

Alphabet K/S postfixed for edema

WHO Classification:

Item	Moderate Undernutrition	Severe Undernutrition
Symmetrical Edema	No	Yes[a]
Weight for Height (Measure of wasting)	SD Score[b] -2 to -3 (70-79% of Expected[c] Wasting)	SD Score <-3 (<70% of Expected Severe Wasting)
Height for Age Measure of stunting	SD score -2 to -3 (85-89% of expected Stunting)	SD Score <-3 (< 85% of Expected Severe Stunting)

(a) This includes Kwashiorkor and Marasmic Kwashiorkor

(b) SD Score = $\dfrac{\text{Observed Value - Expected Value}}{\text{Std Deviation of Reference Population}}$

(c) Median 50th Percentile of CDC Standards

Severe Acute Malnutrition (SAM)

Very low weight/height (Z-Score <-3SD) of Median WHO Child Growth Charts
Mid-Arm Circumference <11.5 cm
Or, Presence of Nutritional Oedema increases the risk of death

Etiology and Social Factors

Conditioning Influences:
Infectious Diseases - Diarrhea, ARI, Whooping Cough, Measles, Malaria, TB

Cultural Influences

Food habits, Customs, Beliefs, Traditions, Attitudes, Religion, Food fads, cooking practices; Child rearing practices

Socio-economic factors

Poverty, Ignorance; Illiteracy; Lack of knowledge on nutrition; Inadequate sanitary environment; Large family size

Food Production

Food production may be adequate but there is uneven distribution of food

Health and Other Services

Nutritional Surveillance; Nutritional Rehabilitation; Nutritional Supplementation; Health Education

Clinical Features

Weight for age can reveal Grade I, II or III malnutrition:

Kwashiorkor	Marasmus
1-4 years	6 mths – 3 years
Emaciation masked by edema	Emaciation pronounced
Edema and Ascitis present	Edema absent
Skin and hair changes	No skin and hair changes
Appetite lost	Appetite good
Mental changes	Mental changes absent
Liver may be palpable, Fatty Liver	Liver not palpable
Serum Albumin reduced	Serum Albumin normal

Treatment

Depends on the severity of PEM
  i.   Mild to moderate cases: Parents are given nutrition education:
       (a) Increase quantity of food,
       (b) Increase frequency of feeding,
       (c) Increase quality of food ie Cereals, pulses, GLV, other vegetables and fruits,
       (d) Add ghee, oil or sugar,
       (e) Give milk, eggs, meat, fish
  ii. Nutritional Rehabilitation
       Mothers are educated on right methods of childcare, feeding, nutrition, demonstration of recipes of quality food with locally available foods in Day Care Centres
  iii. Severe Cases of PEM are admitted for 14 days in Nutrition Rehabilitation Centres in hospitals

Principles of Management:

(a) Energy 200 cals/kg, protein 4g/kg per day
(b) Treatment of Nutritional Deficiencies - Vit A, Anemia
(c) Treatment of Infections - TB, Diarrhea, ARI
(d) Early detection and treatment of complications - Dehydration, Hypothermia, Hypoglycemia
(e) Nutrition Education of parents

Prevention of PEM

i. Breast Feeding

Initiation of breastfeeding within half hour of birth, Exclusive breastfeeding for 6 months (180 days), Continued breastfeeding up to 2 years

ii. Complementary Feeding

After 6 months of age, Education on home-made high-protein energy mixture

Davangere Mix

Ragi	250g
Wheat or Rice	250g
Green Gram	250g
Groundnuts	100g
Til (sesame)	50g
Sugar/Jaggery	300g

Hyderabad Mix

Roasted Wheat	40g
Roasted Bengal Gram Dhal	15g
Roasted Groundnut	10g
Jaggery	30g

iii. Early Detection of PEM through growth monitoring in Anganwadis

If PEM detected, it is treated accordingly

iv. Nutritional Supplementation

In ICDS Centres with mid-day meals

v. Measures taken to increase food production and lower food prices

Land reforms

Improved food technology

Distribution of improved seeds to farmers

Irrigation

Subsidy for fertilizers

Subsidized food through Public Distribution System (PDS)

Creation of buffer stock of foods

vi. Aggressive steps for population control

vii. Poverty Alleviation Measures - Vocational skills training for youth; Loan facilities for setting up business ventures; Community centres for handicrafts; Food for work; Wages for work

viii. Control of Endemic Diseases

Immunizations, ORS Therapy, Periodic De-worming, ARI Control, Protected water supply, Sanitary disposal of excreta

Preventive and Social Measures:

Action at Family Level	Action at Community Level	Action at National Level	Action at International Level
- Nutritional Education - Breast Feeding - Infant & Child Feeding - Antenatal Feeding of Mother - Postnatal Feeding of Mother - IYCF - Care of Adolescent Girl - Hygiene, Hand washing - Kitchen Garden - Poultry Rearing - MCH, FP, Immunization Services utilization	- Nutritional Surveillance - Plan, Monitor, Evaluate Nutritional Programmes - ICDS - Nutritional Supplementation - Applied Nutrition - Control of Infectious Diseases - Safe Water - Sanitation - Socio-economic Development	- Rural Development - Increasing Agriculture - Population Stabilization - Nutritional Intervention - Nutrition Related Health Activities: NMEP, Immunization Family Planning - Water & Sanitation - Food Security - Nutrition Promoting Agriculture - Women Empowerment	- Financial Aid from: UNICEF WHO FAO World Bank UNDP CARE

Vitamin A Deficiency

Xerophthalmia

Vitamin A Deficiency presents with Ocular and Extra-ocular Manifestations.

Ocular Manifestations

Xerophthalmia

WHO Classification:

XN Night Blindness

XIA Conjunctival Xerosis

XIB Bitot's Spots

X2 Corneal Xerosis

X3A Corneal Ulceration/Keratomalacia affecting <one-third corneal surface

X3B Corneal Ulceration/Keratomalacia affecting >one-third corneal surface

XS Corneal Scar

XF Xerophthalmic Fundus

Extraocular Manifestations

Follicular Hyperkeratosis, Anorexia, Growth Retardation

Causative Factors:
Low socio-economic status, Ignorance, Faulty feeding practices, Infections (Diarrhea, Measles), Worm infestation, Rice eating, Children aged 1-3 years

Prevalence criteria for determining Xerophthalmia

Criteria	Prevalence in population at risk (6mths-6 yrs)
Night Blindness	>1%
Bitot's Spots	>0.5%
Corneal Xerosis/Corneal Ulceration/Keratomalacia	>0.01%
Corneal Ulcer	>0.05%
Se Retinol<10mcg/dl	>5%

Prevention

1. Short Term Action: High dose Syr. Vit A At 9mths - 100,000 IU;
    At one and half years till 5 years - 200,000 IU every 6 months
2. Intermediate Term Action: Food fortification eg. Vanaspati, Margarine, Milk, Bread
3. Long Term Action: Nutritional Education, Breast Feeding, Complementary Feeding, Safe Water, Sanitation, Immunization, Health Services
    Vit A rich foods: Animal foods (Liver, meat, fish, fish liver oils, whole milk, butter, cheese, eggs)
    Plant foods: (Dark green leafy vegetables, green yellow and orange vegetables and fruits eg carrots, pumpkin, papaya, mango)

Treatment of Vit A deficiency

3 doses: Day 1, Day 2, Day 14 - 200,000 IU
National Vit A Prophylaxis Program initiated in 1970

Nutritional Anaemia

Definition

A disease where the Haemoglobin content in blood is lower than normal; Iron deficiency is the most common cause

Magnitude of problem in India

Major Nutritional problem, 60 – 70% women and children are affected

Causes

1. Inadequate Intake of iron rich foods
2. Poor Bio-availability of Phytates and Oxalates decrease the absorption of iron
3. Excessive losses – Gastrointestinal losses due to Hook Worm,
   Malaria leads to Hemolytic Anemia,
   Piles with bleeding, Menstrual losses
   Deliveries at close intervals and loss of blood during each delivery

Effects of Anaemia

(a) Pregnancy – Increases maternal and foetal mortality and morbidity
   Anemia associated with abortions, premature births, post-partum hemorrhage, low birth weight
(b) Infection – Parasitic diseases eg Malaria, Intestinal Parasites impair immunity increasing susceptibility to infection
(c) Work Capacity – Reduction in work performance, Easy fatigability

Clinical Features

Repeated Infections, Fatigability, Pallor of Skin, Tongue, Oral Mucosa, Conjunctiva

Investigations

(a)   Hb.

Persons	g/dl (venous blood)
Adult Males	13
Adult Females, Non-Pregnant	12
Adult Females, Pregnant	11
Children 6m-6yrs	11
Children 6-14yrs	12

(b) Se Iron Concentration: < 0.5mg/L (N= 0.8 – 1.8mg/L)

(c) Se Ferritin: <10mcg/L indicates absence of stored iron

(d) Se Transferrin Saturation: Should be >16% (N=30%)

Treatment

Requirements of Iron

Age Group	RDA (mg/day)
Children (1–12yrs)	12-34
Adolescents (13–16yrs)	41-50
	28-30
Adult Males	17
Adult Females:	21
Pregnancy	35
Lactation	21

1. Iron & Folic Acid supplementation:

   Mild Anemia IFA Supplementation – National Nutritional Anemia Prophylaxis programme. Tablet containing Elemental Iron 100 mg and Folic Acid 0.5mg for Prophylaxis 1 Tab od for 100 days; For treatment 1Tab bd for 100 days. It should be continued for 2-3 months after Hb becomes normal.

   For severe anemia – Packed Cell Transfusion

   For children – 1 Tab Paediatric Elemental Iron 20mg and Folic Acid 0.1mg od

2. Iron Fortification

   Food Fortification eg Milk, Bread

   Salt – Twin Fortification with Iron and Iodine

3. Other strategies

   Nutritional Education – Increase intake of Iron rich foods eg Ragi, pulses, soya beans,green leafy vegetables, jaggery, dried fruits (dates, figs), sapota, non veg foods like liver, meat, eggs

Enhancers of Iron Absorption	Inhibitors of Iron Absorption
Vitamin C	Milk
Proteins	Antacids
Haem Iron	Tea, Coffee
	Phytates, Oxalates

Iodine Deficiency Disorders (IDD)

IDD is a major public health problem in India.
Previously thought to be problem of the Sub-Himalayan Goitre belt, Kashmir to Naga hills, but now all the states are affected.

Epidemiology

Agent factors
Iodine deficiency due to decreased intake or decreased utilization
Goitrogens (Chemical substances leading to development of Goitre interfere with Iodine utilization by the Thyroid Gland e.g. Cabbage, cauliflower, radish, cassava, millet)

Host factors
School going children, adolescents and pregnant women are more susceptible to Goitre

Environmental factors
Iodine content in soil and water is low in hilly areas.
Vegetables grown in those regions are poor in Iodine.

Clinical features

Iodine deficiency results in Impaired Synthesis of Thyroxine leading to Goitre

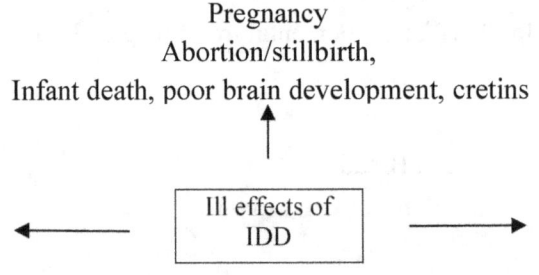

Pregnancy
Abortion/stillbirth,
Infant death, poor brain development, cretins

Ill effects of IDD

Childhood	Adults
Less IQ,mental retardation,	Lack of energy, tired easily,
Milestones delayed,	reduced productivity, goitre
poor performance in schools	Spasticity – spastic diplegia,
growth failure,	spastic quadriplegia,
paralysis, speech defect	neuro muscular weakness in
hearing defect, strabismus	legs, arms, trunk
nystagmus	

Treatment

Lifelong supplementation with Thyroid Hormones

Prevention

1. Iodization of common salt
    50 kg Potassium Iodate is added to 1,000,000 kg salt (50 ppm).
    Potassium Iodate has 60% Iodine therefore, contributes 30kg of Iodine to salt (30PPM of Iodine). Some Iodine is lost during storage and transportation therefore, at consumer level 15PPM of Iodine is sufficient for prevention of IDD.
2. Health Education of the community to use only Iodized salt. Daily requirement is150µg
3. Banning of Non-iodized salt through Prevention of Food Adulteration Act

IDD Control Programme - Refer National Programmes

Fluorosis

Definition

It is a disease affecting the bones and teeth due to excess intake of Fluorine (3-5mg/L) in drinking water

Public Health Problem

It is commonly seen in people whose staple diet is Sorghum (Jowar)
Some of the areas are:
In Andhra Pradesh - Nellore, Nalgonda, Prakasam Districts
In Karnataka - Kolar District
Kerala
Tamil Nadu
Punjab
Haryana

Clinical Features

i. Dental Fluorosis
    Mottling of dental enamel, teeth lose shiny appearance
    chalk white patches —> yellow —> brown/black

ii. Skeletal Fluorosis
    - Deposition of Fluoride in bones, tendons, joints —> Crippling Fluorosis

→ permanent disability. Involvement of vertebral column, affects spinal cord and nerve roots

- Tingling and numbness in limbs, Difficulty in walking, Inability to look sideways. To see what is on his right or left he has to move the whole body to that side.
- On examination, back is curved, joints of lower extremities are fixed and painful.
- Genu Valgum, an abnormal separation of knees and inward bowing of lower extremities.

Prevention

1. De-fluoridation of community water supply by Nalgonda Technique.

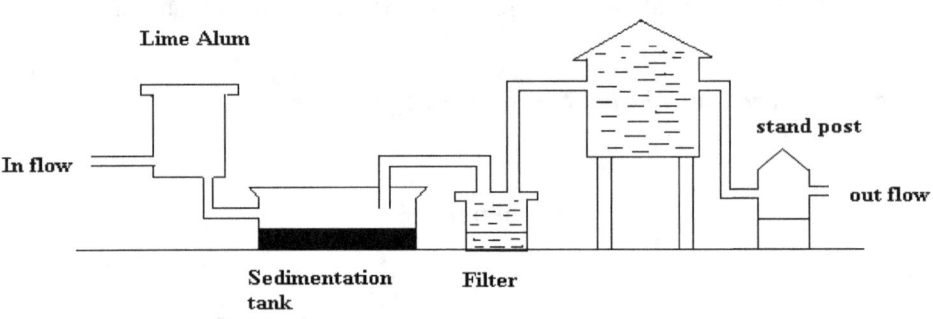

30 mg lime / L, next alum 500mg /L added, stirred 10 mins.

After holding for one hour excess Fluoride precipitates and settles down, supernatant fluid is then drawn and filtered.

2. Changing water source
    Changing to a new source of water with Fluoride content of 0.5-0.8mg/L
3. Fluoride supplements should not be given to children
4. Fluoride toothpaste is not recommended for children up to 6 years.

Lathyrism

Definition

Paralysing disease in humans

Magnitude of the problem

Mainly seen in the poor people of Madhya Pradesh, Uttar Pradesh, Bihar and Orissa

The Pulses - Lathyrus Sativus (Kesari Dal), Chickpea

The Toxin - BOAA (Beta-oxalyl Amino Alanine)

Clinical Features

Seen in poor people

Males > Females

Spastic Paralysis of the lower limbs

(a) Latent stage – Apparently healthy, Exhibits ungainly gait during stress. Important stage for prevention - Withdraw pulse from diet which leads to complete remission
(b) No Stick stage
    Walks with jerky steps
(c) One Stick stage
    Walks with crossed gait, tendency to walk on toes with the aid of a stick
(d) Two Stick stage
    Walks with the aid of two crutches due to excessive bending of knees and crossed legs
(e) Crawler stage
    Crawling because knees cannot support the body weight, Atrophy of thigh and leg muscles

Prevention & Treatment

(a) Vitamin C Prophylaxis – 1000mg Vit C per day for one week
(b) Banning the Crop – PFA Act has banned the Crop
(c) Removal of the Toxin
    i. Steeping Method – Soak in hot water for 2 hours, drain, clean, dry
    ii. Parboiling
(d) Education
(e) Genetic approach - Growing a low toxin variety
(f) Socio Economic change – Improving the socio-economic status and overall development

Food Borne Diseases

Definition

A disease infectious or toxic in nature caused by agents that enter the body through ingestion of food

Classification

Bacterial
Typhoid, Staphylococcal Toxin, Botulism, E. Coli Diarrhoea, Salmonellosis, Cl. Perfringens, B. Cereus, V. Parahaemolyticus, Streptococcal Infection, Shigellosis, Brucellosis

Viral

Viral Hepatitis, Gastroenteritis

Parasites

Taeniasis, Hydatidosis, Ascariasis, Amoebiasis, Trichinosis, Oxyuriasis

Food Toxins

1. Due to naturally occurring toxins in some foods
    (a) Lathyrism (BOAA)
    (b) Endemic Ascitis (Pyrrolizidine Alkaloids)
2. Due to toxins produced by certain bacteria
    (a) Botulism
    (b) Staphylococcal food poisoning
3. Due to toxins produced by fungi
    (a) Aflatoxin
    (b) Ergot
    (c) Fusarium
4. Food borne chemical poisoning
    (a) Heavy metals eg. Mercury (fish), Lead (canned food)
    (b) Oils (Trycresyn Phosphate or TCP), Argemone oil
    (c) Packing material chemicals
    (d) Pesticides (DDT, BHC)

1. Neurolathyrism (refer above)
2. Endemic Ascitis
    Millets contaminated with weed seeds of Crotalaria [Jhunjhunia]. It has Hepatotoxin called
    Pyrrolizidine Alkaloids. Clinically manifests with Ascitis and Jaundice.

Prevention

- Health education about the disease
- De-weeding of weed seeds
- Sieving of Millets

3. Botulism Exotoxin – (Refer Communicable Diseases)
4. Staphylococcal Food Poisoning – Enterotoxin (Refer Communicable Diseases)
5. Aflatoxin (Storage Fungus)
    Fungal Toxin of Aspergillus flavus.
    Food grains attacked – Groundnut, maize, wheat, parboiled rice, rice, sorghum, tapioca

It is a Heptotoxin - Related to Indian childhood Cirrhosis; Is carcinogenic and leads to Hepatic Carcinoma.

Prevention

- Proper storage – moisture < 10%
- Contaminated food should not be consumed
- Health education about the disease

6. Ergotism (Field Fungus)
    Ergot is a field fungus.
    Wheat, bajra, rye, sorghum affected by Claviceps Fusiformis. This leads to Ergotism.

Clinical features
Nausea, vomiting, giddiness, drowsiness, cramps in limbs, Peripheral Gangrene

Prevention
Ergot infested grains can be removed by:
    (a) Floating in 20% salt water
    (b) Handpicking
    (c) Air floatation

7. Fusarium Toxins
    Fusarium is a field fungus.
    Toxic metabolites produced by Fusarium Incamatum attacks rice, sorghum.

8. Epidemic Dropsy
    It is caused by contamination of Mustard Oil with Argemone Oil.
    Toxic Alkaloid Sanguinarine in Argemone Oil.

Clinical Features
Sudden Non-Inflammatory bilateral swelling of legs with Diarrhoea, Dyspnea, Cardiac Failure, Death
Contamination of Mustard Oil with Argemone Oil may be accidental or deliberate.
Seeds of Argemone Mexicana resemble Mustard Seeds and can be harvested together accidently.
Unscrupulous dealers mix Argemone Oil with Mustard Oil.
Tests to detect Argemone Oil:
    (a) Nitric Acid test
    (b) Paper Chematography

Prevention:
(a) Removal of Argemone Weeds
(b) PFA Act (Prevention of Food Adulteration Act)

Food Additives and Food Fortification

Food Additives	Food Fortification
Definition: Non nutritious substances added to food to improve the appearance, flavour, texture, storage properties	Nutrients are added to foods to improve the quality of the diet of a group, community or population
	Eg. Iodization of salt
First category – Not harmful	Fluoridation of water
Colouring Agents (Saffron, turmeric)	Vit A&D to Vanaspati, milk
Flavouring Agents (Vanilla Essence)	Twin fortification of salt with Iodine and Iron
Sweetness (Saccharin)	
Preservatives (Sodium Benzoate)	
Acidity imparting agents (Citric Acid, Acetic Acid)	
Second category – Contaminants from packing, processing, farming practices (Insecticides, Pesticides)	

Food Adulteration

Definition

Food Adulteration entails mixing, substitution, concealing quality, putting up decomposed foods for sale, misbranding, addition of toxicants.

Effects

Economic loss
Ill health
Death

Examples

Food Material	Common Adulterants
Cereals – Rice, Wheat	Mud, Grit
Dals	Kesari Dal
Haldi Powder	Lead Chromate Powder
Black Pepper	Seeds of Papaya
Tea Dust/Leaves	Used Tea Dust, Black Gram Husk
Coffee Powder	Chicory
Mustard Seeds	Argemone Seeds
Edible Oil	Argemone Oil
Sweetmeats	Non-permitted Colours
Milk	Starch, Water

Prevention of Food Adulteration Act (PFA Act)

- Enacted in 1954; Amended in 1964, 1976, 1986
- Objective – To ensure pure and wholesome food to consumers and protection from deceptive trade practices
- Minimum standard for food should be adhered to
- It is implemented with the help of public health laboratories, food analysts and food officers trained for this.

Implementation of the Act

- Fine of Rs1000
- Imprisonment for six months
- If death or grievously hurt fine Rs 5000, Life Imprisonment
- Consumer can take sample to submit for testing
- Voluntary organizations can take sample to submit for testing

Food Standards

1. Codex Alimentarius
2. PFA Standard
3. The Agmark Standard
4. BIS Mark – Bureau of Indian Standards

ZINC

A component of >300 Enzymes
Active in Glucides and Protein metabolism; Required for Insulin Synthesis

Deficiency

Growth failure; Sexual Infantilism, Delayed Wound Healing, Loss of Taste, Liver Disease, Pernicious Anemia, Thalassemia, Myocardial Infarction, Spontaneous Abortions, Congenital Malformation (Anencephaly), IUGR, Low Birth Weight, Pre-term Delivery

Benefits

Decreases severity of Diarrhea, Decreases Malarial Attacks, Improves Immunity, Antioxidant

Sources

Meat, Fish, Milk

RDA
> Males – 17mg/day
> Females – 13mg/day
> Children – 10mg/day
> Infants - 5mg/day

DIETARY ANTIOXIDANTS

Nutrients: Vit A, C, E, Selenium

Non-nutrients: Isothiocyanates; Caffeic, Ferrulic, Gallic, Ellagic Acids

Enzymes: Superoxide Dismutase, Catalase Superoxides Mutase

Benefit

Reduce adverse effect of Reactive Oxygen Species (ROS) and nitrogen species that result in Oxidant Damage

National Nutrition Programmes - Refer National Programmes

CHAPTER 3

EPIDEMIOLOGY

Definition

The study of distribution and determinants of health-related states or events in specified populations and the application of this study to the control of health problems is called Epidemiology.

Incidence

Number of new cases occurring in a defined population during a specified period of time. Incidence measures the rate at which new cases occur in a population

Incidence rate (IR):

$$\frac{\text{No. of new cases of specific disease during a given time period}}{\text{Population at risk during that period}} \times 1000$$

Eg TB
IR=1/1000 population

Eg. If there had been 500 new cases of illness in a population of 30,000 in a year

IR = 500/30,000 X 1000
= 16.7 per 1000 per year

Incidence Rate also refers to:

New spells or episodes of disease arising in a given period of time, per 1000 population
Eg. A person may suffer from common cold more than once a year
If he suffered twice, he would contribute 2 spells of sickness in that year.

$$IR = \frac{\text{No. of spells of sickness in a defined period}}{\text{Mean No. of persons exposed to risk in that period}} \times 1000$$

Special Incidence Rates:

Eg (a) Attack Rate
   (b) Secondary Attack Rate
   (c) Hospital Admission Rate

(a) Attack Rate:

Definition:
It is the Incidence Rate (expressed as %) used when population is exposed to risk for a limited period of time e.g. During an epidemic.
It relates to the number of cases in the population at risk and reflects the extent of the epidemic.

$$\text{Attack Rate} = \frac{\text{No. of new cases of a specified disease during a specified time interval}}{\text{Population at risk during the same interval}} \times 100$$

(b) Secondary Attack Rate (SAR):

Definition:
No. of exposed persons developing the disease within one incubation period following exposure to a primary case

$$SAR = \frac{\text{No. of exposed persons developing the disease within one incubation period}}{\text{Total No. of exposed or susceptible contacts}} \times 100$$

Uses of Incidence Rate

(a) Taking action to control a disease
(b) For research into aetiology, pathogenesis, distribution of diseases and the efficacy of preventive & therapeutic measures

Rising Incidence Rates.

	Might suggest need for new Disease Control/Prevention programmes
Eg. IR AIDS rising	Or, Reporting practices have improved
	Change in the aetiology of a disease – Change in agent, host or environmental characteristics

Prevalence

Definition

All current cases (old and new) existing at a given point in time, or over a period of time in a given population.

Types of Prevalence

Prevalence is of 2 types
(a)   Point Prevalence
(b)   Period Prevalence

(a)   Point Prevalence:

Definition:
No. of all current cases (old & new) of a disease at one point in time in a defined population. "Point" may be a day/several days/weeks depending on the time taken to examine the population sample.

$$\text{Point Prevalence} = \frac{\text{No. of all current cases (old \& new) of a specified disease existing at a given point in time}}{\text{Estimated population at the same point in time}} \times 100$$

Point prevalence can be made specific for age, sex, other factors

(b)   Period Prevalence

Definition:
Frequency of all current cases (old & new) during a defined period of time (eg annual prevalence) expressed in relation to a defined population.

$$\text{Period Prevalence} = \frac{\text{No. of cases (old \& new) of a specified disease during a given period of time interval}}{\text{Estimated mid-interval population at risk}} \times 100$$

Term Incidence and prevalence are illustrated as:

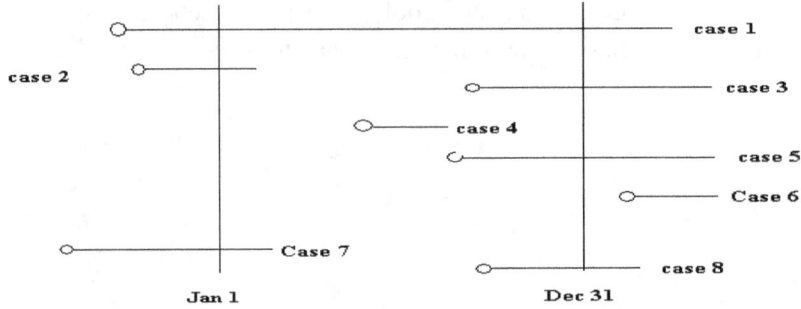

No. of cases of a disease beginning, developing and ending during a period of time.

Incidence would include cases   –   3, 4, 5, 8
Point Prevalence Jan 1 cases   –   1, 2, 7
Point Prevalence Dec 31 cases   –   1, 3, 5, 8
Period Prevalence (Jan-Dec) cases –   1, 2, 3, 4, 5, 7, 8

Relationship between Prevalence and Incidence
Prevalence depends on 2 factors:
   i.   Incidence and
  ii.   Duration of Illness

Assuming that Population (P) is stable and Incidence (I) and Duration (D) are unchanging:
$P = I \times D$
= Incidence x Mean Duration
Eg. Incidence is 10 cases per 1000 population per year
Mean duration of disease 5 years
Prevalence = 10 x 5 = 50 per 1000 population

Conversely it is possible to derive Incidence and Duration as follows:
$I = P/D$
$D = P/I$

The longer the duration of a disease, the greater is its Prevalence
Eg. TB has a high Prevalence Rate because new cases keep cropping up throughout the year and old cases persist for months or years.

If a disease is acute and of short duration either because of rapid recovery or death, the Prevalence Rate will be low compared with the Incidence Rate eg. Food poisoning, Homicides.

Changing Prevalence from one time period to another may be due to changes in:
  i.   Incidence
  ii. Duration, or
  iii. Both

Eg. Improvements in treatment may decrease the duration of a disease therefore, decrease the Prevalence of the disease

If treatment prevents death but does not produce recovery, Prevalence may increase. Eg. Coronary Heart Disease, Diabetes, Hypertension, Cancer.

If Duration is decreased, Prevalence may decrease despite increase in Incidence.

Prevalence has been compared with a photograph (An instantaneous record), incidence with a film (A continuous record)

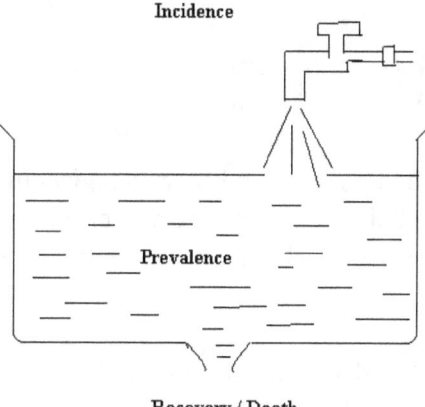

Epidemiological Methods

Introduction

Primary aim of an Epidemiologist is to study the occurrence of disease in people who are exposed to numerous factors and circumstances some of which may play a role in disease aetiology.

Classification of Epidemiological Studies
1. Observational studies
    (a) Descriptive studies

(b) Analytical studies
   i. Ecological or Correlational with populations as unit of study
   ii. Cross Sectional or Prevalence, with individuals as unit of study
   iii. Case Control or Case Reference, with individuals as unit of study
   iv. Cohort or Follow Up, with individuals as unit of study.

2. Experimental studies or Intervention studies
   (a) RCT (Randomized Controlled Trials) or Clinical Trials with patients as unit of study
   (b) Field Trials or Community Studies with healthy people as unit of study
   (c) Community Trials with communities as unit of study

Descriptive Epidemiology

Introduction

The best study of mankind is man.
Eg. Burkitt's Lymphoma was studied by Burkitt in Africa and led to the incrimination of Epstein Barr Virus
Kuru Study in New Guinea led to the discovery of Slow Virus Infections due to chronic degenerative Neurological Disorders in humans.

Descriptive studies are the first phase of an Epidemiological Investigation.
They study the distribution of disease or health related characteristics in human populations and determine the characteristics which the disease seems to be associated with.

Questions asked for the Study:
a. Time Distribution - When does the disease occur?
b. Place Distribution - Where does it occur?
c. Person Distribution - Who is suffering from the disease?

Procedures of Descriptive Studies:

1. Defining the Population
2. Defining the Disease
3. Describing the Disease by
   (a) Time
   (b) Place
   (c) Person
4. Measurement of Disease
5. Comparing with known Indices
6. Formulation of Etiological Hypothesis

1. Defining the Population

A population is defined based on the number, age, gender, occupation and cultural characteristics.

It can be the whole population in a geographic area or representative sample or a specially selected group

(Age/Sex/Group)

Eg Population under 5 years

Occupational Group

Hospital Patients

Small Communities (Framingham Study) or

Wider Groupings

- Population needs to be large so that age, gender and other specific rates are meaningful.
- The community should be stable, without migration into or out of the area.
- Inclusion and exclusion criteria should be clear Eg Visitors & relations should not be included
- There should be community participation.
- Health facilities should be closeby to provide easy access to patients requiring medical services.
- Eg Framingham Heart Study in US – All the above criteria were considered

2. Defining the disease under study

An operational definition is required by which the disease or condition can be identified and measured in the defined population with a degree of accuracy.

Eg Tonsillitis might be clinically defined as an inflammation of the tonsils caused by infection usually through Streptococcus Pyogenes.

However, this definition cannot be used to measure the disease in a community.

Operational definition clearly states the criteria by which the disease can be measured, "The presence of enlarged, red tonsils with white exudates which on throat swab culture grow predominantly S. Pyogenes".

In certain diseases, Eg Neurological Diseases, which do not have pathognomonic symptoms and signs, the Epidemiologist frames his own definition based on the objectives.

3. Describing the Disease

Describing the occurrence and distribution of disease/health related events/ characteristics within the Population by time, place and person, identifying those characteristics associated with the presence or absence of disease in individuals.

Characteristics examined in Descriptive Studies

Time	Place	Person
Year,	Climatic Zones,	Age,
Season,	Country,	Sex,
Month,	Region,	Marital Status,
Week,	Urban,	Occupation,
Day,	Rural,	Social Status,
Hours of onset,	Local,	Education,
Duration	Community,	Birth Order,
	Towns,	Family size,
	Cities,	Height,
	Institutions	Weight,
		Blood Pressure,
		Blood cholesterol,
		Personal habits

Time Distribution

Definition

A disease described by time of occurrence ie. Week, month, year, day of week, hour of onset.

It raises questions whether the disease is seasonal or whether periodic increase or decrease is present or if there is a consistent time trend.

This gives clues about the etiology or source of disease, thereby suggesting preventive measures.

Epidemiologists have identified 3 kinds of time trends
  i.   Short Term Fluctuations
  ii. Periodic Fluctuations
  iii. Long Term or Secular Trends

(I)   Short Term fluctuations

Epidemic:

Definition:
The occurrence in a community or region of cases of an illness or other health related events, clearly in excess of normal expectancy.

Epidemicity is relative to usual frequency of disease in the same area, among the specified population in the same season of the year.

Types of Epidemics:
There are 3 major types of Epidemics:

A. Common Source Epidemics
    (a) Single Exposure or "Point Source' Epidemics
    (b) Continuous or Multiple Exposure Epidemics

B. Propagated Epidemics
    (a) Person to Person
    (b) Arthropod Vector
    (c) Animal Reservoir

C. Slow (modern) Epidemics

The Epidemic Curve is a graph of the time distribution of epidemic cases.

The Epidemic Curve may suggest:
   i. Time relationship with exposure to a suspected source
  ii. Cyclical or Seasonal pattern suggestive of a particular information
 iii. Common Source or Propagated spread of the disease

A. Common Source Epidemics

(a) A common source, single exposure epidemic, also known as "Point Source" epidemic,

Exposure to the disease agent is brief and simultaneous; the resultant cases all develop within one incubation period of the disease (Eg. Epidemic of food poisoning)

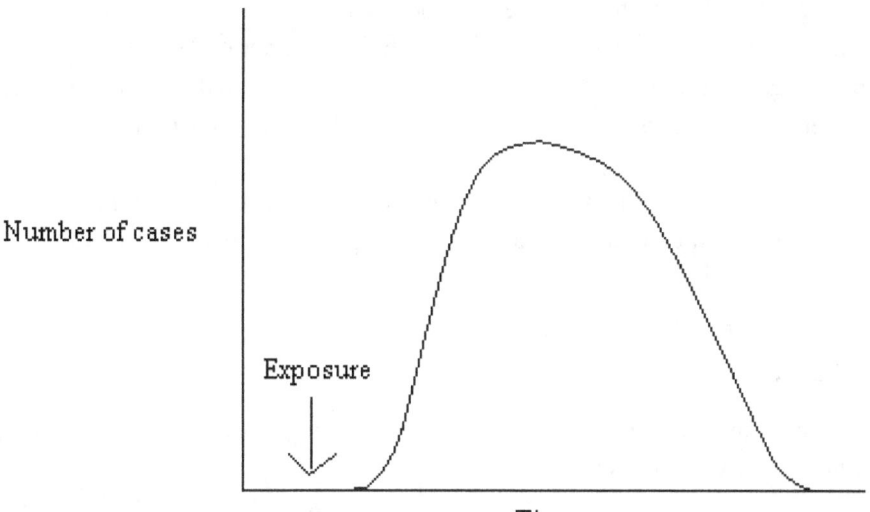

The curve usually has one peak
  i.   The Epidemic Curve rises and falls rapidly with no secondary waves
  ii. The epidemic tends to be explosive (Clustering of cases within narrow intervals of time)
  iii. All cases develop within one incubation period of the disease

Common Source Epidemics are frequently due to exposure to an infectious agent.
They can result from pollution of environment (air, water, food, soil) by industrial chemicals or pollutants.

Eg.
- The Bhopal gas tragedy in India
- Atomic Bomb explosion in Hiroshima, Nagasaki.
- Minamata Disease in Japan from consuming fish

(If the epidemic continues for more than one incubation period, it is either multiple exposure to a common source or propagated epidemic)

(b) Common Source, Continuous/Multiple Exposure Epidemics
   Exposure from the same source may be prolonged, continuous, repeated or intermittent, not necessary at the same time/place.

Eg.
  i.   A prostitute may be the common source in a Gonorrhea Outbreak but as she will infect her clients over a period of time there may be no explosive rise in the number of cases
  ii. A well of contaminated water
  iii. Nationally distributed brand of vaccine (Eg Polio vaccine)
  iv. Food could result in similar outbreaks
       The resultant epidemics tend to be more extended or irregular.
  v.   Eg. Respiratory illness or Legionnaire's Disease in the summer of 1976 in Philadelphia (USA) (it continued beyond the range of one incubation period); There was no evidence of secondary cases among persons who had contact with ill people

A variation to the above model is that an epidemic may be initiated from a common source, Eg. Cholera (water borne), the epidemic reaches a sharp peak but falls off gradually over a longer period of time.

B. Propagated Epidemics

These are mostly of infectious origin and result from person-to-person transmission eg Hepatitis A, Polio, TB, SARS, MERS

The epidemics show a gradual rise and fall over a much longer period of time.

Transmission continues until:
i. The number of susceptibles are depleted, or
ii. Susceptible individuals are no longer exposed to infected persons or intermediary vectors

The speed of spread depends upon:
i.   Herd Immunity
ii. Opportunities of contact
iii. Secondary Attack Rate (SAR)

Propagated Epidemics are more likely to occur where:
(a) Large number of susceptibles are aggregated, or
(b) There is a regular supply of new susceptible individuals (births, immigrants) lowering herd immunity

Course of Typical Propagated Epidemic

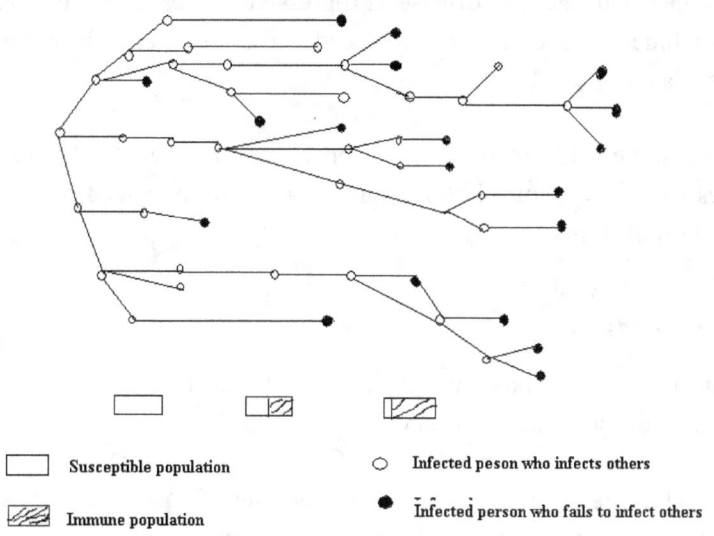

☐ Susceptible population   ○ Infected peson who infects others

▨ Immune population   ● Infected person who fails to infect others

(II) Periodic Fluctuations
      i. Seasonal Trends
      ii. Cyclic Trends

i. Seasonal Trends
- Early Spring - Measles, Varicella
- Summers - Gastrointestinal infections, because of warm weather and rapid multiplication of flies
- Winters - Upper Respiratory Infections

Seasonal variations of disease occurrence may be related to environmental conditions (temperature, humidity, rainfall, life cycle of vectors, overcrowding) which directly or indirectly favour disease transmission.

ii. *Cyclic Trends*

Some diseases occur in cycles spread over short periods of time eg. Days, weeks, months or years.

In Pre-vaccination era:
  i.   Measles peaks every 2-3 years
  ii. Rubella peaks every 6-9 years
       (This is due to naturally occurring variations in herd immunity. A build-up of susceptibles is again required in the herd before there can be another attack)
  iii. Influenza pandemics every 7-10 years due to antigenic variations
  iv. Non-communicable diseases may also show periodic fluctuation eg. Automobile accidents are more frequent on weekends especially Saturdays. Knowledge of cyclicity of diseases is useful for enabling communities to defend themselves.

(III) Long Term or Secular Trends

Changes in occurrence of disease (Progressive increase or decrease) over a long period of time of several years or decades Eg. Coronary Heart Disease, Diabetes Mellitus, Cancer

A consistent upward trend and decline of communicable diseases in developed countries namely Typhoid, Polio, Diphtheria due to improved socio-economic status and standard of living

Uses of Time Trends

- By monitoring Time Trends, the epidemiologist finds out:
    o Which diseases are increasing?
    o Which diseases are decreasing?
    o Which diseases are emerging health problems?
    o What is the effectiveness of control measures?
- He tries to formulate an Aetiological Hypothesis
- He seeks explanation whether the changes were due to changes in the Aetiological agent
- Variations in diagnosis
- Variations in reporting
- Variations in case fatality
- Variations in age distribution, or
- Variations in quality of life, Socio-economic status, Personal habits
- Eg. The time clustering of cases of Adenocarcinoma of vagina in young women led to incrimination of its cause, in-utero exposure to Diethylstilboestrol

Time Trends enable the epidemiologist to provide guidelines to health administrator regarding prevention and control.

PLACE DISTRIBUTION

Distribution of a disease in different populations gives insight to the differences in the disease patterns between countries and within countries.

Migrant studies is one way of distinguishing genetic and environmental factors.
Eg. Punjabi Indians in India vs Punjabi Indians in UK with respect to Coronary Heart Disease.

Geographic patterns provide important clues for causes of the disease.

Variation may be classified as:
(a) International Variations
(b) National Variations
(c) Rural Urban Differences
(d) Local Distributions

(a) International Variations
- Ca Stomach is common in Japan but unusual in US
- Ca Oral Cavity & Ca Cervix is common in India compared to the industrialized countries.
- Breast Ca is the highest in Western countries while it is lowest in Japan

(b) National Variations
- Endemic Goitre, Fluorosis, Lathyrism, Guinea worm disease, Leprosy, Malaria, Nutritional Deficiency diseases are variably distributed throughout India.
- Descriptive Epidemiology helps to provide data regarding the type of disease problems, their magnitude in terms of incidence, prevalence and mortality rates.
- This enables provision of appropriate health care services.

(c) Rural – Urban Variations
Diseases in Urban areas include Chronic Bronchitis, Lung Ca, Cardiovascular Diseases, Mental Illness, Drug Dependence and accidents

Diseases in Rural areas include Skin Diseases, Zoonotic Diseases, Soil Transmitted Helminths, Death rates eg. rural > urban.

Variations are due to population density, education, social class, environmental factors, sanitation, safe water and medical care facilities

The epidemiologist seeks to define groups who are at higher risk for particular diseases and provide guidelines for their prevention and control.

(d)   Local Distribution

Inner and outer city variations in disease frequency are best studied on a spot map or a shaded map.

These maps show at a glance the areas of high or low frequency, boundaries and patterns of disease Distribution.

Eg. John Snow of England on investigating the Cholera Epidemic in 1854 in Golden Square district of London was able to focus attention on the common water pump in Broad Street as the source of the infection.

Based on this, Snow hypothesized that Cholera was a water borne disease long before the birth of Bacteriology.

The clinician is also benefited from the knowledge that a patient brings to him from a certain geographic area which is endemic for certain diseases eg. Leishmaniasis or Yaws.

Geographic distribution of disease may change if changes occur in the agent, host and environmental factors.

Migration Studies

Migration of human populations from one country to another provides opportunity to evaluate the role of genetic and environmental factors.

Migrant studies can be carried out in the following 2 ways:
  i.   Comparison of disease and death rates for migrants with those of their kin who have stayed at home (genetically similar groups living under different environmental conditions)

       If disease and death rates in migrants are similar to the country of adoption over a period of time, it may be due to the change in environment. A special case would be the study of twins who are exposed to different environment of migration.
  ii. Comparison of migrants with local population of the host country provides information on genetically different groups living in similar environment. If migrant's rates of disease and death are similar to the country of origin, the likely explanation would be genetic factors.

Migrant studies have shown that Japanese ancestry men living in USA experience a higher rate of Coronary Heart Disease than those Japanese living in Japan.

Japan has a higher rate of Stomach Ca and lower rate for Colon Ca than USA.

However, third generation descendants of Japanese migrants to USA have rates of Stomach and Colon Ca like those of the USA. These studies suggest that the Japanese were probably adopting the American way of life.

PERSON DISTRIBUTION

The disease is characterized by defining the persons who develop the disease by:
Age
Gender
Ethnicity
Marital Status
Occupation
Social Class
Behavior
Stress
Migration

1. Age

Age is strongly related to a disease.
Eg. Measles in childhood, Cancer in middle age, Atherosclerosis in old age

Bimodality:

Sometimes there may be 2 separate peaks instead of one in the Age Incidence Curve of a disease
Eg. Hodgkin's Disease, Leukemia, Female Breast Ca.

The curve is Bimodal with an initial peak at 15-35 years and the later peak starting at age 50.

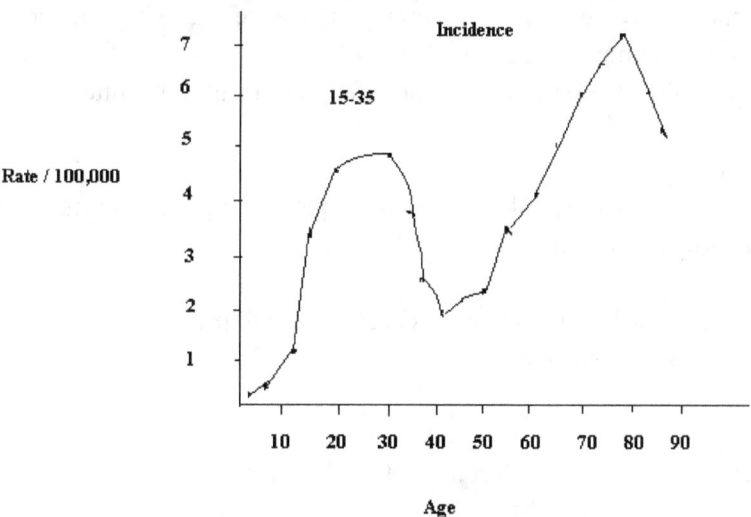

Bimodality in Hodgkin's disease in USA

2. Gender

Women – diabetes, obesity, hyperthyroidism more common

coronary heart disease, lung cancer less common

Variations in disease frequency between genders have been ascribed to:
(a) Basic biological differences including gender
(b) Cultural & behavioral differences
    (Eg Smoking, Alcoholism, Automobile use)

It is the 4:1 Male to Female Ratio in Lung Ca that has helped to identify cigarette smoking as a causal factor.

3. Ethnicity

Differences in disease occurrence have been noted between populations of different racial & ethnic origins.

Eg Hypertension	–	American Blacks
Sickle Cell Anemia	–	Africans
Coronary Heart Disease	–	Indians
Stomach Ca	–	Japanese
Breast Ca	-	Americans
Colon Ca		

4. Marital Status

Mortality is lower for married males & females
Married people are generally more secure, protected and lead sober lives.
Marital status may be a risk for certain diseases eg Ca Cx (Higher with multiple sexual partners and promiscuity)
This in turn raises the possibility of an infectious agent transmitted venereally.

5. Occupation

Occupation may alter the habit pattern of employees eg Night Shifts, Sleep, Smoking, Alcohol, Drug Addiction

Persons working in particular occupations are exposed to particular risks:
Eg. Coal mine workers - Silicosis

Chimney sweeps -	Scrotal Ca
Sedentary occupations -	Coronary Heart Disease
Coal, Asbestos, Beryllium -	Pneumoconiosis
Lead -	Plumbism

6. **Social Class**

   People of higher class enjoy better health, longer life expectancy, better nutritional status, better utilization of medical & health care, but more of Coronary Heart Disease, Diabetes Mellitus

7. **Behaviour (Lifestyle)**

   cigarette smoking, alcohol, sedentary lifestyle, overeating related to coronary heart disease

   Drug abuse

   Betel leaf with Tobacco leads to Oropharyngeal Cancer

   Coffee, tea

8. **Stress**

   Affects a variety of variables

   Eg. Susceptibility to disease

   Exacerbation of symptoms

   Compliance with medical regimen

9. **Migration**

   leprosy, filaria, malaria were rural problems but now in urban areas also due to migration

Variations in distribution of disease in age, sex, occupation and other subgroups of the population can be the starting point of an Epidemiological enquiry leading to formulation of an Aetiological Hypothesis for further study. Knowledge of the frequency of distribution in subgroups of the population has also generated the concept of high-risk groups.

4. *Measurement of Disease:*

   Amount of disease in a population can be studied in terms of:

   Mortality

   Morbidity - Incidence, Prevalence

   Disability etc.

Descriptive Epidemiology may use a cross-sectional or longitudinal design to obtain estimations of the magnitude of health & disease problems in human populations.

5. *Comparing with known Indices*

   By comparing between different populations and subgroups of the same population, it is possible to arrive at clues to the Disease Aetiology.

   We can also define groups at increased risk for certain diseases.

6.   ***Formulation of a Hypothesis***

At the end of a Descriptive Study, it is possible to formulate a hypothesis relating to the Disease Aetiology.

Hypothesis is a supposition, arrived at from observation or reflection.

It can be accepted or rejected using techniques of Analytical Epidemiology.

The Hypothesis should specify the following:

(a)   The population – The characteristics of the persons to whom the hypothesis applies

(b)   The specific cause – Being considered

(c)   The expected outcome – The disease

(d)   The disease-response relationship – The amount of cause needed to lead to a stated incidence of effect

(e)   The time-response relationship - The time period that will elapse between exposure to the cause and observation of the effect.

Eg. Cigarette smoking causes Lung Cancer is an incomplete hypothesis.

Improved Hypothesis:

Smoking 30-40 cigarettes per day causes Lung Cancer in 10% of Smokers, after 20 years of exposure.

The success or failure of a research project depends on the soundness of the Hypothesis.

Uses of Descriptive Epidemiology

(a)   Provide data regarding the magnitude of the Disease Load and Types of Disease problems in the community in terms of Morbidity & Mortality Rates & Ratios

(b)   Provide clues to Disease Aetiology & help in formulation of Aetiological Hypothesis

(c)   Provide baseline background data for planning, organizing and evaluating preventive and curative services

(d)   Contribute to research by describing variations in disease occurrence by time, place and person

ANALYTICAL EPIDEMIOLOGY

Differences between Analytical Epidemiology & Descriptive Epidemiology

Descriptive Epidemiology	Analytical Epidemiology
Looks at the entire population	Subject of interest is the individuals within the population
Objective is to formulate a Hypothesis	To test the Hypothesis
	Although individuals are evaluated, inference is not to individuals but to the population

Analytical Studies:

These are of 2 major types:
   i.   Case Control Study
   ii. Cohort Study

It can determine:

(a) Whether or not a statistical association exists between a disease and the suspected factor

(b) If one exists, the Strength of Association

CASE-CONTROL STUDY

Factor(s)   ◄-------------   Individuals with a   } Cases
Present   Particular Disease

or   ◄-------------   Individuals without   }
Absent   any particular Disease   } Controls

PROSPECTIVE STUDY/COHORT STUDY

Individual Exposed to   ------►   Presence or
Particular Factor(s)   Absence of
                                             Disease

Individual Unexposed to   ------►
Particular Factor(s)

                    ------►
          Time

CASE CONTROL STUDY (Retrospective Study)

There are 3 distinct features in Case Control Study:
  i.   Both Exposure & Outcome (Disease) have occurred before the start of study
  ii. Study proceeds backwards from Effect to Cause
  iii. It uses a Control/Comparison Group to support or refute an inference

Cases and controls must be comparable with respect to the Confounding Factors eg. Age, gender, occupation, social status

Questionnaire includes personal characteristics and antecedent exposure which may be responsible for the condition

Examples of Case Control Studies:

Cancers eg. Lung Cancer, Adenocarcinoma of Vagina, Oral Contraception and Thromboembolic Disease, Thalidomide Tragedy, Liver Cirrhosis, Congestive Heart Failure, Lupus Erythematosis

Basic Design of Case Control Study:

Suspected or Risk factors	Cases (Disease Present)	Control (Disease Absent)
Present	a	b
Absent	c	d
	a + c	b + d

2 X 2 Table

Eg. If we want to test the Hypothesis that Cigarette Smoking causes Lung Cancer using Case Control Method, the investigation begins by assembling a group of Lung Cancer cases (a+c) and a group of suitably matched controls (b+d).
Past history of the 2 groups is gathered for presence or absence of smoking.

If the frequency of smoking a/a+c is higher in cases than in controls b/b+d, an association is said to exist between Smoking & Lung Cancer.

Case Control Studies are most useful in chronic disease problems when the causal pathway may span many decades.

Basic steps:
There are 4 basic steps in conducting a Case Control Study:
1.   Selection of Cases & Controls

2. Matching
3. Measurement of Exposure
4. Analysis & Interpretation

1. Selection of Cases & Controls

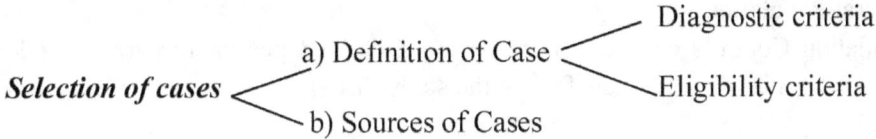

Selection of cases
  a) Definition of Case
    Diagnostic criteria
    Eligibility criteria
  b) Sources of Cases

(a) **Definition of Case:**

It involves 2 specifications:
  i. Diagnostic Criteria
    Diagnostic Criteria & Stage of Disease (Eg. Breast Ca Stage 1) must be specified.
  ii. Eligibility Criteria
    Only Incident Cases
    (Newly Diagnosed Cases within the specified period of time are eligible than Prevalent Cases (Old cases/cases in the advanced stage of the disease)

(b) **Sources of Cases:**
  i. Hospitals – Convenient to select cases from hospitals (from a single hospital/network of hospitals) admitted during a specified period of time; the entire case series or a random sample is selected
  ii. General Population – In Population-Based Study, all cases occurring within a defined geographical area, during a specified period of time – the entire series/random samples are selected for the study

Selection of Controls
Controls must be free from disease under study, they must be as similar to cases as possible.

Sources of Controls
  i. Hospital Controls
  ii. Relatives
  iii. Neighborhood Controls
  iv. General Population

  i. Hospital Controls
    These controls may be selected from the same hospital as cases but with different Illnesses
    Eg. If we are going to study Ca Cx patients, the Control Group may comprise of Breast Ca, GIT Ca, or patients with Non-Cancerous Lesions and other patients

ii. Relatives – Spouses/Siblings
(Sibling Controls are unsuitable where genetic conditions are under study)
iii. Neighborhood Controls
Persons living in the same locality as cases or persons working in the same factory or children attending the same school
iv. General Population
Population Controls can be obtained from a defined geographic area by taking a random sample of individuals free of the study disease.

How many controls are needed?

If many cases are available and the cost for collecting case and control is about equal, then one control for each case.

If the study group is small then as many as 2, 3 or 4 controls can be selected for each study subject.

2. Matching

Controls may differ from Cases in a number of factors eg. Age, gender, occupation, social status.

Comparability between cases and controls must be ensured.

This involves "Matching"

Matching:

It is a process by which Controls similar to Cases are selected with regard to certain variables (Eg. Age), which are known to influence the outcome of the disease, which if not adequately matched, could distort or confound the results.

Confounding factor is defined as one which is associated with both, Exposure and Disease.

A Confounding factor is one which is associated with exposure and is itself a Risk Factor for the disease.

Eg. 1) In the study of Role of Alcohol in the Aetiology of Oesophagal Cancer, smoking is a confounding factor because
(a) It is associated with the consumption of alcohol, and
(b) It is an independent Risk Factor for Oesophagal Cancer

2. Age can be a confounding variable
When investigating the relationship between Steroid Contraceptive and Breast Cancer, if women taking contraceptives were younger than those in the Comparison Group, they would definitely be at lower risk of Breast Ca since the disease is more common with increasing age.
The confounding factor of "Age" can be neutralized by matching such that both the groups have equal proportion of each age group.

While matching we should be careful that the suspected Aetiological Factor we wish to measure should not be matched because by matching its Aetiological Role is eliminated.

Eg. In the above case it would be useless to match cases and controls on Steroid Contraceptive use because by doing so the Aetiological Role of the Steroid Contraceptive cannot be investigated.

Matching Procedures:

(a) Group Matching – Assigning cases to Sub-Categories (Strata) based on characteristics eg. Age, gender, occupation, social class and then establishing appropriate controls. The Frequency Distribution of the matched variable must be similar in the study and in the Comparison Group

(b) Pairs Matching – For each case a control is chosen. It can be matched quite closely eg. If we have a patient, a 50-year-old mason, with a particular disease we will search for a 50-year-old mason without the disease as control. Thus, one can obtain pairs of patients and controls of the same age, gender, duration and severity of illness

3. **Measurement of Exposure**
   Information about exposures should be obtained for Cases and Controls.

   Procedures Used:
   (a) Interviews
   (b) Questionnaires
   (c) Past Records eg. Hospital records, Employment records

4. **Analysis**
   To find out:
   (a) Exposure Rates among cases and controls to suspected factor
   (b) Estimation of the risk to disease associated with exposure (Odd's Ratio)

(a) **Exposure Rates**
   Case Control Study provides direct estimation of Exposure Rates to a suspected factor among cases and controls.

Case Control Study of Smoking and Lung Cancer

	Cases (with Lung Ca)	Controls (without Lung Ca)
Smokers		
(< 5 cigarettes/day)	33	55
Non-smokers	2	27
Total	35 (a+c)	82 (b+d)

Exposure Rates:

(a) Cases = a/a+c = 33/35 = 94.2%

(b) Controls = b/b+d = 55/82 = 67.0%

P < 0.001

Inference:
The Frequency Rate of Lung Cancer was higher among smokers than non-smokers.

To ascertain whether there is a statistical association between exposure and occurrence of Lung Ca, we calculate the P value. Here it is < 0.001 therefore, it is significant at 0.1% level.
The Test of Significance will depend upon the variables under investigation.

Discrete variables
The results are presented as Rates or Proportions of those present or absent in the study or control group.
Test of Significance is applied - Standard Error of Difference between 2 proportions or Chi Square Test.

Continuous Variables

(Eg. Age, BP) The data will have to be grouped & Test of Significance is likely to be the Standard Error of Difference between 2 Means or T-test.

According to convention, if $P \leq 0.05$, it is statistically significant.
The smaller the P value, the greater the statistical significance or probability that the association is not due to chance alone.

However, Statistical Association (P value) does not imply Causation.

(b) Estimation of Risk
    This is obtained by calculating
        i. Relative Risk
        ii. Odd's Ratio

Relative Risk (RR)
It is the Ratio between Incidence of Disease among exposed persons and non-exposed persons.

$$RR = \frac{\text{Incidence among exposed}}{\text{Incidence among non-exposed}} \times 100$$

$$= \frac{a}{a+b} \div \frac{c}{c+d} \times 100$$

Case Control Study does not provide Incidence Rates from which RR can be calculated directly because there is no appropriate denominator or population at risk.

(RR can be determined exactly only through Cohort Study)

Odd's Ratio (Cross Product Ratio)

Odd's Ratio (OR) is a measure of Strength of Association between Risk Factor and Outcome. Odd's Ratio is closely related to RR.

Derivation of OR is based on 3 assumptions:

(a) Disease being investigated must be relatively rare (Eg. Chronic Diseases)
(b) Cases must be representative of those with the disease
(c) Controls must be representative of those without the disease

OR is the Cross Product Ratio:

	Disease	
	Yes	No
Exposed	a	b
Not Exposed	c	d

$$\text{Odd's Ratio} = \frac{ad}{bc}$$

$$= \frac{33 \times 27}{55 \times 2}$$

$$= 8.1$$

Inference:

Smokers of < 5 cigarettes per day had an 8:1 times the risk of Lung Ca as compared to Non-Smokers.

Bias in Case Control Study

Bias is any systematic error in the determination of association between Exposure and Disease. The RR Estimate may increase or decrease as a result of Bias.

Varieties of Bias

(a) Interviewer's Bias

When the interviewer knows the Hypothesis and knows the cases, he may interview the cases more thoroughly than the controls regarding a positive H/O, the suspected Causal Factor.

To check this, the time taken for interview can be noted for cases and controls.

To eliminate this Bias, double blinding can be done.

(b) Memory or Recall Bias

Cases may recall the past history better than controls eg. Patient who has suffered Myocardial Infarction may recall certain habits or events better than those who have not.

(c) Selection Bias

Cases and Controls may not be representative of Cases and Controls in the general population.

(d) Berkesonian Bias

Dr Joseph Berkson recognized this problem.

Bias arises because of different rates of admissions in hospitals for people with different diseases

(e) Confounding Bias

It is an important source of Bias, controlled by Matching in Case Control Study.

Advantages & Disadvantages

Advantages	Disadvantages
Easy to carry out	Bias problems
	Eg. Relies on memory or past records
Rapid	
Inexpensive	Validation of information is difficult
No risk to subjects	
	Selection of Control Group may be
No attrition problems	difficult
Ethical problems minimal	
	Representativeness of Cases & Controls is
Requires few subjects	a concern
Suitable for investigating rare diseases	
	Does not distinguish between Causes &
Allows study of several different	Associated Factors
Aetiological Factors eg. Smoking, diet,	
physical activity, personality in	Not suited for evaluation of therapy or
Myocardial Infarction	Prophylaxis of Disease
Risk factors can be identified and	Incidence cannot be measured
Prevention & Control Programmes can	
be established	Relative Risk can only be estimated

Examples of Case Control Studies:
- Cigarette Smoking & Lung Cancer
- Maternal Smoking & Congenital Malformations
- Radiation & Leukemia
- Oral Contraceptive use & Hepatocellular Adenoma
- Induced Abortion & Spontaneous Abortion
- Physical Activity & Coronary Death
- Artificial Sweeteners & Bladder Cancer
- Herpes Simplex & Bell's Palsy

I. Adenocarcinoma of the vagina

Unusual occurrence of this Tumour in 7 young women (15–22 years), born in a Boston Hospital between 1966-1969

Time clustering of cases
7 occurring within 4 years at a single hospital led to the enquiry.
Cause was investigated by a Case Control Study in 1971.
For each case, 4 Matched Controls were selected.

Controls were identified from the Birth Records of the hospital in which each case was born.
Female births occurring closest in time to each patient were selected as Controls.

Information was collected through:
Personal interviews regarding
(a) Maternal Age
(b) Maternal Smoking
(c) Antenatal Radiology
(d) Diethyl Stilboestrol (DES) exposure in Foetal Life

Results revealed that 7 out of 8 cases were exposed to DES in Foetal Life to prevent possible miscarriage during the first Trimester of pregnancy.
None of the mothers in the Control Group had received DES.

Association between Maternal DES Therapy & Adenocarcinoma of Vagina Amongst Female Offspring

Information Acquired Retrospectively	Cases (8)	Controls (32)	Significance Level
Maternal Age	26.1	29.3	NS
Maternal Smoking	7	21	NS
Antenatal Radiology	1	4	NS
Oestrogen Exposure	7	-	$P < 0.00001$

Case Control Method revealed that exposure to DES In Utero caused Vaginal Adenocarcinoma in the exposed child 10-20 years later.

2. Oral Contraceptives & Thromboembolic Disease

The Study was conducted by Vassey & Doll (1968 – 1969)

Interviewed women admitted to hospitals with Venous Thrombosis or Pulmonary Embolism and compared with women admitted to the same hospitals with other diseases and matched for age, marital status and poverty.

Out of 84 (42) 50% of those with Thrombosis and Pulmonary Embolism had used Oral Contraceptives as compared with 14% of Controls.

Relative Risk of users to non-users was 6.3:1. Users of OCPs were 6 times as likely as non-users to develop Thromboembolic Disease.

Case Control Studies on the Safety of Oral Contraceptives

	No.	% of OCPs
Cases (Venous Thrombosis & Pulmonary Embolism)	84	50
Controls	168	14

3. Thalidomide Tragedy

In 1958, Thalidomide was marketed as a safe Non-Barbiturate Hypnotic in Britain.

In 1961, at a Congress of Gynaecologists, attention was drawn to a large number of births with Congenital Abnormalities.

A retrospective study of 46 mothers who had delivered deformed babies showed that 41 had taken Thalidomide during their early pregnancy.

None of the Control 300 mothers with normal babies had taken Thalidomide.

COHORT STUDY

(Prospective Study, Longitudinal Study, Incidence Study, Forward Looking Study)

Introduction

It is another type of Analytical Observational Study undertaken to obtain evidence to support or refute the existence of an association between suspected cause and disease.

Definition of Cohort

A group of people who share a common characteristic or experience within a defined time period eg. Age, occupation, exposure to drug or vaccine, pregnancy, insured persons

Birth Cohort

A group of people born on the same day or in the same period of time (usually 1 year) eg. Birth Cohort of 2010 includes all those born in the year 2010

Marriage Cohort

A group of males or females married on the same day or the same period of time

Exposure Cohort

Persons exposed to a common drug/vaccine/infection within a defined period

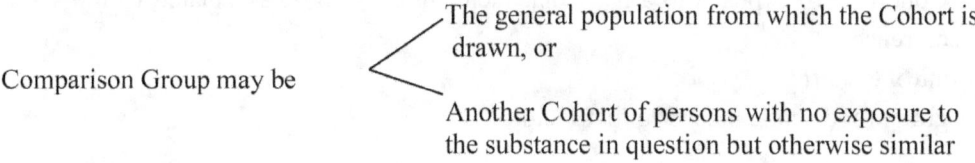

Comparison Group may be
- The general population from which the Cohort is drawn, or
- Another Cohort of persons with no exposure to the substance in question but otherwise similar

Distinguishing Features of Cohort studies

(a) Cohorts are identified prior to the appearance of the disease
(b) Study Groups are observed over a period of time to determine the frequency of disease among them
(c) Study proceeds from Cause to Effect

Indications for Cohort Studies

(a) When there is good evidence of association between Exposure and Disease
(b) When exposure is rare but incidence of disease is high among exposed
   Eg. Special Exposure Groups in industries; Exposure to X-rays etc.
(c) When attrition of study population can be minimized eg. Follow-up easy, cohort is stable, cooperative and easily accessible
(d) When ample funds are available

When study is initiated in Cohort Study, exposure has occurred but disease has not.

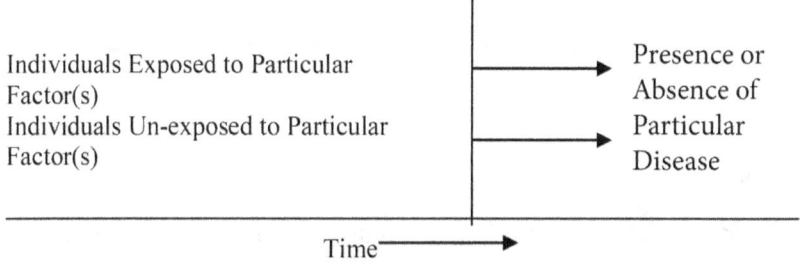

Individuals Exposed to Particular Factor(s)
Individuals Un-exposed to Particular Factor(s)

Presence or Absence of Particular Disease

Time

Framework of a Cohort Study

Cohort	Disease		Total
	Yes	No	
Exposed to Putative Aetiological Factor	a	b	a+b
Not exposed to Putative Aetiological Factor	c	d	c+d

We begin with:

i. Study Cohort

A Cohort (a+b) exposed to a particular factor thought to be associated with disease occurrence

ii. Control Cohort

A group (c+d) not exposed to that factor

General considerations:

i. Cohorts must be free from disease under study eg. We are studying Coronary Heart Disease, the Cohort members are examined and those who already have the disease are excluded

ii. Both groups (Study & Control Cohorts) should be equally susceptible to the disease under study eg. Males >35 years would be appropriate for studies on Lung Cancer

iii. Both groups should be comparable in all variables

iv. Diagnostic and Eligibility Criteria of the disease must be defined beforehand

The groups are followed up under same identical conditions over a period of time to determine the outcome of exposure   Disease
Disability or
Death

In the above Table, (a+b) persons were exposed to the factor out of which 'a' developed the disease; (c+d) persons were not exposed out of which 'c' became cases.

At the end of the follow-up period, the Incidence Rate of the disease was determined in both groups.

If incidence of disease in the exposed group (a/a+b) is significantly higher than in non-exposed group (c/c+d) it would suggest that the disease and suspected cause are associated.

Types of Cohort Studies

There are 3 types of Cohort Studies based on time of occurrence of disease in relation to time at which investigation is initiated and continued:

i. Prospective Cohort Studies
ii. Retrospective Cohort Studies
iii. Combination of Retrospective & Prospective Cohort Studies

i. *Prospective Cohort Study*
The outcome (eg. Disease) has not occurred at the time when investigations began
Prospective Studies begin in the present and continue into future.
Eg. Uranium miners & Lung Cancer (Uranium miners had an increased frequency of Lung Ca compared to non-miners)

Framingham Heart Study
Doll & Hill's Prospective Study on Smoking & Lung Ca
Study of Oral Contraceptive & Health

ii. *Retrospective Cohort Studies*
Also called Historical Cohort Study; Prospective Study in Retrospect; Non-Concurrent Prospective Study
In this, outcomes have all occurred before the start of the investigation.

Investigator goes back in time, 10-30 years, and selects the study groups from existing records (past employment, medical or other records) & traces them through time from a past date to the present.
Eg. Foetal Monitoring & Neonatal Health (The Neonatal Death Rate was 1-7 times higher in unmonitored infants)

Study of Role of Arsenic in Human Carcinogenesis

Physician's exposure to Radiation & Mortality experience
PVC (Polyvinyl Chloride) & Angiosarcoma of Liver

Retrospective Cohort Studies are more economical and produce results more quickly than Prospective Cohort Studies.
iii. *Combination of Retrospective & Prospective Cohort studies*
The Cohort is identified from past records & is assessed to date for the outcome and then followed up prospectively into the future for further assessment of outcome.

Eg.
Court-Brown & Doll in the Study on Effects of Radiation
They assembled a Cohort in 1955 consisting of 13,352 patients who had received large doses of
Radiation Therapy for Ankylosing Spondylitis between 1934–1954
Outcome evaluated was death from ⟵ Leukemia or
Aplastic Anaemia

Results showed that Death from Leukemia or Aplastic Anaemia was higher in their cohort than in the general population. A Prospective Component was added to the study and the cohort was followed up to identify deaths occurring in subsequent years.

Elements of A Cohort Study

1. Selection of Study Subjects
2. Obtaining Data on Exposure
3. Selection of Comparison Groups
4. Follow up
5. Analysis

1. Selection of study subjects

(a) General Population – Eg. Framingham Heart Study. If the population is very large a Representative Sample is taken.

(b) Special Groups (i) Select Groups eg. Professional groups (Doctors, nurses, lawyers, teachers, civil servants)
   Eg. Doll's Prospective Study on Smoking and Lung Ca was carried out on British Doctors

ii. Exposure Groups
   Special exposure to physical, chemical and other disease agents
   Workers in industries, those employed in high-risk situations
   Eg. Radiologists exposed to X-rays

2. Obtaining Data on Exposure

Information about exposure is obtained from:

(a) Cohort Members – Through personal interviews or mailed questionnaires eg. Doll and Hill used mailed questionnaires to collect smoking histories from British Doctors

(b) Review of Records – Medical Records eg. Dose of radiation, kinds of surgery, medical treatment

(c) Medical Examination/Special Tests – Some type of information obtained by Medical
   Examination/Special Tests eg. BP, ECG, Serum Cholesterol

(d) Environmental Surveys – Information on exposure levels of suspected factor in the environment where the cohort lived/worked

Information about exposure

(a) According to whether or not they have been exposed to the suspected factor
(b) According to the degree of exposure

Basic information about Demographic Variables should also be collected.

3. *Selection of Comparison Groups*
    Obtained in the following ways:
    (a) Internal Comparison: Cohort Group can be classified into several Comparison Groups according to degree of exposure to risk (Smoking, BP, Se Cholesterol) before the development of the disease
        The groups so defined are compared in terms of subsequent
        Morbidity and Mortality Rates
    (b) External Comparisons: When information on degree of exposure is not available, it is necessary to do external comparison to evaluate experience of the Exposed Group eg. Smokers & non-smokers; Cohort of
        Radiologists & Ophthalmologists. The Study & Control Cohorts should be similar in demographic & important variables
    (c) Comparison with General Population rates:
        If none is available, Mortality Experience of the Exposed
        Group is compared with Mortality Experience of the general population in the same area
        Eg. Comparison of the frequency of Lung Ca among Uranium
        Mine Worker with Lung Ca Mortality in the general population where the miners reside or comparison of frequency of Ca among Asbestos Workers in the general population in the same geographic area

4. *Follow-up*
    (a) Periodic Medical Examination of each member of the cohort
    (b) Reviewing Physician & Hospital Records
    (c) Routine Surveillance of Death Records
    (d) Mailed questionnaires, telephone calls, periodic home visits, preferably on annual basis

Attrition, a certain % of losses to follow up are inevitable due to death, change of residence, migration, occupation change

Should have a system for obtaining Basic Information on the outcome of those who cannot be followed up for full duration of the study as it may Bias the results.

It is recommended to achieve as close to 95% follow up if possible.

5. *Analysis*
    The Data is analysed in terms of:
    (a) Incidence Rates of outcome among exposed and unexposed
    (b) Estimation of Risk

    (a) Incidence Rates
        Can be calculated in the exposed and unexposed members

Cigarette smoking and Lung Cancer

Cigarette smoking	Developed Lung Ca	Did Not Develop Lung Ca	Total
Yes	70 (a)	6930 (b)	7000 (a+b)
No	3 (c)	2997 (d)	3000 (c+d)

Incidence Rates

(a)   Among smokers = 70/7000 = 10 per 1000

(b)   Among non-smokers = 3/3000 = 1 per 1000

Statistical Significance: P< 0.001

(b)   Estimation of Risk

Estimation of Risk of the outcome (eg. Disease or death) in the exposed and unexposed Cohorts is based on:

   i.   Relative Risk (RR),
   ii.   Attributable Risk (AR)

Ratio of Incidence of Disease or Death among exposed & incidence among non-exposed.

$$RR = \frac{\text{Incidence of Disease or Death among exposed}}{\text{Incidence of Disease or Death among non-exposed}}$$

RR of Lung Cancer = 10/1 = 10

Inference: Smokers are 10 times at greater risk of developing Lung Ca than non-smokers.

RR is a direct measure of Strength of Association between suspected cause and effect.

RR of 1 = No association

RR of 2 indicates that Incidence Rate of disease is 2 times higher in Exposed Group as compared with Un-Exposed.

The larger the RR the greater the Strength of Association between suspected factor and disease.

RR of 0.25 indicates a 75% reduction in Incidence Rate in exposed individuals as compared with un-exposed (eg. Screening of houses & malaria, those who are living in houses which are screened have 75% reduction in the incidence rate of malaria)

It is useful to consider 95% confidence interval of RR since it provides an indication of the likely maximum levels of risk.

Risk does not necessarily imply causal association.

Attributable Risk (Risk Difference)
The difference in Incidence Rate of Disease or Death between an Exposed Group & Non-Exposed Group expressed as a %.

$$AR = \frac{\text{Incidence of Disease Rate among exposed-Incidence of Disease Rate among non-exposed}}{\text{Incidence of Disease Rate among exposed}} \times 100$$

In the above eg:
$$AR = \frac{10-1}{10} X100 = 90\%$$

Inference:
It indicates to what extent the disease can be attributed to the exposure

In the above, 90% of Lung Ca among smokers was attributable to their smoking.

It suggests the amount of disease that might be eliminated if that factor could be controlled.

Population Attributable Risk
Definition: Incidence of Disease or Death in the total population minus the Incidence of Disease or Death among those who were not exposed to the suspected causal factor.

Lung Cancer Death Rates among Smokers and Non-Smokers: UK Physicians

Deaths per 100,000 person years			
Heavy Smokers	224	Exposed to suspected factor	(a)
Non-Smokers	10	Un-Exposed to suspected factor	(b)
Total population	74		(c)
Individual RR	a/b 22.40		
Population Attributable Risk (c-b)/c = 86%			

Population AR provides estimate of the amount by which the disease could be reduced in that population if the suspected factor was eliminated or modified.

In the given example, 86% of deaths from Lung Cancer could be avoided if the Risk Factor of cigarettes was eliminated.

Difference between Relative Risk & Attributable Risk

RR	AR
Indicates Strength of Association the larger the RR the stronger the association between cause & effect But RR does not reflect the potential public health importance as AR does	AR gives a better idea than RR of the impact of successful Preventive/Public Health Programme in reducing the problem

RR & AR of Cardiovascular Complications in Women Taking Oral Contraceptives

Cardiovascular Risk 100,000 patient years	Age(years)	
	30 – 39	40 – 44
Relative Risk	2.8	2.8
Attributable Risk	3.5	20.0

The RR of Cardiovascular Complications in users of OCPs is independent of age whereas, the AR is > 5 times higher in the older age groups.

This Epidemiological Observation is the basis for not recommending OCPs in those ≥ 35 years of age.

Risk Assessment for Smokers Vs Non-Smokers

Cause of Death	Death Rate/1000		RR	AR (%)
	Smokers	Non smokers		
Lung Cancer	0.90	0.07	12.86	92.2
CHD	4.87	4.22	1.15	13.3

Smoking is attributable to 92% of Lung Cancer & 13.3% of CHD.

In CHD, both RR & AR are not very high, suggesting not much of the disease could be prevented as compared to Lung Cancer.

Advantages & Disadvantages of Cohort Studies

Advantages	Disadvantages
(a) Incidence can be calculated	(a) Large No. of people involved, unsuitable for investigating rare diseases
(b) Relative Risk & Attributable Risk can be calculated	(b) Takes long time to complete the study eg. 20-30 years.
(c) Dose Response Ratios can be calculated	(c) Expensive, lot of funding is required
(d) Bias is minimized since Comparison Groups are formed before the disease develops	(d) Administrative problems eg. Loss of experienced staff, extensive record keeping, loss of funding
(e) Several outcomes related to exposure can be studied simultaneously eg. Cohort Studies for Association between Smoking & Lung Ca also showed Association of Smoking with CHD, Ca Oesophagus, Peptic Ulcer	(e) Attrition – Persons lost to follow up due to change of residence, migration or death
	(f) Study itself may change people's behaviour eg. In smoking & Lung Ca the study subjects may decrease or stop smoking
	(g) There may be changes in the Standard Methods or Diagnostic Criteria of the disease over prolonged follow up. Once Study Protocol is finalized it is difficult to introduce new knowledge or new tests later
	(h) Selection of Comparison Groups which are representative of the exposed & non-exposed segments of the population is a limiting factor. Volunteers may not be representative of all individuals with the characteristic interest
	(i) Ethical problems as evidence accumulates about the implicating factor in Aetiology of Disease, we are obliged to intervene & if possible, decrease or eliminate this factor
	(j) Practical considerations dictate that we must concentrate on a limited No. of factors related to the disease outcome

Differences Between Case Control & Cohort Studies

Case Control Study	Cohort Study
1. Proceeds from Effect to Cause	1. From Cause to Effect
2. Starts with the Disease	2. Starts with people exposed to the Risk Factor
3. Tests whether suspected cause occurs more frequently in those with disease than among those without disease	3. Tests whether disease occurs more frequently in those exposed than those not exposed
4. Usually the first approach to testing of a Hypothesis, but also useful for Exploratory Studies	4. Reserved for testing of precisely formulated Hypothesis
5. Involves fewer No. of subjects	5. Larger No. of subjects
6. Yields relatively quick results	6. Long follow-up period therefore, delayed results
7. Suitable for study of rare diseases	7. Inappropriate when the disease or exposure is rare
8. Yields only estimate of RR (Odds Ratio)	8. Yields Incidence Rates, RR & AR
9. Cannot yield information about diseases other than those selected for study	9. Several outcomes can be studied
10. Relatively inexpensive	10. Expensive

Examples of Cohort Studies

Eg 1. Smoking & Lung cancer
Conducted in 1951
Conducted by Doll & Hill
Questionnaire sent to 59,600 Doctors listed in the medical register of UK
Enquired about their Smoking Habits
This enabled them to form 2 Cohorts

Smokers & nonsmokers were selected
They were similar in all other respects eg. Age, education, social status
Received usable replies from 40,701 Physicians (34,494 Men) & (6,207 Women)
Follow up for 4 years & 5 months by obtaining notification of Physician's deaths

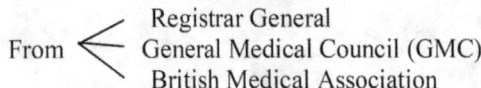

From
Registrar General
General Medical Council (GMC)
British Medical Association

For every death due to Lung Cancer, confirmation was obtained by writing to the Physicians certifying the death & also when necessary to the hospital or consultant to whom the patient had been referred.

Lung Cancer Death Rate among Smokers & Nonsmokers – UK physicians

Deaths per 100,000 person years			
Heavy Smokers	224	Exposed to suspected factor	(a)
Non-Smokers	10	Un-Exposed to Suspected Factor	(b)
Total population	74	(c)	
Individual RR	a/b	22.40	
Population attributable risk (c-b)/c = 86%			

Eg 2. The Framingham Heart Study

The Study was conducted in 1948

The Framingham Heart Study, initiated by US Public Health Service to study the relationship of a number of Risk Factors (Eg. Smoking, Serum Cholesterol, Blood Pressure, Weight) with the development of Cardiovascular Disease.

Framingham town in Massachusetts had a population of 28,000
The Study was planned for 20 years
The Study subjects were of 30 – 59 years of age.

Out of 10,000 in this age group, 6,507 were invited to participate
Out of which 5,209 volunteered

The Initial Examination revealed that 82 had clinically evident CHD, therefore, they were excluded

Finally, the No. of persons who participated were 4,469

Follow up was done every 2 years for 20years ⟨ Biennial Examinations &
Death Certificate Records

Information obtained on Se Cholesterol
BP
Cigarette smoking
Weight

The study identified the following Risk Factors:

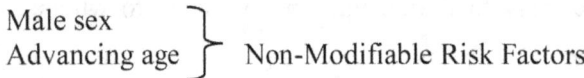

Male sex
Advancing age } Non-Modifiable Risk Factors

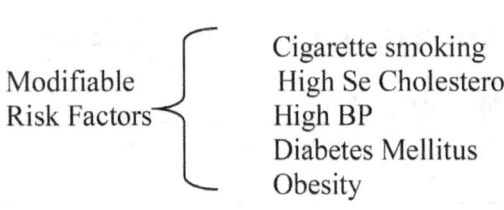

Modifiable
Risk Factors {
Cigarette smoking
High Se Cholesterol
High BP
Diabetes Mellitus
Obesity

Eg 3. Oral Contraceptives & Health

The Study was initiated in 1968
It was conducted by the Royal College of General Practitioners in England

Study Subjects were aged between 15 – 49 years (Reproductive Age Group)

There were 23,000 users of the pill
23,000 comparison groups using Other Methods/No Method were brought under observation of 1400 General Practitioners

Follow-up was for: Episodes of Illness
Pregnancies, and
Death

Results – Risks & Benefits of OCP use

The study showed that:
  i.   Risk of Hypertension increased
  ii. Mortality increased from diseases of Cardiovascular System
  iii. Risk of Benign Breast Disease decreased with the dose of Norethisterone Acetate (Progestogen)

RANDOMIZED CONTROLLED TRIALS (RCT)

Gold standard for evaluation of new therapies or new programmes

Steps:
1. Drawing up a Protocol
2. Selecting Reference & Experimental Populations
3. Randomization
4. Manipulation

5. Follow-up
6. Assessment of Outcome

Design of RCT

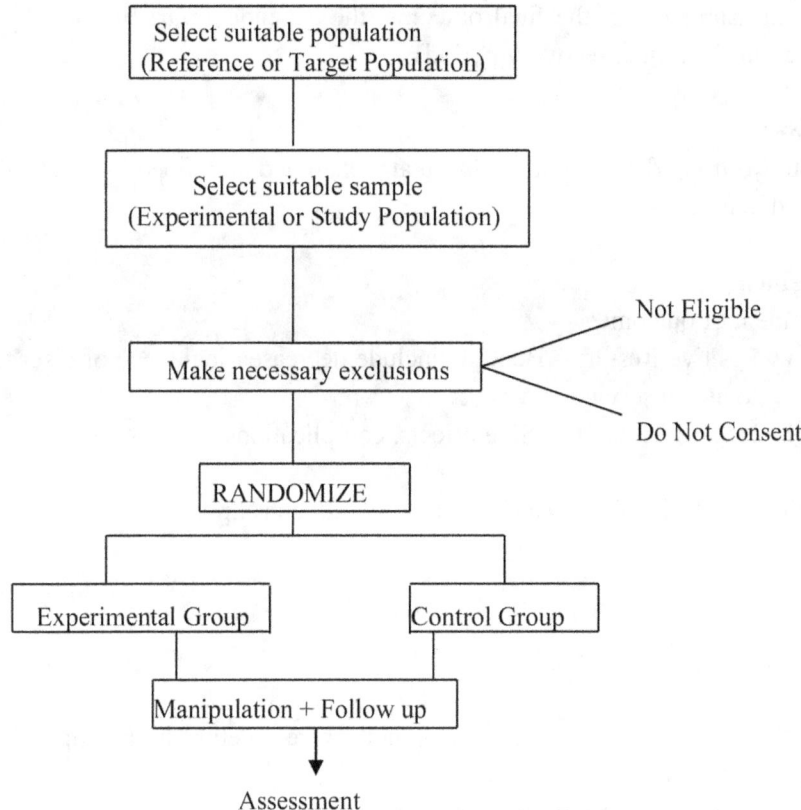

1. **Protocol**

   It helps to specify the aims, objectives, methods of study, selection of study group, control group, inclusion & exclusion criteria, manipulation, evaluation

2. **Selecting Reference & Experimental Population**
      i. Reference Population – Population to which findings of the trial are expected to be applicable
      ii. Experimental Population – Actual population which participates in the study

3. **Randomization**

   The heart of a Control Trial
   It is a statistical procedure by which participants are allocated either to the Study Group or the
   Control Group, to receive or not to receive a drug or a preventive procedure

4. **Manipulation**

Manipulation of the Study Group with drug, vaccine, dietary component, a habit

The manipulation creates:

An Independent Variable – Drug, vaccine, new procedure whose effect is determined by the measurement of the final outcome, the dependent variable (Eg. Incidence of disease, survival time, recovery period)

5. **Follow-up**

The Study Group & the Control Group are examined at defined intervals of time in a standard manner.

6. **Assessment**

Assessment of outcome:

   i. Positive Results – Benefits include decreased incidence of disease and cost to health service
   ii. Negative Results – Side effects, complications

Statistical Analysis of the Data is done in both the groups.

Blinding

To prevent Bias:

(a) Single Blind Trial – The participant is not aware whether he belongs to the Study Group or the Control Group
(b) Double Blind Trial - Neither the participant nor the Doctor knows the group allocation & the treatment received
(c) Triple Blind Trial - The participant, the Doctor & the Data Analyzer do not know the group allocation

Types of RCT

(a)	Clinical Trials	– Eg. Aspirin on Cardiovascular Mortality Betacarotene on Cancer incidence, Efficacy of Tonsillectomy for recurrent throat infections
(b)	Preventive trials	– Vaccines
(c)	Risk Factor Trials	– North Karelia Project in Finland, Stanford 3 Community Study, the Oslo Study, Multiple Risk Factor Interventions Trial (MRFIT) in USA to assess the effect of intervention on Coronary Heart Disease
(d)	Trial of Aetiological Agents	–Eg. Retrolental Fibroplasia & administration of Oxygen to premature babies

(e) Cessation Experiments   –Eg. Smoking & Lung Ca
(f) Evaluation of Health Services –RCT is used to assess the effectiveness & efficiency of health services
Eg. Domiciliary treatment of PTB is as effective as the more costly hospital/sanatorium treatment

ASSOCIATION & CAUSATION

Types of Association:
   a) Spurious Association
   b) Indirect Association
   c) Direct (Causal) Association   ⟨One-to-one Causal Association
                                          Multifactorial Association

(a) Spurious Association

It is an Observed Association between disease & suspected factor which may not be real eg. A study in UK showed that Perinatal Mortality was greater in hospital deliveries than home deliveries

(b) Indirect Association

It is an Association between a variable & the disease due to the presence of another factor (Confounding factor) which is common to both the variable & the disease
Eg. Association of Altitude & Endemic Goitre
Endemic Goiter is not due to altitude but due to environmental deficiency of Iodine.

(c) Direct (Causal) Association
   i.   One to one causal relationship

A ⟶ B, when factor A is present, disease B must result, but this is not always the case eg. TB
   ii. Multifactorial Causation

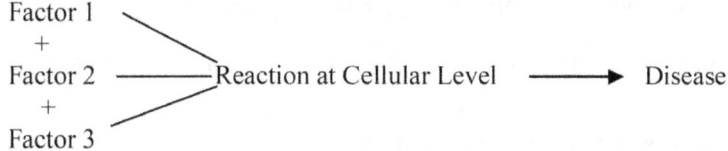

Eg. Smoking, diet, sedentary leads to Myocardial Infarction

Additional Criteria for Judging Causality

Eg. Association between Cigarette Smoking & Lung Cancer

1. Temporal Association

Causal Association requires that exposure to a cause must temporarily precede the onset of the disease.

Eg. Smoking precedes Lung Cancer

2. **Strength of Association**
    There is a likelihood that the causal relationship is more if Relative Risk, Dose Response & Duration Response is higher
    Eg. Risk of Lung Cancer is 8 times more among smokers than non-smokers

3. **Specificity of Association**
    It implies a one-to-one relationship between Cause and Effect.
    Attributable Risk shows that 80-90% of Lung Cancer can be attributed to Cigarette Smoking.

4. **Consistency of Association**
    The results can be replicated in different settings.
    Eg. 50 Retrospective Studies and 9 Prospective Studies in different countries showed a Consistent
    Association between Cigarette Smoking & Lung Cancer

5. **Biological Plausibility**
    There should be a Biological Credibility to the association.
    Eg. Inhalation of hot smoke into lungs & deposition of chemical carcinogen over a number of years initiating Neoplastic changes in the Lungs

6. **Coherence of Association**
    Coherence with known facts which are thought to be relevant
    Eg. Rise in cigarette consumption leading to rise in Lung Cancer.
    Fall in relative risk of Lung Cancer when cigarette smoking ceased.

Uses of Epidemiology

1. To study the rise & fall of a disease in the population

Epidemics of Coronary Heart Disease, Cancer, Diabetes, Accidents, AIDS have been studied.
It helps in making future projections & identifying the emerging health problems.

2. **Community Diagnosis**
    Identification & quantification of health problems in a community in terms of Mortality, Morbidity,
    Disability Rates & Ratios to find out the health care needs
    It helps to:

    (a) Prioritize Disease Control & Prevention Programmes
    (b) Serve as a benchmark for evaluation of Health Services

(c) Source of new knowledge about Disease Causation, Distribution & Prevention

3. **Evaluation of Individuals' Risks & Chances**
    Relative Risk & Attributable Risk helps to quantify the Degree of Risk eg. Smokers & Non-smokers for selected causes of death eg. Lung Cancer, Coronary Heart Disease or risk of bearing a Mongol child

4. **Syndrome Identification**
    Medical syndromes have been identified through Observational Studies eg. AIDS

5. **Completing the Natural History of a Disease**
    Disease patterns in the community studied and its relationship to agent, host, environmental factors help to fill the gaps in the natural history of disease eg. recognition that one-third to two-third of all deaths due to coronary heart disease occur within one hour; therefore ICUs sprang up

6. **Searching for Causes & Risk Factors**
    Case Control & Cohort Studies help in identifying the Causes and Risk Factors.
    Eg. Rubella ⟶ Congenital Defects in newborn
    Thalidomide ⟶ Phocomelia
    Cigarette Smoking ⟶ Lung Cancer

7. **Planning & Evaluation**
    Planning is essential for rational allocation of limited resources.
    Epidemiological information regarding distribution of health problems over time & place helps in planning, developing programmes & assessing impact of the services.

Infectious Disease Epidemiology

Definitions

Infection – The entry & development/multiplication of an Infectious Agent in the body of a man or animals.
Infection does not always cause illness.

Several levels of Infection:
(a) Colonization eg. Staph Aureus on Skin & Nasopharynx
(b) Sub-Clinical Infection eg. polio,
(c) Latent Infection eg. Virus of Herpes Simplex
(d) Clinical Infection.

Contamination – The presence of an Infectious Agent on a body surface, on clothes, beddings, toys, surgical instruments, dressings, inanimate articles eg. Water, milk, food.

Pollution – The presence of offensive but not necessarily infectious matter in the environment.

Infestation – Lodgement, Development, Reproduction of Arthropods on the surface of a body or in clothing eg. Lice, Itch Mites

Host – The person or animal, birds, arthropods that afford lodgement to an Infectious Agent

Obligate Host –The only host eg. Man in Measles, Typhoid

Definitive Host – The host in which the parasite undergoes the Sexual Stage

Intermediate Host – The host in which the parasite undergoes Asexual Stage

Transport Host – A carrier in which the agent remains alive but does not undergo development

Infectious Disease – A clinically manifest disease of man/animals resulting from an infection

Contagious Disease – A Disease that is transmitted through contact eg. Scabies, Trachoma, STD, Leprosy

Communicable Disease – An illness due to a specific Infectious Agent or its Toxic Products capable of being directly/indirectly transmitted from man to man, animal to animal, or from the environment (through air, dust, soil, water, food) to man/animal

Epidemic – (epi = upon, demos = people)
The unusual occurrence in a community of disease, health related behaviour (eg. Smoking) or health related event (eg. Traffic accidents) clearly in excess of the expected occurrence

Endemic – (en = in, demos = people)
The usual or expected frequency of a disease within a geographic area or population group

Sporadic – It means scattered about; cases occur irregularly, infrequently from time-to-time eg. JE, Polio, Tetanus, Herpes Zoster

Pandemic – An epidemic affecting a large proportion of the population, over a wide geographic area such as a section of a nation, entire nation, a continent or the world. eg. Cholera, Influenza, SARS, COVID-19

Exotic Diseases – These are imported into a country in which they do not occur eg. Rabies in UK

Zoonosis – An Infectious Disease, transmissible from vertebrate animals to man eg. Rabies, Hydatidosis, Plague, Bovine TB, Brucellosis, Anthrax, Salmonellosis, Endemic Typhus, KFD, Monkeypox, Lassa Fever

Epizootic – An epidemic of disease in an animal population
Eg. Anthrax, Brucellosis, Rabies, Influenza, Rift Valley Fever, Q Fever, JE, Equine Encephalitis, Plague

Enzootic – An endemic occurring in animals eg. Anthrax, Brucellosis, Rabies, Bovine TB, Endemic Typhus, Tick Typhus

Epornithic – An epidemic of disease in a bird population

Nosocomial Infection (Hospital Acquired Infection)
An infection originating in a patient while in a hospital or health care facility. Eg. Surgical Wound Infection, Hepatitis B, Urinary Tract Infections

Opportunistic Infection
Infection by an organism which takes the opportunity due to defect in host defence to infect the host & hence cause disease
Eg. AIDS, Herpes Simplex, CMV, T Gondii, M Avium Intracellulare, Pneumocystis

Iatrogenic (Physician-Induced) Disease
An adverse consequence of a Therapeutic, Diagnostic or Preventive procedure that causes Impairment, Disability, Handicap or Death resulting from a Physician's professional activity or professional activity of other Health Care Workers which are preventable

Eg. Anaphylaxis due to drugs like Penicillin, Reactions to Immunizing Agents, Aplastic Anaemia following Chloramphenicol Therapy, Childhood Leukemia due to Prenatal X-rays, Hepatitis B following Blood Transfusion.

Surveillance
The continuous scrutiny of factors that determine the Occurrence & Distribution of a Disease or health related events. Surveillance is essential for effective Control & Prevention.

It also means the continuous scrutiny of Health Indices, Nutritional Status, Environmental Hazards, Health Practices & Factors that may affect health. Eg. Epidemiological Surveillance, Nutritional Surveillance, Demographic Surveillance, Serological Surveillance

Eradication
Termination of all transmission of infection by extermination of the Infectious Agent through Surveillance & Containment. Eg. Smallpox, Guinea Worm.

Diseases amenable to Eradication are Measles, Polio, Diphtheria.

Dynamics of Disease Transmission

Communicable Diseases are transmitted from sources/reservoirs to the Susceptible Host.

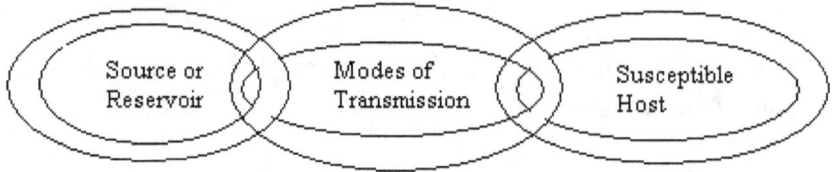

Components:
(a) Reservoir
(b) Transmission
(c) Host

(I) Reservoir:

Any person, animal, arthropod, plant, soil or substance in which an Infectious Agent lives & multiplies, reproduces itself & can be transmitted to a Susceptible Host is called a Reservoir.

Source – Any person, animal, object or substance from which an Infectious Agent passes to the host

Type of Reservoirs
1. Human Reservoir
2. Animal Reservoir
3. Non-Living Reservoir

1. *Human Reservoir*
(a) Cases – Clinical Illness – A person having the disease with symptoms & signs
    Sub-Clinical Cases – The Disease Agent may multiply but no symptoms & signs seen; Can be detected only by Laboratory Tests
    Latent Infection– The host does not shed the Infectious Agent which lies dormant in the host without symptoms. Eg. Herpes Zoster
    Primary Case – The first case introduced into the population. The Index Case which first comes to the attention of the Investigator
(b) Carriers - An infected person or animal that harbours an Infectious Agent in the absence of Clinical Disease & serves as a potential Source of Infection for others

Classification

A. By Type
   (a) Incubatory
   (b) Convalescent
   (c) Healthy

B. Duration
    (a) Temporary
    (b) Chronic

C. Portal of Exit
    (a) Urinary
    (b) Intestinal
    (c) Respiratory
    (d) Others

Incubatory Carriers	– Those who shed the Infectious Agent during the Incubation Period eg. Measles, Mumps, Pertussis, Diphtheria, Polio, Influenza, Hepatitis B
Convalescent Carriers	– Those who shed the Disease Agent in the Convalescence Period eg. Typhoid, Dysentery, Cholera, Diphtheria, Pertussis
Healthy Carriers	– They appear healthy but shed the Disease Agent eg. Polio, Diphtheria, Cholera, Typhoid Mary, Salmonellosis, Meningococcal Meningitis
Temporary Carriers	– Those who shed the Infectious Agent for short periods of time. Eg. Incubatory, Convalescent, Healthy Carriers
Chronic Carriers	– One who excretes the Infectious Agent for indefinite periods eg. Typhoid, Dysentery, Hepatitis B, Cerebrospinal Meningitis, Malaria, Gonorrhoea
Urinary Carriers	– Eg. Typhoid
Intestinal Carriers	– Eg. Polio, Viral Hepatitis, Dysentery
Respiratory Carriers	– Eg. Diphtheria
Others	– Skin Eruptions (Staph Aureus), Open Wounds, Blood

2. ***Animal Reservoir***
    Animals & birds which may be cases or carriers
    Zoonosis – Diseases from vertebrates to man
    Eg. Rabies, Yellow Fever, Influenza, JE through wild birds (Herons, Ardeid birds) & pigs

3. ***Non-living Reservoir***
    Eg. Soil may harbour Tetanus, Anthrax, Coccidiodomycosis, Mycetoma

(II) Transmission
    Communicable diseases may be transmitted from the Reservoir to the Host in the following ways:

A. *Direct Transmission*
    1. Direct Contact
    2. Droplet Infection

3. Contact with Soil
4. Inoculation into Skin/Mucosa
5. Transplacental

B. Indirect Transmission
(Five Fs – Fluid, Food, Flies, Fomite, Finger)
1. Vehicle Borne
2. Vector Borne
3. Airborne
4. Fomite Borne
5. Fingers

A. Direct Transmission

1. Direct Contact
The contact is through skin to skin, mucosa to mucosa or mucosa to skin of the same or another person
eg. STD, AIDS, Leptospira, Leprosy, Skin Infections, Eye Infections

2. Droplet Infection
The direct projection of spray of droplets of Saliva or Nasopharyngeal Secretions during Coughing, Sneezing, Speaking, Spitting, Talking into the atmosphere. The droplets may fall on the Conjunctiva, Respiratory Mucosa or skin of host within 30-60 cm thus, he may acquire the infection eg. Respiratory Infections, Eruptive Fevers, Common Cold, Diphtheria, Pertussis, TB, Meningococcal Meningitis

3. Contact with Soil
Disease acquired through contact with soil eg. Hookworm, Tetanus, Mycosis

4. Inoculation into Skin or Mucosa
Disease Agent is inoculated directly into the Skin or Mucosa eg. Rabies virus by dog bite, Hepatitis B through contaminated Needles, Syringes

5. Transplacental Transmission
Disease Agents transmitted Transplacentally eg. HIV, TORCH (Toxoplasma, Rubella, Cytomegalovirus, Herpes Virus), Varicella, Syphilis, Hepatitis B, Coxsackie B.
Non-living Agents eg. Thalidomide, Diethylstilboestrol

B. Indirect Transmission
1. Vehicle Borne
Transmission of Infectious Agent through water, food, ice, blood, tissues, organs eg. Staph Aureus Through food, Hepatitis A, Acute Diarrhoea, Typhoid, Cholera, Polio, Food Poisoning,

Intestinal Parasites;

Through blood, Hepatitis B, Malaria, Syphilis, Brucellosis, Trypanosomiasis, Infectious Mononucleosis, Cytomegalovirus Infections;

Through Organ Transplantation which may lead to CMV Infection

2. *Vector Borne*

    These are spread through a Vector such as Arthropod (eg. Fly) or any living carrier (eg. Snail) that transports the Infectious Agent to the Host Mechanical Transmission

Biological transmission

  i.   Propagative – The Agent multiplies in the Vector eg. Plague

  ii. Cyclo-propagative – The Agent changes in form and number eg. Malaria

  iii. Cyclo-developmental – The Agent undergoes only development, no multiplication eg. Filaria

  iv. Transovarial Transmission – The Agent is transmitted vertically from infected female to progeny in the Vector eg. KFD, Dengue

  v.   Trans-stadial Transmission – The Disease Agent is transmitted from one stage of life cycle to another eg. Nymph to adult in the Vector eg. KFD

3. *Air Borne*

    (a) Droplet Nuclei

    Particles of 1-10µ which are dried residue of droplets

    These are formed by

    (a) Evaporation of droplets Coughed/Sneezed

    (b) Atomizing Devices (Aerosols)

    (c) Microbiological Laboratories in Abattoirs, float in air & may be disseminated by air currents eg. Respiratory Infections – TB, Influenza, Chicken Pox, Measles, Pertussis, Toxic Air Pollutants.

(b) Dust

During talking, coughing, sneezing, the larger droplets expelled settle on the floor, carpets, furniture, clothes, bedding, linen, eg. Streptococci, Viruses, Fungal Spores, Skin Squamae, TB Bacilli,

Staph Infection, Pneumonia, Psittacosis.

During sneezing, dusting, bedmaking the dust becomes airborne.

Dust particles may be from Soil through Wind eg. Fungal Spores – Coccidioidomycosis.

This type of transmission is most common in Hospital Acquired (Nosocomial) Infection.

4. *Fomite Borne*

Fomites are inanimate articles eg. Clothes, towels, linen, handkerchiefs, cups, spoons, pencils, books, toys, drinking glasses, door handles, taps, lavatory chains, syringes, instruments, surgical dressings which are contaminated by Infectious Discharges from patients.

Diseases Transmitted – Diphtheria, Typhoid, Dysentery, Diarrhoea, Hepatitis A, Eye Infections,
Skin Infections – Scabies, Pediculosis

5. *Unclean Hands & Fingers*

Hands harbour Disease Agents from skin, nose, bowel etc. due to poor personal hygiene.
Diseases Transmitted – Staphylococcal Infection, Streptococcal, Typhoid Fever, Dysentery, Hepatitis A, Intestinal Parasites, SARS COV-2

(III) Host

Susceptible Host

For successful Parasitism the Disease Agent must find:
1. Portal of Entry – Eg. Respiratory Tract, Alimentary Tract, Genitourinary Tract, Skin
2. Site of Election – Where the agent can multiply & survive
3. Portal of Exit – For reaching a new host & propagating its species
   If there is no portal of exit, it becomes Dead End Host
   Eg. Rabies, Tetanus, Bubonic Plague, Hydatid Disease, Japanese Encephalitis, Dengue, Trichinosis
4. Survival in External Environment – Until a new host is found

Incubation Period (IP)

The Time Interval between invasion by Infectious Agent & appearance of the first sign or symptom, when multiplication of Infectious Agent takes place.

Median Incubation Period:
The time required for 50% of the cases to occur following exposure

Factors determining incubation period:
(a) Generation Time
(b) Infective Dose
(c) Portal of Entry
(d) Individual Susceptibility

Length of incubation period characteristic of each disease:
(a) Short Incubation Period - Few hours to 3 days – Staph Food Poisoning, Cholera, Dysentery, Influenza
(b) Medium Incubation Period 10 days to 3 weeks – Typhoid, Chicken Pox, Measles, Mumps

(c) Long Incubation period - Weeks to months/years – Hepatitis A, Hepatitis B, Rabies, Leprosy, TB, Slow Virus Diseases

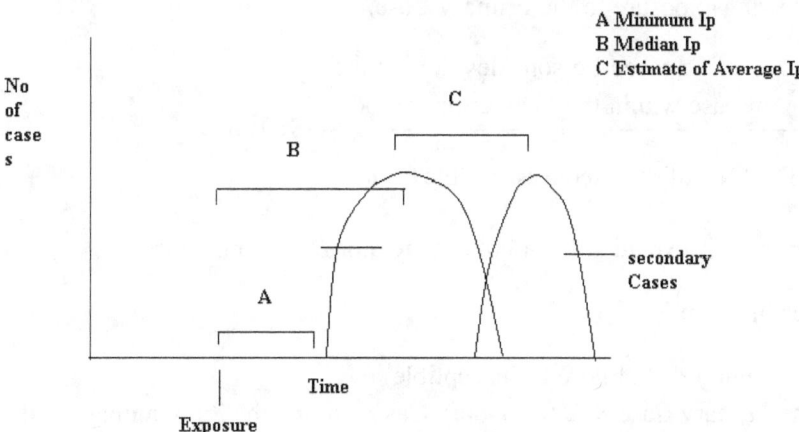

Uses of Incubation Period
1. Tracing the Source of Infection & Contacts
2. Period of Surveillance (Quarantine) – For maximum Incubation Period of the Disease
3. Immunization – The knowledge of IP helps in prevention of the Disease with Human Immunoglobulins and Antisera
4. Identification of Point Source – In Point Source Epidemic, all cases occur within one IP
5. Identification of Propagated Epidemics – Cases occur later than IP
6. Prognosis – Short IP, worse prognosis eg. Rabies, Tetanus

Latent Period
The period from Disease Initiation to Disease Detection
Eg. Cancer, DM, Coronary Heart Disease
In Communicable Diseases the Latent Period is equivalent to IP.

Serial Interval
The period from onset of Primary Case to onset of Secondary Case
Eg. In a family there is a Primary Case & then 2 – 3 Secondary Cases

The gap in time between onset of Primary Case and Secondary Case is called the Serial Interval. From this Incubation Period can be guessed.

Generation Time
The Time Interval between Receipt of Infection & Maximal Infectivity of the host, roughly equal to Incubation Period.

Communicable Period
Period of Infectivity – The time during which the Infectious Agent may be transferred directly/indirectly from person to person, animal to person, person to animal/arthropods.

It can be measured by Secondary Attack Rate (SAR).

Secondary Attack Rate (SAR)

The number of exposed persons developing the disease within the range of the Incubation Period, following exposure to the Primary Case.

$$SAR = \frac{\text{No. of Exposed Persons developing the disease within the Incubation Period}}{\text{Total No. of Exposed/Susceptible Contacts}} \times 100$$

The primary case is excluded from both numerator & denominator.

Eg. Measles in a family of 6:

2 parents (Immune) & 3 children (Susceptible)
There is one Primary Case & 2 Secondary Cases among the 3 remaining children.

$$SAR = \frac{2}{3} = 66.6\%$$

Uses:

1. To measure the spread of an Infection within a family, household or a closed aggregate of persons
2. To determine whether the Disease of unknown Etiology (eg. Hodgkin's Disease) is communicable or not
3. To evaluate the effectiveness of Control Measures such as Isolation, Immunization

Host Defences

1. Active Immunity
   (a) Humoral Immunity
   (b) Cellular Immunity
   (c) Combined
2. Passive Immunity
   (a) Normal Human Ig
   (b) Specific Human Ig
   (c) Animal Antitoxins or Antisera

I Active immunity

Definition
The Immunity which an individual develops as a result of Infection or Immunization & is associated with the presence of Antibodies against the Microorganism or its Toxin.

Active Immunity is acquired in 3 ways:

(a)   Following Clinical Infection - Rubella, Measles, Chicken Pox

(b)   Following Sub-Clinical Infection - Polio, Diphtheria

(c)   Following Immunization with an Antigen which may be a Killed Vaccine, Live Attenuated Vaccine or a Toxoid

The Immune Response

(a)   Primary Response

When the Antigen is administered for the first time to a person, IgM appears after 3-10 days, reaches a peak then declines as fast as it has developed.

Later when IgG appears, it reaches a peak in 7-10 days then declines gradually over a period of weeks or months.

"Memory Cells" or "Primed Cells" by B & T Lymphocytes are produced.

(b)   Secondary (Booster) Response

Differs from Primary Response in the following ways:

    i.   Shorter Latent Period

    ii.   Production of Antibody is more rapid

    iii. Antibodies are more abundant

    iv.   Antibody Response is maintained at higher levels for longer period

    v.   Antibody has greater capacity to bind to the Antigen

1.   *Humoral Immunity*

B – Cells (Bone Marrow Derived Lymphocytes) produce Humoral Immunity. Immunoglobulins belong to 5 main classes – IgG, IgM, IgA, IgD and IgE.

Antibodies circulate in the body & neutralize the microbe, the toxin or render the microbe susceptible to attack by Polymorphonuclear Leukocyte & Monocyte.
The antibodies are specific, they react with the same Antigen which provoked their production.

2.   *Cellular Immunity*

It is mainly by T-Lymphocytes. On contact with the Antigens, T-Cells cause activation of macrophages, release of Cytotoxic Factors, Mononuclear Inflammatory Reactions, Delayed Hypersensitivity Reactions, Secretion of Immunological Mediators eg. Immune Interferon.

Cellular Immunity is important in TB, Leprosy, Brucellosis & body's reaction to foreign material eg. Skin Grafts.

3. *Combined*
    B Cells & T-Lymphoid Cells, Macrophages, K (killer) Cells are involved in Immune Reactions.
    Vaccines elicit both Humoral & Cell Mediated Immunity.

    Many factors are involved in the maintenance of such Immunity such as Fatigue, Diet, Drugs, Strange Surroundings, Emotional Shock which decrease Immunity.

Immunizing Agents

VACCINES	BCG	
	Typhoid Oral	Bacterial
	Plague	
Live AttenuatedVaccines	Sabin (Oral Polio)	
	Yellow Fever	
	Measles	
	Rubella	Viral
	Mumps	
	Influenza	
	Epidemic Typhus	Rickettsial
Inactivated or		
Killed Vaccine	Typhoid	
	Cholera	Bacterial
	Pertussis	
	CS Meningitis	
	Plague	
	Rabies	
	Salk (Polio)	
	Influenza	Viral
	Hepatitis B	
	JE	
	KFD	
Toxoids	Diphtheria	Bacterial
	Tetanus	

IMMUNOGLOBULINS

Human Immunoglobulins	Hepatitis A	Human Normal Ig
	Measles	
	Mumps	
	Rabies	
	Tetanus	
	Hepatitis B	Human Specific Ig
	Varicella	
	Diphtheria	
Non-Human (Antisera)	Diphtheria	
	Tetanus	Bacterial
	Gas Gangrene	
	Botulism	
	Rabies	Viral

II Passive Immunity

Antibodies produced in one body (human or animal) are transferred to another to induce protection against disease.

Passive Immunity may be induced:
(a) By administration of an Antibody containing preparation (Immunoglobulin or Antiserum)
(b) By transfer of Maternal Antibodies across Placenta. Human milk also contains antibodies.
(c) By transfer of Lymphocytes to induce Passive Cellular Immunity

Difference between Passive and Active Immunity:
  i. Immunity is rapidly established
 ii. Immunity is only temporary
iii. There is no education of Reticulo-Endothelial System

Uses
  i. It is useful for individuals who cannot form antibodies
 ii. It is useful for a normal host who takes time to develop antibodies following Active Immunization

Herd Immunity

Immunity of a group or community - Resistance of a group to invasion and spread of Infectious Agent because of resistance of a high proportion of individual members of the group.

When an Infectious Disease is introduced into a "Virgin" Population, it becomes a major Epidemic.

As time passes, affected people die or recover.

Recovered individuals become Immune & the percentage of Susceptible Individuals in the community decreases.

When Susceptible Individuals are < 20% the Epidemic dies out.

The Susceptible Individuals escape infection because of immunity in the rest of the community, called Herd Immunity.

Herd Immunity is due to:
(a) Clinical & Sub-clinical Infection in the Herd
(b) Immunization of the Herd eg. Diphtheria, Polio
(c) Herd Structure which includes animals & insects

Immunoglobulins

Human Immunoglobulin System is composed of 5 major classes – IgG, IgM, IgA, IgD, IgE & Sub-classes.

IgG	Ig M	Ig A	Ig D	Ig E
- Major Immunoglobin - 85% of Ig largely Extravascular - Transported across Placenta - Eg. Antibodies to Bacteria - Antiviral, - Antitoxic Antibodies - Indicates past Infection	- 10% of Ig - Antibody which is immediately formed with exposure to Antigen - Indicates recent infection	- 15% of Ig Antiviral, - Antibacterial activity - In body secretions eg. Saliva, Milk, Tears, Bronchial Secretions, Vaginal Secretions, Intestinal Secretions - Provides Local Immunity	- Function not yet determined	- Major Antibody - Responsible for Immediate Allergic Anaphylactic Reactions

Immunoglobulin preparations

(a) Normal Human Ig:
    It is an Antibody Rich Fraction obtained from a pool of at least 1000 donors
    Eg. To prevent Measles, Hepatitis A, Protection for travellers, and Control Institutional &
    Household outbreaks of Hepatitis A Infection

(b) Specific Human Ig:
    Preparations made from patients who have recently recovered from an infection or
    have been immunized against a specific infection. It is used in Chicken Pox, Hepatitis
    B, Rabies, Tetanus

Antisera or Antitoxins

They are materials prepared in animals.

Passive Immunization is done by administration of Antisera or Antitoxins prepared from
Non-Human Sources (Horses) for Tetanus, Diphtheria, Botulism, Gas Gangrene, Snake
Bite, Rabies

Disadvantages

Anaphylactic Shock, Serum Sickness

Common Ig used	*Common Antisera used*
Hep B HBIG 0.07 ml/kg for prevention (2nd dose after 30 days)	ADS 1000 IU IM
Measles HIG 0.25 ml/kg for prevention	Gas Gangrene 10,000 IU Botulism 10,000 IU IM
Rabies RIG 20 IU/kg for prevention	ARS 40 IU/kg IM
Tetanus TIG 250 units for prevention 6,000 units for therapy	ATS 1500 units SC or IM

Cold Chain

A system of Storage & Transport of Vaccines at low temperature from manufacturer to
vaccination site.

It is important because Vaccine Failure may occur due to failure to Store & Transport under
Strict Temperature Controls. Vaccines are Thermolabile, therefore, they should be Stored
& Transported between 2 - 8^{0}C.

Cold Chain Equipment

1. *Walk-in Cooler (WIC)*
    A refrigerated room which is present at the manufacturer's place, state & regional headquarters and can store Vaccines upto 3 months.

2. *Freezers, Refrigerators, Ice-lined Refrigerators (ILR)*
    They are available at District HQ & PHCs

    The Freezer is used for freezing icepacks.

    The Refrigerator has a Freezing Compartment on top & space below where the temperature is maintained at 2 - 8°C.

    ILR has long tubes with frozen water along its sides. It can maintain the temperature during electricity breakdown for 10 hours/day.

3. *Cold Box*
    The Cold Box is used for transportation of Vaccines from District HQ to PHCs.
    Ice packs are placed along the four sides & the bottom to keep it cool.

4. *Vaccine Carrier*
    It is used to carry small quantities of Vaccines (16-20 vials) for Out-Reach sessions. Fully frozen 4 Ice Packs are used for lining the sides and vials of DPT, DT, TT & Diluents should not be placed in direct contact with the frozen ice packs.

5. *Day Carriers*
    These are used to carry small quantities of vaccines (6-8 vials) for a nearby session.
    Fully frozen 2 Ice Packs are used only for a few hours for a time period of 4-6 hours

An ordinary Thermos Flask can also be used instead of a Day Carrier.

6. *Ice Packs*

    Ice Packs contain water. No salt should be added to it. Ice Packs are frozen in the Deep Freezer.
    Risk of Cold Chain failure is highest at Sub-centre or Village Level, therefore, these should be supplied from the PHC only on the day of Immunization.

Adverse Event Following Immunization (AEFI)

Definition
Any untoward medical occurrence which follows Immunization

1. Vaccine Quality Related Reactions
Reaction related to the quality of the Vaccine which is now rare because of Good Manufacturing Practices.

Vaccine Reactions:
   (a) Common Minor Vaccine Reactions
      Local - Pain, Swelling, Redness at Injection Site
      Systemic Reaction - Fever, Irritability, Malaise, Loss of Appetite
      Measles - Fever, Rash, Conjunctivitis
      Mumps - Swollen Parotid Glands
      Rubella - Joint Pain, Swollen Lymph Nodes
      OPV- <1% Diarrhea, Headache, Muscle Pain

   (b) Rare, more serious Vaccine Reactions
      Serious - Death, Life Threatening, Requires Hospitalization or Prolongation of Hospitalization, Persistent Disability, Congenital Anomaly or Birth Defect
      Severe - Refers to intensity of a specific event eg. Mild or moderate Fever
      Anaphylaxis - Severe reaction causing Circulatory Collapse.
      Signs - General Erythema, Urticaria upper and lower limbs, Respiratory Tract Obstruction, Limpness, Pallor, Loss of Consciousness.
      CNS - Seizures, Persistent Inconsolable Screaming, Encephalopathy
Advisable for Vaccinee to be observed for 20 mins at least after injection.

2. Immunization Error Related Reactions
Injection handling, Prescribing and Administration of Vaccine associated with particular provider or health facility or a single vial of vaccine that has been inappropriately prepared or contaminated.

Due to Non-sterile Injection, Local Reaction (Suppuration, Abscess), Systemic Reaction (Sepsis, Toxic Shock Syndrome, Blood Borne Virus Infection - HIV, Hep B, Hep C) can be seen

Nowadays auto-disabled syringes are used therefore, Infection has decreased.

Contaminated Vaccine - Eg. Bacterium Staphylococcus Aureus - Sick within a few hours, Local Tenderness, Tissue Infiltration, Vomiting, Diarrhoea, Cyanosis, High Temperature.

Bacteriological Examination of Vial should be done.

3. Immunization Anxiety Related Reactions
It is unrelated to vaccination.
Fainting (Adults/Adolescents and rare in young children)
Anxiety can lead to Hyperventilation, Breath Holding

4.   Coincidental Events
Manifestations of Congenital or Neurological Condition.

Precautions to be taken:
1.   Test dose to be given prior to administration of Antiserum.
       Intradermal Injection of 0.2ml Antiserum diluted 1:10 with Saline.
2.   Adrenaline and Chlorpheniramine Maleate should be kept as standby in case of Anaphylaxis.
3.   Proper Sterilization of Syringes & Needles
4.   Measles & BCG to be reconstituted only with Diluent supplied
5.   Reconstituted Vaccines should be discarded at the end of each Immunization Session
6.   Only Vaccines should be stored in the Refrigerator
7.   Training of Immunization Worker & Close Supervision is important
8.   Epidemiological Investigation of any AEFI should be done to find out the Cause & Preventive Action should be taken

Disease Prevention & Control

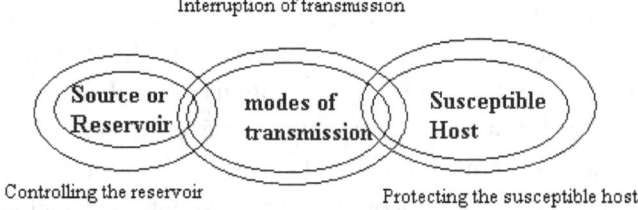

I.   Controlling the Reservoir
  1.   Early Diagnosis & Treatment
       Prompt detection of Cases & Carriers and their Treatment.
       Eg. Malaria, TB – Early diagnosis & treatment helps to prevent the spread of the Diseases.

       Treatment can be individual or mass treatment.
       Mass Treatment is given in Trachoma, Scabies, Pediculosis, Malaria, Filaria, Helminthiasis.

  2.   Notification
       Notifiable Diseases – Polio, Cholera, Plague, Yellow Fever, Malaria, Viral Influenza, Louse Borne Typhus Fever, Relapsing Fever

       The diseases should be notified to Health Authorities National International level – WHO.

3. *Epidemiological Investigation*

Investigation of an Epidemic should be done as soon as a Disease is notified to the Health Authorities to find out the Agent, Reservoir, Vectors, Mode of Transmission & the Susceptible Host.

4. *Isolation*

Separation for the period of communicability of the infected persons from others should be done to prevent Direct or Indirect Transmission of the Infectious Agent from those Infected to those who are Susceptible.

Purpose - To protect the Community by preventing Transfer of Infection from the Reservoir to the Host.

Isolation can also be achieved by "Ring Immunization" ie. Encircling the Infected Persons with a barrier of Immune Persons through whom the infection is unable to spread eg. Used in Small Pox Eradication, Measles Control & Eradication in North America, Polio Eradication.

Recommended Periods of Isolation

Disease	Duration of Isolation
Chicken Pox	Until all Lesions are crusted; 6 days after onset of rash
Herpes Zoster	6 days after onset of rash
Measles	Catarrhal Stage to day 3 of the rash
German Measles	None
Cholera, Diphtheria	3 days after Tetracycline is started; 48 hours of antibiotics or negative cultures after treatment
Salmonellosis Shigellosis	Until 3 consecutive negative stool cultures
Hepatitis B	3 weeks
Polio	2 weeks for adults; 6 weeks for pediatrics
TB	Until 3 weeks of Effective Chemotherapy
Mumps	Until swelling subsides
Pertussis	4 weeks or until Paroxysms cease
Meningococcal Meningitis Strept. Pharyngitis	Until first 6 hours of Effective Antibiotic Therapy

5. *Quarantine*

The limitation of freedom of movement of healthy persons or domestic animals exposed to a
Communicable Disease for a period of time not longer than the longest incubation period of the Disease in such a manner so as to prevent effective contact with those not exposed.

Types

(a) Absolute Quarantine – Defined above

(b) Modified Quarantine – Selective partial limitation of freedom of movement eg. Exclusion of children from school

(c) Segregation – Separation for special consideration eg. Removal of Susceptible Children to homes of Immune persons

Recent Trends

Quarantine is outdated, it has been replaced by Active Surveillance

II Interruption of Transmission (Fs)

1. Fluid - Treatment of water through Filtration, Chlorination
2. Food - Proper cooking, storing, refrigeration, reheating
3. Fingers - Regular Hand washing
4. Flies - Flies, Mosquitoes, Rats, Dogs to be controlled
5. Fomite - Disinfection of Fomites, Sterilization
6. Faeces - Sanitary Latrines – Proper Disposal of Faeces

III Protecting the Susceptible Host

1. Active Immunization
Immunization protects the maximum number of persons.
It augments Herd Immunity, making the Infection more difficult to spread.

National Immunization Schedule

Beneficiaries	Vaccines
Birth	BCG, OPV-0 Dose (Institutional Deliveries)
6 weeks	BCG (If not given at birth) Pentavalent-1, OPV-1, IPV-1
10 weeks	Pentavalent-2, OPV-2
14 weeks	Pentavalent-3, OPV-3, IPV-2
9 months	MR (Measles, Rubella), Syrup Vit A (1 Lakh)
16 - 24 months	DPT, OPV, MR, Vit A (2 Lakh)
5 - 6 years	DT (2nd Dose DT to be given 1 month later if not previously immunized)
10 years	TT (2nd Dose TT after 1 month if not previously immunized)
At 16 years	TT (2nd Dose TT after 1 month if not previously immunized)
For pregnant Women Early in Pregnancy One month after TT–1	TT-1 or Booster TT-2

2. *Passive Immunization*
   There are 3 types of preparations:
   (a) Normal Human Immunoglobulin eg. Hepatitis A, Measles vaccine
   (b) Specific Human Immunoglobulin eg. Chicken Pox, Hepatitis B vaccine
   (c) Antisera eg. ATS, ADS, Botulism, Gas Gangrene

3. *Combined Passive & Active Immunization*
   In Tetanus, Rabies, Diphtheria, Passive & Active Immunization is done simultaneously to provide immediate (temporary) Passive Immunity & long-lasting Active Immunity.

4. *Chemoprophylaxis*
   Protection of individuals from disease which may be:
   (a) Causal Prophylaxis, or
   (b) Clinical Prophylaxis

Disease	Chemoprophylaxis
Cholera	Tetracycline or Furazolidone for household contacts
Conjunctivitis Bacterial	Erythromycin Ophthal ointment
Diphtheria	Erythromycin & 1st Dose of vaccine
Influenza	Oseltamivir
Malaria	Chloroquine, Fansidar for travelers
Meningitis, Meningococcal	Ciprofloxacin & Minocycline for household & close community contacts; Immunization in all cases against Serogroups A & C
Plague	Tetracycline for contacts of Pneumonic Plague

5. ***Non-Specific Measures***

Better housing, better socio-economic status, education, safe water supply, community participation in
National Health Programmes, Disease Surveillance

Surveillance

Continuous scrutiny of all aspects of Occurrence & Spread of Disease pertinent to Effective Control.
Objective – Ultimate objective is prevention of the Disease

Components

Surveillance includes Reporting of Cases, Laboratory Confirmation, Finding the Source of Infection, Routes of Transmission, Identification of all Cases, Susceptible Contacts & those at risk in order to prevent the spread of the disease.

Method
- Systematic collection of Morbidity, Mortality Data,
- Orderly consolidation of this Data
- Special field investigations
- Rapid Dissemination of the Information to those responsible for Control & Prevention
- Evaluation of the Control Measures instituted
- If Control Measures are not successful, identification of reasons for failure, Control Measures are then modified & re-evaluation is done later

Types

Individual Surveillance – Surveillance of Infected persons till they are no longer a risk to other individuals

Local Population Surveillance – Eg. Surveillance of Malaria

National Population Surveillance - Eg. Surveillance of Smallpox after the disease has been eradicated

International Surveillance – WHO maintains Surveillance of important Diseases like Malaria, Influenza, Polio

Emporiatrics

Definition

Emporiatrics is the science of Health of travellers

Recommendations to Travellers

1. Diarrhoeal Diseases – While travelling be careful of what you eat & drink

   As far as possible eat cooked food and take hot drinks

   Use Mineral water or Boiled water for drinking

2. Hepatitis A – Normal Human Immunoglobulin 0.02 – 0.05ml/kg to be taken every 4 months

3. Hepatitis B – Vaccine in 3 doses. To avoid infections, use only sterile syringes & needles

4. Malaria – Prophylaxis with Chloroquine tablets should be taken one week before travelling to any Endemic area up to 4-6 weeks after returning home.

5. STD, HIV – Avoid sex or use a condom. Avoid injections and if unable to avoid, use sterile syringes & needles.

6. To prevent Insect Bite use DEET Application

7. Avoid bathing in contaminated water as it may cause eye, ear or skin infections

8. Yellow Fever vaccine should be taken for those travelling to such Endemic areas

9. Tetanus Immunization should be done if > 10 years have elapsed since the last injection

10. Carry sufficient stock of all medicines if the traveler has any Chronic Diseases

Disinfection

Definition

The killing of Infectious Agents outside the human body by Physical & Chemical agents through Antiseptics & Disinfectants is known as Disinfection.

Difference Between Disinfection and Antiseptic

Disinfection	Antiseptic
Kills Outright	Prevents Growth
Immediate action, short duration	Mild action, Prolonged duration
Can be antiseptic in weaker strength	
Bactericidal	Bacteriostatic

Types

(a) Concurrent Disinfection – Throughout the illness Sputum, Vomitus, Stool, Urine, Linen, Hands, Clothes, Apron, Gown should be Disinfected

(b) Terminal Disinfection – After the patient has been removed by Death or to hospital, infective material, utensils should be disinfected

(c) Prophylactic Disinfection

    Chemical – Water Purification by Chlorine

    Boiling water during the Cholera Epidemic

    Milk Pasteurization

    Hand Washing

       i. After Defaecation

      ii. After cleaning child who has Defaecated

     iii. Before preparing food

     iv. Before eating

      v. Before feeding a child

Test

$$\text{Rideal Walker Coefficient (RW)} = \frac{\text{Minimum concentration of Phenol which kills 24 hours B Typhosa}}{\text{Minimum concentration of disinfectant which kills 24 hours B Typhosa}}$$

Methods

Natural Agents

1. Sunlight
2. Air

Physical Agents

Burning   – Swab, Dressing

Hot Air   – Glassware, Syringes, Swabs, Dressing, Oils, Vaseline, Sharp Instruments

Boiling   – In 10 mins the Bacteria is killed

               In 30 mins the Spores are destroyed on Linen, Utensils, Instruments, Glassware

Autoclaving   – At 120° C 20 lbs/sq m in 5 mins kills Spores on Linen, Dressings, Gloves, Syringes, Instruments, Culture Media

Radiation   – Bandages, Dressing, Catgut, Surgical Instruments

Chemical Agents

Solids:

Lime – Faeces, urine (10–20%, 2 hours),

CaOCl2 – Stool 400 g/L 2 hours

Urine 5 g/L 10 hours

Sputum 200 g/L 1 hour

KMnO4 – Wash Fruits, Vegetables

Bleaching powder – 1-3% water

Faeces, Urine 5% for 1hour

Halazone Tabs – 4mg for 1L for 1hour

Liquid:

Formalin – 40%, 2-3% wall, room furniture

Phenol - 10% Faeces, 5% floor, drain

Cresol - 5-10% Faeces, Urine, room, sputum

Lysol – Emulsion with Cresol

Chlorhexidine (Hibitane) – Skin Antiseptic

Cetrimide - 1-2% Cetavlon

Ethyl Alcohol (Methylated Spirit) - Skin disinfection, Hand Washing

Dettol – Chlorxylenol 5% - 15 mins for Instruments, Plastic Equipment

Savlon (Cetavlon + Hibitane) – Lippes Loop, Thermometer

Gas

Formaldehyde – Room-12hrs

Ethylene Oxide – Used for Fabrics, Plastic Equipment, Cardiac Catheters, Books

Recommended Disinfection Procedures

1.   Faeces & Urine

To be collected in impervious vessels

Equal volume of Disinfectants

Bleaching powder	50g (5%)
Cresol	50ml (5%)
Phenol	100ml (10%) or
Formalin	100ml (10%) per litre water
Quicklime	25%
Boiling Water for 2-hours.	

After disinfection, the excreta should be emptied into a water closet or buried.
Bedpans, Urinals to be autoclaved

2. Sputum (Eg. TB)
    Sputum received in Gauze/Paper Handkerchiefs to be destroyed by burning or
    Disinfected by boiling/autoclaving for 20 minutes at 20 lbs pressure or
    Patient to spit in Sputum Cup half filled with 5% Cresol.
    Cup should be allowed to stand for 1-hour then the contents to be disposed off.

3. Room
    Usual – Cleaning, Airing, Sunlight
    Chemical Disinfection – Floors, hard surfaces to be sprayed or mopped with 25%
    Chlorinated Lime or Formalin 1% or Cresol 2.5 % for 4 hours contact or Fumigation
    with Formaldehyde eg. OT
    Disinfection to prevent Tetanus by boiling Formalin
    500 ml Formalin + 1 L water per 30 cu m space, or
    500 ml Formalin + 1L water + 170-200 g KMnO4 for 6-12 hours.

Investigation of an Epidemic

Definition

Epidemic is the unusual occurrence in a community of disease, health related behaviour
(Eg. Smoking) or health related event (Eg. Traffic Accidents) clearly in excess of expected
occurrence

Objectives of Investigation

(a) To define the magnitude of Outbreak (time, place, person)
(b) To determine the factors responsible for the Epidemic (Agent, Host, Environment)
(c) To identify the Cause, Source(s) of Infection, Modes of Transmission for determining
     measures to control the epidemic
(d) To make recommendations to prevent recurrence

Steps in Investigation

1. *Verification of Diagnosis*
    When a lay person or a health worker reports a case of Polio, the Medical Officer of
    PHC has to verify the diagnosis with clinical symptoms, signs and lab investigations.

2. *Confirmation of Existence of an Epidemic*
    By comparing the Disease frequencies during the same period of the previous years,
    the Epidemic can be confirmed;

Two standard errors from Endemic occurrence.

In Polio even a single case is considered Epidemic because we are trying to eradicate the Disease.

3. **Defining the Population at Risk**
   (a) Obtaining a map of the area
       Map must be prepared with landmarks and houses drawn on it.
   (b) Counting the Population
       Complete door to door survey including age, gender of the population. This identifies the
       Denominator ie. Population at Risk.

4. **Rapid search for all cases & their characteristics**
   (a) Medical Survey –House-to-house survey is carried out, looking for symptoms and signs.
   (b) Epidemiological Case Sheet – Information about Name, age, gender, occupation, social class, travel, H/o exposure, Time of onset of Disease, signs, symptoms, parties attended, food eaten, H/o Injections is gathered.
   (c) Searching for more cases - Patient is asked if he knows any one at home or workplace with similar symptoms and signs.
   (d) Search for new cases is done every day till the area is free of the Epidemic ie. Twice the Incubation Period.

5. **Data Analysis**
   Data analysis is done with respect to time, place, person wherein the Agent, Host, Environmental Factors are identified

6. **Formulation of Hypothesis**
   Based on time, place, person distribution or Agent, Host, Environmental Factors a Hypothesis is
   Formulated with regard to source, causative agent, modes of transmission, environmental factors which are causing the Epidemic.

7. **Testing of Hypothesis**
   All Hypotheses should be considered and comparing the Attack Rates among those exposed and not exposed to the Suspected Factors a possible Hypothesis is determined.

8. **Evaluation of Ecological Factors**
   Ecological Factors for Sanitary status of eating establishments, water, milk supply, human population movements, atmospheric changes (temperature, humidity), air pollution, insects, rodents, animal reservoirs are evaluated.
   Case – Control Method can be used for studying the Epidemic.

9. *Further Investigation of Population at Risk*

Population at risk or a sample should be studied:

Medical examinations, screening tests, suspected food examined, faeces or blood samples, biochemical studies and immunity status should be assessed.

10. *Writing the Report*

The Report should be completed and should include the following information:

(a) Background

(b) Historical Data

(c) Methodology of Investigations

(d) Analysis of Data & Interpretation

(e) Control measures recommended

CHAPTER 4

MENTAL HEALTH

WHO Definition

Health is a state of complete physical, mental and social well-being and not merely the absence of disease or infirmity.

Mentally Healthy Person

Accepts himself as secure, adequate, neither underestimates nor overestimates his ability, accepts his shortcomings, has self-respect, gets along with other people, takes responsibility for neighbours and fellow countrymen, is able to meet the demands of life and has problem solving capacity.

Mentally Ill Person

A mentally ill person worries, has no concentration, is unhappy, loses his temper easily, has loss of sleep, mood swings, dislikes people, is bitter, has fear, is nervous and has aches and pains.

Mental Illness

1. Psychosis
    i. Schizophrenia (Split Personality)
    ii. Manic Depressive Psychosis
    iii. Paranoia
2. Neurosis/Psychoneurosis – Morbid fears, Compulsions, Obsessions
3. Personality/Character Disorder

Causes

1. Organic Conditions – Cerebral Atherosclerosis, Neoplasms, Neurological Diseases, Endocrine Diseases, TB, Leprosy, Epilepsy
2. Heredity – Schizophrenia, Depression

3.   Social Factors – Stress, Worries, Anxiety, Unhappy Marriage, Broken Homes
4.   Economic Factors – Poverty, Poor Standard of Living
5.   Environmental Factors –
   a.   Toxic Substances - Lead;
   b.   Drugs - Alcohol, Barbiturates;
   c.   Trauma - Road Accidents, Occupational Accidents;
   d.   Infective Agents - Measles, Rubella;
   e.   Radiation
6.   Crucial life points uncared
   i.   Pregnancy
   ii.   Under 5 years
   iii.   School Child
   iv.   Adolescence
   v.   Elderly

Prevention

   i.   Primary Prevention
        Improving social environment, better living conditions, Improved health care services
   ii.   Secondary Prevention
        Early diagnosis of mental illness and treatment, Counseling services
   iii.   Tertiary Prevention
        Rehabilitation

Mental Health Services

1.   Early Diagnosis & Treatment
2.   Rehabilitation
3.   Group & Individual Psychotherapy
4.   Psychoactive Drugs
5.   After Care Services
6.   Mental Health Education

Alcoholism and Drug Dependence

Definition

Drug Dependence - A psychic or physical state characterized by behavioural responses and compulsion to take the drug.

Agent Factors

1.   Alcohol
2.   Tobacco

3. Opioids
4. Cannabinoids
5. Sedatives/Hypnotics
6. Cocaine
7. Other Stimulants including Caffeine
8. Hallucinogens
9. Volatile Solvents
10. Others used in combination

Host Factors

1. Age – Young Age
2. Sex – M>F
3. Social Factors
4. Economic Factors
5. Environmental Factors

Clinical features

- Loss of interest in daily activities, Sports
- Loss of appetite, Weight
- Unsteady gait, Tremors
- Eyes – Red, Puffy
- Speech – Slurred
- Skin – Injection marks
- GIT – Nausea, Vomiting
- CNS - Drowsiness, Sleeplessness, Lethargy
- Mood – Changing moods, Temper
- Depersonalisation, Emotional Detachment
- Impaired Memory, Concentration
- Presence of needles, syringes, strange packets at home

Factors associated with Drug Abuse

- Unemployment
- Living away from home
- Urbanization
- Relaxed parental control
- Early exposure to drugs
- Broken homes
- One-parent families
- Occupation eg Tourism
- Drug production or sale

- Areas with high crime rates or vice
- Delinquency

Prevention

1. Legislation – Control on manufacture, sale, prescription
   Eg. No smoking in public places or public vehicles, Prohibition of sale to minors, Statutory warning on cigarette packets
2. Health Education – Eg. WHO's 10 Life Skills Education in Schools (Problem solving, Decision making, Critical thinking, Creative thinking, Communication skills, Interpersonal relationships, Self-awareness, Empathy, dealing with stress, Dealing with emotions)
3. Community Approach – Alternative activities eg. Teen centres for athletics, Sports, Music, Art
4. NGOs

Treatment

- De-addiction Programmes
- Post-detoxication Counseling and Follow up
- Rehabilitation
- Breakaway from Peer Group

CHAPTER 5

GENETICS & HEALTH

Genes

Genes are units of heredity.
They contain hereditary information for transmission from generation to generation.
They may be Homozygous (AA) or Heterozygous (aA).
They are located on Chromosomes which are Autosomes (22 pairs) and Sex Chromosomes (1 pair).

Mitosis

Ordinary cell division

Meiosis

Reduction division, Diploid to Haploid (46 to 23)

Classification

 i. Chromosomal Abnormalities
 ii. Unifactorial (Single gene or Mendelian disease)
iii. Multifactorial Disorders

i. *Chromosomal Abnormalities*
 • Klinefelter's Syndrome
 • XYY Syndrome
 • Turner's Syndrome
 • Super Females

ii. *Mendelian Diseases*

Autosomal Dominant	Autosomal Recessive	Sex-Linked Disorders
Polyposis Coli Huntington's Chorea Neurofibromatosis Marfan Syndrome Retinoblastoma ABO Blood Group Hyperlipoproteinemia I, II, III, IV Polycystic Kidney	Phenylketonuria Alkaptonuria Maple Syrup Urine Disease Cystic Fibrosis Fibrocystic Disease of Pancreas Agammaglobulinemia Haemoglobinopathies Galactosaemia Hirschsprung Disease	Recessive: Haemophilia Type A & B Duchene Muscular Dystrophy Colour Blindness G6PD Deficiency Retinitis Pigmentosa Hydrocephalus Agammaglobulinemia - Bruton Type Dominant: Vit D Resistant Rickets

iii. Multifactorial Disorders
- Hypertension
- Diabetes
- Coronary Heart Disease
- Congenital Heart Malformations
- Schizophrenia
- Mental Retardation
- Duodenal Ulcer

Preventive & Social Measures

I   Primary Prevention

(a) Health Promotion
i. *Eugenics* – The science which improves genetic endowment
Negative Eugenics
Aim: To reduce the frequency of Hereditary Diseases and Disability
Eg. To improve the German race, Hitler killed the weak and defective people who had serious hereditary diseases. They could have been sterilized instead.

Positive Eugenics
Aim: To improve the Genetic Composition of the population by encouraging carriers of desirable genotypes to assume parenthood.

ii. *Euthenics*
Environmental manipulation is Euthenics.

An environment which will enable the genes to express themselves.
Dr Glen Doman did research on mentally subnormal children and found that their IQ could be improved with Environmental Stimulation.

iii. Genetic Counseling
    (a) Prospective Genetic Counselling
       If Heterozygous Marriage can be prevented, the risk of giving birth to children with Genetic Disease reduces.
       Eg. Sickle Cell Anemia, Thalassemia.
       Screening to identify Heterozygous individuals is beneficial.

    (b) Retrospective Genetic Counselling
       After the occurrence of a disorder in the family, Counselling is sought to prevent further abnormalities in siblings
       Eg. Congenital Abnormalities, Mental Retardation, Psychiatric Illness, Inborn Errors of Metabolism, Sickle Cell Anemia, Thalassemia.

    Genetic counseling centres should be established.

    Methods
    i.   Contraception
    ii. MTP
    iii. Sterilization

iv. Consanguinous Marriages
There is an increased risk of abnormal offspring when blood relatives marry eg. Diabetes, Hypertension, Coronary Heart Disease, Hypercholesterolemia, Alkaptonuria, Phenylketonuria, Albinism, Retinitis Pigmentosa

v. Late Marriages
Mongolism is more frequent in children of elderly mothers therefore, early marriages are favoured.

vi. Specific Protection
    (a) X-Ray – Protection from unnecessary X-rays or protection of Gonads during X-ray investigation.
    (b) Anti-D Globulin is given to Rh Negative mother after delivery of Rh Positive baby.

II. Secondary Prevention
Early Diagnosis and Treatment

(a) *Detection of Genetic Carriers*
Healthy carriers can be identified
Eg Duchenne Type Muscular Dystrophy, Hemophilia, PKU, Galactosaemia.

(b) *Prenatal Diagnosis*
Amniocentesis at 14-16 weeks can be done for diagnosis
Eg Down's Syndrome, Galactosemia, Maple Syrup Urine Disease, Tay-Sachs Disease, Alpha Thalassemia, Neural Tube Defects.

Indications for Amniocentesis:
  i.   Mother ≥ 35 years
  ii. Parents with Down's Child
  iii. Parents with Chromosomal Anomaly Child
  iv. Parents with Metabolic Defect Child eg. Neural Tube, Anencephaly, Spina Bifida
  v.   Parents with Chromosomal Translocation
  vi. For sex determination in Sex-linked Genetic Disease eg. Muscular Dystrophy

Indications & Methods for Prenatal Diagnosis

Indications	Methods
Advanced maternal age, previous child with Chromosomal Abnormality, Intrauterine Growth Delay	Cytogenetics (Amniocentesis, Chorionic Villus Sampling)
Biochemical Disorders	Protein Assay, DNA Diagnosis
Congenital Anomaly	Sonography, Foetoscopy
Screening for Neural Tube Defects and Trisomy	Maternal Serum Alpha Fetoprotein & Chorionic Gonadotropin

(c) **Screening of Newborn Infants**
   Screening tests on newborns eg. Sex Chromosome Abnormalities, Congenital Dislocation of Hip,
   PKU, Congenital Hypothyroidism, Sickle Cell Disease, Cystic Fibrosis, Duchenne Muscular
   Dystrophy, Congenital Adrenal Hyperplasia, G6PD Deficiency

(d) **Recognizing Pre-clinical Cases**
   Screening tests for diagnosis of PKU, Urine Sugar for Diabetes, Se Uric Acid for Gout, Sickle Cell Trait by subjecting Red Cells to Reduced Oxygen Tension, Thalassemia Minor by Blood Picture

III. Tertiary Prevention
   Rehabilitation

   Medical, social, educational and vocational measures to train and retrain a person to the highest level of functional ability.

CHAPTER 6

OCCUPATIONAL HEALTH

Definition

Occupational Health is the promotion of physical, mental, social, well-being of workers, prevention of diseases, protection from risks, adaptation of work for man and of each man to his job.

Ergonomics

Greek Ergon = Work

    Nomos = Law

This means fitting the job to the worker.

Ergonomics includes the designing of machines, tools, equipment, manufacturing processes and layout of work places for efficiency of man and machine.

The Objective of Ergonomics is to achieve the adjustment of man and his work for human efficiency and well-being.

Occupational Diseases

I Diseases due to Physical Agents

1. Heat - Heat Hyperpyrexia, Heat Exhaustion, Heat Syncope, Heat Cramps, Burns, Prickly Heat
2. Cold - Trench Foot Frostbite, Chilblains
3. Light - Occupational Cataract, Miner's Nystagmus
4. Pressure - Caisson's Disease, Air Embolism
5. Noise - Occupational Deafness
6. Radiation - Cancer, Leukemia, Aplastic Anemia, Pancytopenia
7. Electricity - Burns
8. Mechanical Factors – Injuries, Accidents

II Diseases due to Chemical Agents

1. Gases - CO_2, CO, HCN, CS_2, NH_3, N_2, H_2S, HCl, SO_2 cause Gas Poisoning
2. Dusts (Pneumoconiosis)
   i. Inorganic Dusts:
   - (a) Coal Dust – Anthracosis
   - (b) Silica – Silicosis
   - (c) Asbestos – Asbestosis, Lung Cancer
   - (d) Iron – Siderosis
   ii. Organic Dusts:
   - (a) Cane Fibre – Bagassosis
   - (b) Cotton Dust – Byssinosis
   - (c) Tobacco – Tobacosis

    (d) Hay or Grain Dust – Farmer's Lung

3. Metals & their compounds
   - Toxic Hazards from Lead
   - Mercury
   - Manganese
   - Cadmium
   - Beryllium
   - Arsenic
   - Chromium
4. Chemicals – Acids, Alkalis, Pesticides
5. Solvents – Benzene, Trichloroethylene, Chloroform

III Diseases due to Biological Agents
   - Brucellosis
   - Leptospirosis
   - Anthrax
   - Actinomycosis
   - Hydatidosis
   - Psittacosis
   - Tetanus
   - Encephalitis
   - Fungal Infections

IV Occupational Cancers
   - Skin Cancer
   - Lung Cancer
   - Leukemia
   - Bladder Cancer
   - Scrotal Cancer

V Occupational Dermatosis
   - Dermatitis
   - Eczema

VI Diseases of Psychological Origin
   - Neurosis,
   - Hypertension,
   - Peptic Ulcer

Pneumoconiosis
Definition

Inhalation of Organic or Inorganic Dust of 0.5μ produces Pneumoconiosis causing inflammatory changes in lungs, infections, fibrosis & reduces work capacity.

Types
- Silicosis
- Anthracosis
- Byssinosis
- Bagassosis
- Asbestosis
- Farmer's Lung

	Silicosis	Anthracosis	Byssinosis	Bagassosis	Asbestosis	Farmer's lung
Cause	Inhalation of dust containing SiO_2	Coal Dust	Cotton Fibre Dust	Bagasse - Sugar Cane Dust - Thermoactinomyces Sacchari	Asbestos Fibre	Mouldy Hay/Grain Dust - Micropolyspora Faeni (Thermophilic Actinomycetes)
Occupation	Miners (in Coal, Mica, Gold, Silver, Lead, Zinc), Iron & Steel Industry, Pottery, Ceramic Industry, Sand Blasting, Metal Grinding, Building & Construction work.	Coal Miners			Manufacturing Industry for Asbestos Cement, Fireproof Textiles, Roof, Brake Lining	Farmers
Cl. Features	Cough, Breathlessness, Chest Pain, Decreased Lung Capacity	(a) Simple Pneumoconiosis (b) Progressive Massive Fibrosis (PMF), Severe Respiratory Disability, Death	Cough, Breathlessness, Chronic Bronchitis, Emphysema	Cough Breathlessness, Haemoptysis, Fever, Fibrosis, Emphysema, Bronchiectasis	Cough, Clubbing, Cyanosis, Respiratory Insufficiency, Bronchogenic Ca, Mesothelioma Ca of GIT, Risk of Ca increased with Smoking, Fibrosis, Death	Cough, Breathlessness, Impairment of Pulmonary Function, Cor Pulmonale
CXR / X-ray	Snowstorm Appearance, Silicotuberculosis			Mottling Shadow, Impairment of Pulmonary Function	X-ray – Ground Glass Appearance	
Rx	No treatment, Dust control measures eg. Enclosure, Substitution, Isolation, Hydroblasting, Good House Keeping, Personal Protection	No Rx Notifiable Disease, Compensable Under Workmen's Compensation Act	No Rx Prevention – Dust Control, Periodic Examination	Dust Control, Personal Protection, Medical Control, Bagasse Control	No Rx Prevention – Safe Types of Asbestos, Use Substitution, Dust Control	No Rx

Lead Poisoning

Definition

Disease due to the Inhalation or Ingestion of Lead.

Source

Occupational – Industries which manufacture Batteries, Glass, Shipbuilding, Printing, Pottery, Rubber

Non occupational – Gasoline, Drinking Water through Lead Pipes, Chewing Lead Paint on window sills, toys

Mode of Absorption

(a) Inhalation – Inhalation of Lead Dust in industries
(b) Ingestion – Food, Drinks, Water
(c) Skin – Absorption of Tetraethyl Lead (Organic Compound)

Clinical Features

Inorganic Lead causes GIT Symptoms - Abdominal Colic (Lead Colic), Constipation, Loss of Appetite, Blue Line on Gums (Lead Line), Stippling of Red Cells, Anemia, Wrist Drop, Foot Drop

Organic Lead causes CNS Symptoms - Headache, Mental Confusion, Delirium, Insomnia

Investigations

CPU – Coproporphyrin in Urine > 150μg/L
ALAU – Amino Levulinic Acid in Urine > 5mg/L

Lead in Blood & Urine - Lead in Urine > 0.8mg/L
                     - Lead in Blood > 70μg/100ml
Basophilic Stippling of RBCs

Prevention

*   Substitution
*   Isolation
*   Local Exhaust Ventilation
*   Personal Protection
*   Good Housekeeping
*   Working Atmosphere Lead

- Periodic Examination of Workers
- Personal Hygiene – Hand Washing
- Health Education

Management

- Saline Purge
- D-Penicillamine
- Notifiable Disease

Occupational Cancers

Types

Skin cancer

Cancer of Scrotum has been observed among Chimney Sweepers by Percival Pott
Cancer of Scrotum and skin is caused by Coal Tar, X-rays, certain Oils and Dyes

Occupations: Gas Workers, Coke Oven Workers, Tar Distillers, Oil Refiners, Dye Makers, Road Makers, Industries where Mineral Oil, Pitch and Tar is used

Lung Cancer

Occupations: Gas Industry, other Industries where Asbestos, Nickel, Chromium is used, Arsenic Roasting Plants, Mining of Radioactive Substances eg. Uranium

Bladder Cancer

Occupations: Aniline Industry, Rubber Industry, Dye stuffs and Dyeing Industry, Gas Industry, Electric Cable Industry

Leukemia

Occupations: Roentgen Rays, Benzol, Radioactive Substances

Characteristics of Occupational Cancer

- They appear after prolonged exposure
- 10-25 years after exposure
- They may appear even after cessation of exposure
- Age Incidence < In general for cancer
                    Localization of Tumours

Control

1. Control of Industrial Carcinogens
2. Medical Examination
3. Notification
4. Inspection of Factories
5. Licensing of Establishments
6. Personal Hygiene
7. Health Education
8. Research

Occupational Dermatitis

Causes

- Physical: Heat, Cold, Moisture, Friction, Pressure, X-rays
- Chemical: Acids, Alkalis, Dyes, Solvents, Grease, Tar, Pitch, Chlorinated Phenols
- Biological: Viruses, Bacteria, Fungi
- Plant Products: Leaves, Vegetables, Fruits, Flowers

Prevention

1. Preselection
   Medical examination before employment
2. Protection
   Protective clothing, gloves, aprons, boots, barrier creams
3. Personal Hygiene - Hand washing
4. Health Education
5. Periodic Inspection

Occupational Hazards of Agricultural Workers

Zoonotic Diseases

Brucellosis, Anthrax, Leptospirosis, Tetanus, Tuberculosis (Bovine), Q Fever

Respiratory Diseases

Causes:
Dusts of Grains, Rice Husks, Cotton Fibres, Sugar Cane, Tea, Tobacco, Hay, Wood

Diseases:
Byssinosis, Bagassosis, Farmer's Lung, Occupational Asthma

Chemical Hazards:
Fertilizers, Insecticides, Pesticides may result in Poisoning

Physical Hazards:
Heat, Solar Radiation, High Humidity, Cold, Noise, Vibrations, Inadequate Ventilation, Uncomfortable Positions

Accidents:
Agricultural machinery may lead to accidents. Insect or Snake Bites are also possible.

Sickness Absenteeism

Causes

- Medical – Accidents, Respiratory Illness, Alimentary Illness
- Non-Occupational – Nutritional Disorders, Alcoholism, Drug Addiction
- Economic – Sick Leave with Pay
- Social – Weddings, Festivals, Repair of House

Prevention

1. Good factory management and practices
2. Good human relations
3. Adequate preplacement examination
4. Ergonomics

Prevention of Occupational Diseases

I Medical Measures	II Engineering Measures	III Legislation
i. Communicable Dis. Control	Design of Building	Factories Act
ii. Nutrition	Good Housekeeping	ESI Act
iii. Environmental Sanitation	General Ventilation	
iv. Mental Health	Mechanization	
v. MCH Measures	Substitution	
vi. Family Planning	Dusts	
vii. Preplacement Examination	Enclosure	
viii. Periodical Examination	Exhaust Ventilation	
ix. Medical & Health Care Services	Isolation	
x. Notification	Protective Devices	
xi Supervision of working Environment	Environmental Monitoring	
xii. Health Education & Counselling	Statistical Monitoring	
xiii. Records Maintenance & Analysis Research		

I   Medical Measures

i.   *Communicable Disease Control*
Early Diagnosis and Treatment or removal from the working environment or both.
Eg. TB, Typhoid, Hepatitis, Amoebiasis, Malaria, STDs, Intestinal Parasites, Immunization
Programmes

ii.   *Nutrition*
Canteen to provide balanced diet at reasonable cost under sanitary control.
Storage space for workers' lunch packs and designated place for eating.

iii.   *Environmental Sanitation*
- Water supply – Safe water for drinking; Drinking water fountains
- Food – Sanitary preparation, Storage, Handling, Education of food handlers.
- Toilet – Latrines and Urinals
- Garbage and waste disposal
- General Plant Cleanliness – Vacuum cleaning, Mopping
- Sufficient space – 500 cu ft for every worker
- Lighting – Natural, Artificial or both
- Ventilation – Sufficient
- Temperature – Comfortable
- Protection against Hazards eg. Dusts, Fumes, Toxic Hazards
- Housing – Near a plant with community amenities

iv.   *Mental Health*
- Early Diagnosis and Treatment of Mental Illness, Stress
- Rehabilitation
- Promote Health and Happiness

v.   *MCH Measures*
- Maternity leave for 6 months
- Free antenatal, natal and postnatal services
- Prohibits night work 7pm-6am
- Prohibits work underground
- Provides for Creches
- Prohibits employment of women & children in dangerous occupations

vi.   *Family Planning*
Family Planning to improve the quality of life, Promote the small family norm

vii. Preplacement Examination

It is done at the time of employment.

Medical history of the worker, Family, Occupational, Social history, Physical Examination, Systemic Examination, vision, hearing carried out.

Blood tests, urine, CXR, ECG, special tests for endemic diseases.

Candidate may be rejected or given a suitable job.

Purpose of Preplacement Examination

To place the right man in the right job so that the worker will be efficient – Ergonomics.

List of occupations where it is risky employing men from certain diseases:

Hazard	Undesirable Conditions
Lead	Anemia, Hypertension, Nephritis, Peptic Ulcer
Dyes	Asthma, Skin, Bladder, Kidney Diseases, Precancerous Lesions
Solvents	Liver & Kidney Disease, Dermatitis, Alcoholism
Silica	TB, Chronic Lung Disease
Radium X-ray	Ill Health, Blood Disease

Preplacement Examination – It is a benchmark for the future.

viii. Periodical Examination
- Daily, monthly or yearly depending on the occupation
- Normally once a year
- Daily, when exposed to Irritant Chemicals eg. Dichromates
- Monthly, when exposed to Lead, Toxic Dyes, Radium
- Occupational diseases may take months, years to develop
- Periodical Examination helps in early detection

ix. Medical & Health Care Services
- ESI provides medical care for the worker and his family
- First Aid is available at the workplace
- Vaccinations against Diseases

x. Notification
Registration – Eg Factories Act, Mines Act, Required for cases of Occupational Diseases.

xi. Supervision of Working Environment
Physician should inspect the working environment of the workers to know about temperature, lighting, ventilation, noise, humidity, space, air pollution, sanitation, water

xii. Health Education & Counselling

Health Education should be given about the risks in the industry and their protective measures

Eg. - Masks, gloves, boots, hand washing

xiii. Maintenance of Records & Analysis

Records are necessary for planning, monitoring, evaluation of Occupational Health Service

Eg. - Workers Health Records, Disability Records

II   Engineering Measures

i.   Design of Building

At the Blue Print stage, the details of walls, floor, ceilings, roof, doors, windows, cubic space should receive attention so that the required changes may be made.

ii. Good Housekeeping

Washing once a year - Walls, ceiling, passages.

Vacuum cleaning - To remove dust from floors, ledges, beams.

Protective Devices - Masks, gloves, aprons, should be kept clean and in good condition.

iii. General Ventilation

Good general ventilation is necessary for a healthy environment.

iv. Mechanization

Mechanization reduces contact with harmful substances thus, decreasing Dermatitis.

v.   Substitution

Replacement of harmful material by harmless ones

Eg. - White Phosphorus to be replaced by Phosphorus Sesquisulphide in the Match Industry to eliminate the possibility of Phossy Jaw.

Lead paints should be substituted by Zinc or Iron paints.

vi. Dusts

Can be controlled by Water Sprays like Wet Drilling of Rock.

vii. Enclosure

Harmful materials and processes can be enclosed to prevent the escape of dust and fumes into the factory atmosphere

viii. Exhaust Ventilation

An exhaust ventilation extracts dust, fumes, injurious substances before they escape into the factory atmosphere

ix. Isolation

Offensive processes can be isolated in a separate building or the operations can be done at night.

x. **Protective Devices**
   Protective Devices such as Respirators, Gas Masks, Ear Plugs, Ear Muffs, Helmets, Safety Shoes, Aprons, Gloves, Gum Boots, Barrier Creams, Screens, Goggles to be provided by the owner.

xi. **Environmental Monitoring**
   Monitoring of atmosphere for dusts and gases should be done to check if they are within permissible limits.
   Monitoring of Temperature, Ventilation and Lighting should be done regularly.

xii. **Statistical Monitoring**
   Analysis of Data on Health and Environmental Exposure should be done regularly to evaluate the adequacy of Preventive Measures

xiii. **Research**
   Study on Permissible Limits of Exposure to Dusts, Toxic Fumes, Occupational Cancers,
   Accident Prevention, Industrial Fatigue, Vocational Psychology should be conducted.

Legislation

1. **The Factories Act 1948**

Scope:
   Factory - An establishment employing ≥ 10 workers where power is used or ≥ 20 workers where power is not used
- The Act applies to whole of India except Jammu and Kashmir.
- Personnel - Chief Inspector of Factories, Additional Chief Inspectors, Joint Chief Inspectors, Deputy Chief Inspectors and Inspectors for implementation.

Health, Safety and Welfare

- Cleanliness, temperature, lighting, ventilation, treatment of waste, drinking water, cleaners to keep water closets clean, personal protective measures, crèches.
- Employment of Young Persons
  - o Prohibits employment of children < 14 years.
  - o Restriction of employment to women and children in dangerous occupations
- Hours of work
  - o 48 hours/week (8hrs X 6days)
- Leave with wages
  - o Weekly holidays
  - o One day every 20 days of work, accumulated up to 30 days
- Occupational Diseases

    o   Notification of accidents or occupational diseases, deaths, serious bodily injury
- Employment in Hazardous Processes
    o   Service conditions of employees in factories involving hazardous processes to be appraised and recommendations given.

2. *The Employees State Insurance Act 1948*
Important Social Security and Health Insurance

Scope
- Small power used in factories employing 10-19 persons, and non-power in factories employing ≥ 20 persons
- Shops
- Hotels, Restaurants
- Cinemas, Theatres
- Road Motor Transport Establishment
- Newspaper Establishments
- Manual, clerical, supervisory, technical employees getting up to Rs10,000 per month.

Administration
ESI Corporation
Chairman (Union Minister for Labour)
Vice Chairman (Secretary to GOI – Ministry of Labour)
Members
Standing Committee

Beneficiaries
828 lakhs have been benefited
ESI Dispensaries provide Medical Facilities

Finance
Employers contribute 4.75% of the Wage Bill
Employees contribute 1.75% of their wages
1/8 Expenditure is done by state, 7/8 by ESI

Benefits
(a) Medical
(b) Sickness
(c) Maternity
(d) Disability
(e) Dependent
(f) Funeral
(g) Rehabilitation

(a) Medical benefits

Direct Pattern – Full Time Service Dispensaries
(≥1000 employees, Medical and Paramedical personnel for Family Units)
(< 750 employees ESI Dispensaries)

Indirect pattern - Panel System - Registered Medical Practitioners are designated as Insurance Medical Practitioners

(b) Sickness Benefit
This is for 91 days in a year, if sickness is certified by an Insurance Medical Officer

Extended Sickness Benefit
In addition to 91 days of Sickness Benefit, in certain long-term diseases the Sickness Benefit is extended for 2 years

   i.   Infectious Diseases – TB, Leprosy, AIDS
   ii. Neoplasms – Malignant Diseases
   iii. Endocrine, Nutritional, Metabolic diseases – DM with Retinopathy, Nephropathy, Diabetic Foot
   iv. CNS – Monoplegia, Hemiplegia, Paraplegia, Parkinson's Disease, Neuromuscular Dystrophy, Myasthenia Gravis
   v.   Eye - Immature Cataract with vision 6/60 or less, Detachment of Retina, Glaucoma
   vi. CVS – Coronary Heart Disease, Unstable Angina, MI with Ejection Fraction < 45%, Congestive Heart Failure, Cardiac Valvular Disease with failure or complications, Cardiomyopathies, Heart Disease with Surgical Intervention with Complications
   vii. Chest Disease – Bronchiectasis, COPD with Cor Pulmonale
   viii.GIT – Liver Cirrhosis, Chronic Active Hepatitis
   ix. Orthopedic Disease – Prolapse Intervertebral Disc, Non-union or delayed union of fracture, Compound Fracture with Chronic Osteomyelitis
   x.   Psychosis – Schizophrenia, Endogenous Depression, MDP, Dementia
   xi. Others - > 20% Burns with Complications, Chronic Renal Failure, Reynaud's Disease

Cash benefit for undergoing Sterilization:
Tubectomy – 14 days,
Vasectomy – 7 days

(c) Maternity Benefit

Cash – 26 weeks for Confinement
6 weeks for Miscarriage
30 days for Sickness during Confinement

(d) Disablement Benefit
Cash for temporary and permanent disablement caused by employment injury and occupational diseases

(e) Dependent's Benefit
Pension – 70% of wages

(f) Funeral Expenses
Cash of Rs 10,000 for funeral

(g) Rehabilitation

Insured person and family is entitled for Medical Treatment, Rehabilitation after permanent disablement or retirement on monthly payment of Rs 10.

Benefits to Employers
1. Exemption from Workmen's Compensation Act
2. Exemption from Maternity Benefit Act
3. Exemption from paying Medical Allowance
4. Rebate under Income Tax
5. Healthy Workforce

CHAPTER 7

URBAN HEALTH

Health Problems

1. Environmental Sanitation
    Lack of facility for sewage disposal causes soil pollution and water pollution
2. Water pollution
    Toxic wastes from industries may pollute water with acids, alkalis, oils, organic, inorganic chemicals
3. Air pollution
    Toxic fumes, gases, smoke, dusts discharged into the air can lead to Chronic Bronchitis, Lung Cancer
4. Housing
    Slums with insanitary dwellings, poor ventilation and lighting
5. Communicable diseases
    Food borne and water borne infections, TB, Filariasis, STDs, Leprosy
6. Food Sanitation
    Typhoid, Cholera, Viral Hepatitis
7. Accidents
    Factory accidents, road traffic accidents
8. Mental Health
    Psychoneurosis, Behaviour Disorders, Delinquency, Suicides
9. Social Problems
    Alcoholism, Drug Addiction, Gambling, Prostitution, Divorces, Broken Families, Crime
10. Mortality
    Death Rates and Infant Mortality Rates are increased

CHAPTER 8

SCREENING

Definition

The search for an unrecognized disease or defect by means of rapidly applied tests, examinations or other procedures in apparently healthy individuals is known as Screening.

Screening & Diagnostic Tests

Screening Test	Diagnostic Test
On healthy people	On sick people
On groups	On single patient
One cut off point used	Symptoms, Signs, Laboratory Results used
Not costly	Costly
Not for treatment	For treatment
Not demanded by patient	Demanded by patient
Once done is final	Repeated, other tests done
Accuracy not justified	Is justified
It is an Epidemiological Procedure	It is a Therapeutic Tool

Lead Time

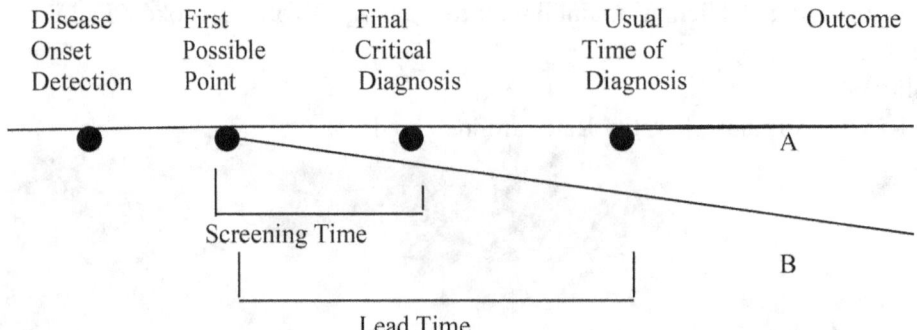

Disease Onset Detection   First Possible Point   Final Critical Diagnosis   Usual Time of Diagnosis   Outcome

A

Screening Time

B

Lead Time

Model for Early Detection Programmes

Detection Programmes should concentrate on conditions where there is a long time-lag between Disease Onset and Final Critical Point.

Lead Time is the advantage gained by Screening ie. the period between diagnosis by early detection and diagnosis by other means.

A – The usual outcome of the disease
B – Outcome to be expected when disease is detected early by Screening
BA – Benefits of the Programme

Cost of Detection programmes should be compared with the Benefits (Outcomes)

Types

1. **Mass Screening**
   Everyone in the community is subjected to the Screening Test eg. Night Blood Smear for Microfilaria.

2. **Selective or High-risk Screening**
   Only high-risk groups for the disease are Screened. eg. ELISA Test of Sex Workers for AIDS; Symptomatic Surveys of Slum Dwellers for TB.

3. **Uniphasic, Biphasic or Multiphasic Screening**
   Uniphasic Screening – Detection of a single condition eg. Urine analysis for diabetes of middle-aged persons
   Biphasic Screening – Detection of two diseases simultaneously. eg. Urine examination of pregnant women for Diabetes and Preeclampsia.
   Multiphasic Screening – Screening Tests for ≥3 applied to the community.

Pre-requisites

Screening is undertaken only if the following conditions are satisfied:

(a) Disease Characteristics
   i.   Disease is of public health importance with significant Morbidity and Mortality
   ii. It is curable eg. Malaria
       Prognosis is improved by treatment eg. Drugs prevent complications and improve survival in Breast Cancer
       If not readily curable, its spread is amenable to control eg. AIDS

     iii. It has a long Latent Period

     iv. It is neither too rare nor too common

(b) Test Characteristics

     i. Appropriate and safe Screening Test is available

     ii. It is acceptable to Physicians and the people

     iii. It is not too costly

Others

     i. Persons found positive are willing to undergo further evaluation

     ii. Medical Care is available for those found positive

Uses of Screening Tests

(a) Case Detection

People are screened to detect the disease among apparently healthy individuals.
Eg. Diabetes Mellitus, Hypertension, Bacteriuria in Pregnancy, Cervical Cancer, Breast Cancer, Deafness in Children, PKU, Hemolytic Disease of Newborn, Hypothyroidism, Iron Deficiency Anemia, Pulmonary TB.

(b) Control of Disease

People are examined for the benefit of others for early diagnosis and treatment, thus reducing the spread of the disease.
Eg. Screening Immigrants for TB, Syphilis to protect the home population.
Screening for Streptococcal Infection to prevent Rheumatic Fever.

(c) Research Purposes

Screening for Research Purposes.
Eg. For obtaining the natural history of a disease - Cancer, Hypertension, or
For obtaining Incidence and Prevalence eg. TB.

(d) Educational Purposes

Creating public health awareness and educating health professionals eg. Screening for Diabetes.

Evaluation of a Screening Test

Disease

Test	+	-	Total
+	a	b	a+b
-	c	d	c+d
	a+c	b+d	a+b+c+d

Sensitivity – Ability of a test to identify correctly all those who have the disease ie True Positive

$$= \frac{a}{a + c} \times 100 = \text{True Positive}$$

Specificity – Ability of a test to identify correctly those who do not have the disease ie True Negative

$$= \frac{d}{b + d} \times 100 = \text{True Negative}$$

$$\text{False +ve} = \frac{b}{b + d} \times 100$$

$$\text{False – ve} = \frac{c}{a + c} \times 100$$

Predictive Value of a +ve test indicates the probability that a patient with a positive test result, has the disease

$$= \frac{a}{a + b} \times 100$$

Prediction Value of a –ve test indicates the probability that a patient with a negative test result, does not have the disease

$$= \frac{d}{c + d} \times 100$$

Unimodal and Bimodal Distribution

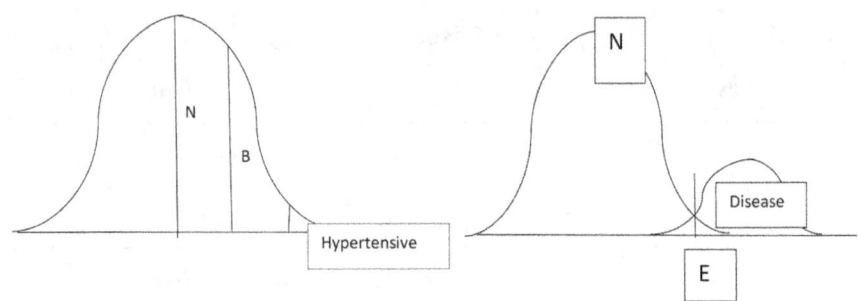

Unimodal distribution
Eg hypertension
follows normal curve, and criteria
fixed, helps to identify Normal(N),
Borderline(B)and & Diseased

Bimodal distribution
Eg phenylketonuria
E is cut-off level
between Normal
& Diseased

Common Screening Tests

In pregnancy	– Hb, Blood Group, Rh Factor
	VDRL
	HIV
	HbsAg
Women	– Pap Smear
Middle Age	– BP
	Cancer
	Blood Sugar
	Obesity
	Se Cholesterol
	PEFR in Lung Disease
	Mass Miniature Radiography in TB
Children	– Audiometry
	Congenital Dislocation of Hip
	Visual Defects
	Congenital Heart Disease
	Hypothyroidism
	Undescended Testis
	PEFR in Lung Disease
Elderly	– Nutritional Disorders
	Cancer
	TB
	Chronic Bronchitis
	Cataract
	Glaucoma

CHAPTER 9

SOCIAL SCIENCES & HEALTH

Definition

Sociology: Socio = Society; Logos = Science
The study of relationships between human beings and human behaviour.

Society: A group of individuals who have organized themselves and follow a given way of life.

Medical Sociology: A specialization in sociology dealing with the study of Health, Health Behaviour and Medical Institutions

Community – A group of individuals and families living together in a defined geographic area, eg. Village, Town or City

Customs

The right way of doing things (folkways); Stringent customs are called Mores.

Culture

A Learned Behaviour which has been socially acquired

Acculturation

Acculturation means culture contact
Diffusion of culture occurs when people of different cultures come together.
Culture contact takes place through:
• Trade and Commerce
• Industrialization
• Propagation of Religion
• Education, and
• Conquest

British culture brought to India through conquest
- Good aspects of culture contact – Introduction of Scientific Medicine, Industrialization and Improvement in Socio-economic Status
- Bad aspects – Introduction of Tobacco, Alcohol, Drugs, Fast Foods, Sedentary Lifestyle, TV, Cinema

Social Security

Security that a society gives to its members during crises such as Loss of work, sickness, invalid state, maternity, old age, death.

Introduction

1881- The first Social Security Act for Industrial Workers was formulated.
Sweden is the only country where the entire population is under Social Security Schemes

Importance

People who are not given security may cause social harm in fulfilling their basic needs of food, shelter, housing.

Social security includes:

(a) Social Insurance
(b) Social Assistance

(a) Social Insurance
It provides Income Security (Cash benefits)
- For Industrial Workers
  Factory's Act
  ESI Act 1948
  Workman's Compensation Act 1923
  Central Maternity Benefit Act 1961
  Family Pension Scheme 1971

- For Civil Servants
  Employees of Central & State Government have:
  Pension
  Gratuity
  Provident Fund
  Family Pension Scheme
  CGHS provides Comprehensive Medical Care

- General Public
  Risk of death, accident and fire are covered by Insurance Schemes
  LIC
  Public Provident Fund (PPF) Scheme

- Rural
  Rs 400 per month in Karnataka for BPL and $\geq$ 65years

Atal Pension Yojana (APY)

For Indian citizens of 18-40 years of age.

Rs 1000-5000 pension is distributed.
If a person chooses Rs 5,000/month guaranteed pension option, his contribution will be between Rs 210-1454 per month depending on the age of entry, till 60 years. Following his death, the pension will go to his spouse and later a corpus of about Rs 8.50 lakh goes to the nominee.

Pradhan Mantri Jeevan Jyoti Bima Yojana (PMJJBY)

A premium of Rs 330 per annum per member is to be paid and it is renewable yearly.
It is a one-year Life Insurance Scheme with a cover of Rs 2 lakh.
The coverage is for death due to any reason and is available to 18-50 years and life cover up to 55 years.

(b) Social Assistance
There is no contribution for this.
The Fund is from general revenues.

Beneficiaries - Unemployed, disabled, old, widows, orphans, handicapped.

Social problems

These include poverty, crime, starvation, alcoholism, drug addiction, STD, street children.

Social Obstetrics

Study of the interplay of social and environmental factors with human reproduction and their influence on the organization, delivery and utilization of Obstetric Services by the community.
Eg. Age at marriage, child bearing, child spacing, family size, education, role of women in society.

Social Pediatrics

Study of social and environmental factors which play a part in a child's health and their influence in the organization, delivery and utilization of Pediatric Services
Eg. Child feeding, immunization, child rearing.

Socialization

A man learning the customs, traditions and beliefs through his interaction with other fellow beings:
(a) Primary Socialization – A newborn learning under his mother's care
(b) Secondary Socialization – Learning in school
(c) Re-socialization – Learning to survive when a person goes to a foreign country

Family

Definition

A group of biologically related individuals living together and eating from a common kitchen.

Types of Families

Nuclear Family	Joint Family	3-Generation Family
Married Couple & their children	No. of married couples & their children. Men are related by blood & women are their wives, unmarried girls, widows	Grand Parents, parents & children

Functions

1. Residence

   A decent home for its members

2. Division of Labour

   Male – Duty is to earn a living and support the family

   Female – To take care of children and run the household

3. Reproduction and bringing up children

   This is an important function.

   Mother's role – To take care of children

   Father's role – To provide education and teach traditions and customs

4. Socialization

    Family teaches children the cultural aspects of eating, dressing, cleanliness, speech, language and behaviour

5. Economic Functions

    Property eg. Farm, shop, dwelling which is handed over to the children

6. Social Care

    Giving a social status to its members; Protecting from insults, defamation; Regulating marital activities

Family in Health & Disease

1. Familial susceptibility to disease

    Hereditary Diseases eg. Diabetes, Hypertension, Coronary Heart Disease, Hemophilia, Colour Blindness, Mental Illness, Schizophrenia, Depression, Congenital Malformations

2. Child Rearing

    Feeding – Breast feeding, complementary feeding; hygiene; sleep; clothing; discipline; habit training which is passed on from one generation to another

3. Socialization

    Teach Socialization to the newborn. Teach the young ones the values of society and culture, beliefs, codes of conduct.

4. Personality Formation

    Lays the foundation of physical, mental and social health of the child.

5. Care of Dependent Adults

    (a) Care of the Sick & Injured

    (b) Care of women during Pregnancy & Childbirth

    (c) Care of Aged & Handicapped

6. Stabilization of Adult Personality

    Family is like a shock absorber eg. Stress of life - injury, illness, births, deaths, tension, emotional upsets, worry, anxiety, economic insecurity.

7. Broken Family

    Where parents have separated or death of one or both the parents.

    Paternal separation (Separation of child from father) or Dual parental separation (Separation of child from both the parents) leads to mental deprivation and affects child development.

    Such children show Psychopathic Behaviour, Immature Personality, Retardation of Growth, Intellect and Speech.

    They may turn to prostitution, crime, vagrancy.

8. Problem Families

    Families which lag behind the rest of the community.

    Such families face problems such as poverty, low standard of living, mental and emotional instability, character defects, alcoholism, child battering, wife battering, marital disharmony.

    Children from such environment may turn to prostitution, crime, vagrancy.

    The Medical Officer, ANM, Social Worker, Health Inspector can identify and render service to such families.

Cultural Factors in Health & Disease

1. *Concept of Aetiology & Cure*

    People believe that diseases are due to:

(a) Supernatural Causes – Wrath of Gods & Goddesses eg. Smallpox, Chickenpox
    Breach of Taboo eg. Venereal Disease due to illicit sexual intercourse with low caste women;
    Past sins eg. Leprosy, TB, Evil eye (children's diseases);
    Spirits or Ghosts eg. Epilepsy, Hysteria, Mental Illness

(b) Physical Causes
    Effects of weather – Heat Attack of Loo (Heat Stroke)
    Water – Disease caused due to Impure Water
    Impure Blood – Skin Diseases eg. Boils, Scabies

2. *Environmental Sanitation*
    Disposal of Human Excreta in rural areas – Open Defaecation
    Disposal of Wastes – Solid Waste thrown in front of the house
    Waste Water – collects around the house where mosquitoes breed
    Animal Dung – Used as manure or fuel
    Water supply – Well water, tanks, ponds which people use for bathing, washing clothes, ablution. Holy water eg. Ganga water
    Housing – Katcha, poor lighting, ill ventilated

3. *Personal Hygiene*
    Oral Hygiene – Twigs of Neem used as toothbrushes in rural areas.
    Ash, Charcoal is used for cleaning teeth

    Bathing - Regular baths, Purifying baths eg. After menstruation, childbirth or oil baths are good practices

    Shaving – Done by traditional barber with no idea of sterilization

Smoking

Hubble – Bubble smoking, a social custom can lead to Oral Cancer

Smoking can cause Lung Cancer, Cancers of Mouth, Pharynx, Larynx, Esophagus, Bladder, Pulmonary TB, Chronic Bronchitis, Emphysema, Coronary Heart Disease, Peptic Ulcer.

Mother's smoking or chewing tobacco may cause Intrauterine Growth Retardation.

Purdah – Muslims are deprived of the beneficial effects of sunlight and have a higher incidence of TB.

Sleep – On the ground, exposed to insect bites

Footwear – Villagers don't wear Footware therefore, Hookworm Infection is possible.

Circumcision – A Muslim custom

4. *Mother & Child Health*

(a) Good Customs – Prolonged breast feeding, oil bath, exposure to sun's rays.

(b) Bad Customs – Non-veg food eg. Eggs, meat, fish are forbidden during pregnancy; Deliveries conducted by untrained Dai; Colostrum not given to the baby; Branding of skin eg. Jaundice, Purgatives eg. Castrol Oil

(c) Unimportant customs - Ear piercing, nose piercing, application of oil on Anterior Fontanelle.

5. *Food Habits*

Vegetarianism – Some people do not take even onion or garlic

Hindus do not eat Beef; Muslims do not eat Pork

Hot Foods – Egg, meat, fish, jaggery, mango

Cold Foods - Curd, milk, lemon

Milk adulterated with water

Ganja, Bhang, Charas consumed frequently

6. *Sex & Marriage*

Marriage is a sacred institution.

Universality of marriage.

Marriage is mostly Monogamy; but Polygamy, Polyandry exists in some societies.

Socio Economic Classification

BG Prasad's Classification (2020) per capita Rs/Mth (Rural and Urban)	Modified Kuppuswamy's Classification (Urban)	Udai Parikh's Classification (Rural)
Social Class I ≥7533 II 3766-7532 III 2260-3765 IV 1130-2259 V ≤1129	a) Education of Family Head Professional/Honours 7 Graduate/PG 6 Intermediate/Post high school diploma 5 High school certificate 4 Middle school certificate 3 Primary or literate 2 Illiterate 1 (b) Occupation Legislators, Senior Officials, Managers 10 Professionals 9 Technicians, Associate Professionals 8 Clerks 7 Skilled, Shop & Market Sales Workers 6 Skilled Agricultural & Fishery Workers 5 Craft & Related Trade Workers 4 Plant & Machine Operators, Assemblers 3 Elementary Occupation 2 Unemployed 1 (c) Monthly income of family (Rs/Mth) ≥199,862 12 99931-199861 10 74755-99930 6 49962-74755 4 29973-49961 3 10002-29972 2 ≤10001 1 Calculation (a+b+c) 26-29 I 16-25 II 11-15 III 5-10 IV <5 V	Criteria based on: Caste Education of HOF Occupation of HOF Social Participation Land holding Housing Farm Power (Owning bullocks, camel, horses, Elephants, tractor) Material Possessions (TV, Radio) Type of family (Joint/ Nuclear)

CHAPTER 10

HEALTH EDUCATION

Definition

The process that informs, motivates and helps people to adopt and maintain healthy practices and lifestyles, advocates environmental changes as needed to facilitate this goal and conducts professional training and research to the same end is known as Health Education.

The Communication Process

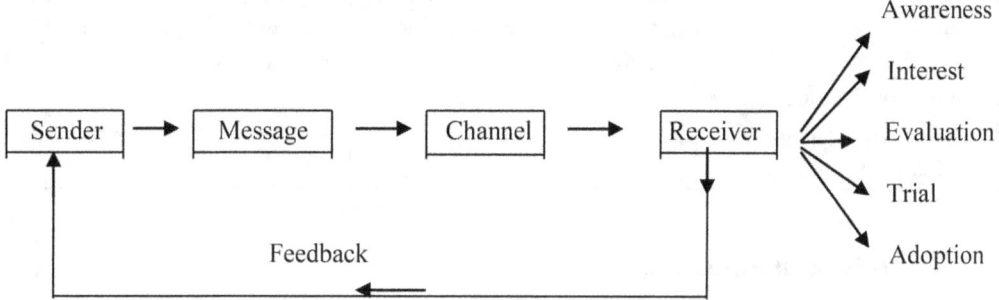

Types of Communication

1.   One-way Communication – Didactic Lecture
2.   Two-way Communication – Socratic Method
3.   Verbal Communication
4.   Non-verbal Communication – Body Language, Facial Expressions
5.   Formal Communication – Follows lines of authority
6.   Informal Communication – Grapevine Communication
7.   Visual Communication – Charts, graphs, pictograms, tables, maps, posters
8.   Telecommunication & Internet – Radio, TV

Barriers of Communication

1. Physiological – Hearing Difficulty, Visual Problems
2. Psychological – Emotional disturbances, Neurosis, Levels of Intelligence, Language Comprehension
3. Environmental – Noise, Visibility
4. Cultural – Illiteracy, knowledge, understanding customs, beliefs, religion, socio-economic differences, language differences

IEC (Information, Education, Communication)

Information	Education	Communication
One or more facts that are received by a human which have some form of worth to him	Process by which behavioural change takes place in an individual as a result of the experiences he has undergone.	Process of exchanging news, facts, opinions, messages between individuals, to help in changing behaviour of others.
Information on Disease: Causes of disease, symptoms, consequences, benefits of treatment	Education is a learning process through which an individual informs and orients himself to develop skills and intelligent action.	A Communicator's job is to help people at things in a new way by sharing ideas and information.
Information on Service: Where are facilities available, Cost of Services		

Approach to Health Education

| (1) Regulatory Approach: Governmental intervention to alter human behavior, laws Eg. Child Marriage Restraint Act No smoking in public places

Helmet Law | (2) Service Approach: Government provides free of cost latrines, yet people do not use them because they did not feel the need | (3) HE Approach: Health Education – The best method to change behaviour

Awareness → Interest →Evaluation → Trial →Adoption

Eg. ORS for Diarrhoea |
|---|---|---|

4. Primary Health Care Approach:
   Health of the people, by the people, for the people where the Principles of Community Participation and Intersectoral Coordination is stressed.

Health Education Vs Propaganda

Health Education	Propaganda
Knowledge Actively Acquired	Instilled in the minds
Skills Actively Acquired	Instilled
Primitive Desires Disciplined	Aroused
Action Reflective Behaviour	Reflexive Behaviour
Emotion Does not appeal to emotion but to reason	Appeals to Emotion
Behaviour Self-Expression	Set Pattern
Process Behaviour Centred	Information Centred

Contents of Health Education

1. Human Biology
2. Personal Hygiene
3. Environmental Hygiene
4. Nutrition
5. Family Health
6. Disease Prevention & Control
7. Mental Health
8. Accident Prevention
9. Use of Health Services

Principles of Health Education

1. Interest – People learn what they are interested in. Must find out their needs.
2. Credibility – Message should be trustworthy and compatible with scientific knowledge
3. Motivation – Must awaken the desire to learn
4. Participation – In Adults, active learning (participation) is important
5. Comprehension – It is necessary to know the level of understanding of the people
6. Reinforcement – Repetition at necessary intervals
7. Learning by Doing – Learning is an action process.
   Chinese proverb "If I hear, I forget; If I see, I remember; if I do, I know."
8. Known to Unknown – In Health Education we must start from Concrete to Abstract; from easy to more difficult
9. Setting an Example – Must practice what we preach.
   If we don't want a patient to smoke cigarettes, we should not smoke
10. Good Human Relations – Good relations of communicator with people helps Health Education

11. Feedback – Health Educator can modify the message or channels according to feedback

12. Leaders – People learn best from local leaders who are role models.

Audio Visual Aids

Auditory Aids:	Visual Aids:	Combined A-V Aids:
Radio	(a) Not requiring projection - Chalk board, leaflets, posters, charts, flannel graphs, exhibits, models, specimens	TV, Films, Videos, CDs, DVDs
Tape Recorder		
Microphones		
Amplifiers	(b) Requiring Projection - slides, film strips	
Earphones		

Methods of Health Communication

Health Communication

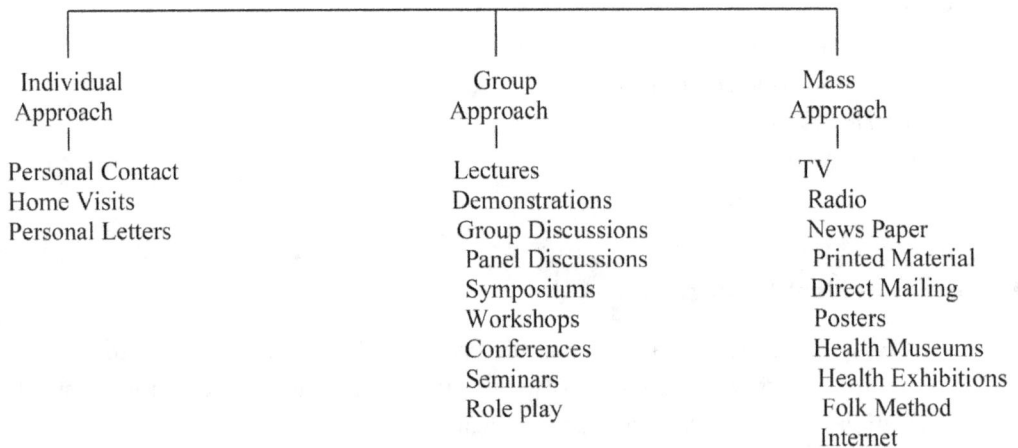

Individual Approach	Group Approach	Mass Approach
Personal Contact	Lectures	TV
Home Visits	Demonstrations	Radio
Personal Letters	Group Discussions	News Paper
	Panel Discussions	Printed Material
	Symposiums	Direct Mailing
	Workshops	Posters
	Conferences	Health Museums
	Seminars	Health Exhibitions
	Role play	Folk Method
		Internet

1. *Individual Approach*

One-to-one approach, highly effective, can be used by doctors, nurses, health workers
Disadvantage – Reaches only a small number of people.

2. *Group Approach*

Advantages	Disadvantages
i. Lecture About 30 people reached at a time, made effective by combining flipcharts, flannel graphs, exhibits, charts & films	One-way Communication can be boring Health behaviour may not be affected Takes time, Personnel should be trained
ii. Demonstrations Highly Effective eg. ORS for Diarrhoea	Some dominating persons Some shy
iii. Group Discussion Very effective method, free exchange of ideas, group of 6-12 members, participants seated in circle, group leader, recorder, reaching decisions	Some deviate from the subject If panel unacquainted with method, preliminary preparation is required
iv. Panel Discussion – Effective, 4-8 qualified persons discuss a topic in front of an audience. The Chairman introduces the topic, speakers, keeps discussions going Audience is invited to participate	
v. Symposium A series of speeches on one subject, each expert on one aspect. No discussion among symposium members. Audience may ask questions at the end. Chairman makes comprehensive summary.	
vi. Seminars & Conferences Regional, State or National level conferences & seminars. Duration ½ day to 1 week. May cover single topic in depth or is broadly comprehensive	
vii. Workshops Series of meetings, emphasis on individual work within the group with the help of consultants. Total workshop is divided into small groups. Each group - One chairman and one recorder. Solve part of the problem and contribute to group work and group discussion and leave workshop with a plan of action.	
viii. Role playing Sociodrama enacted by members. Audiences are actively concerned with drama. Role play followed by discussion of the problem.	

3. ***Mass Approach***

   i. Television

     Popular media which can also reach the Illiterates. Interesting to audience, creates awareness on many topics, good for IEC

   ii. Radio

     Popular media which can reach the illiterates.

     Doctors and health workers can give health talks on radio.

   iii. Internet

     Computer based communication throughout the world. Immediate access to information, literature from WHO and other health agencies and medical journals.

   iv. Newspapers

     Widely disseminated form of literature for literates; articles on health

   v. Printed Material

     Magazines, pamphlets, handouts, booklets used for literates

   vi. Direct Mailing

     Newsletters, booklets on immunization, nutrition, family planning sent to village leaders, literate persons, panchayats, local bodies, opinion leaders

   vii. Posters, Billboards, Signs

     Create awareness by catching the eye. Message simple, short, catchy, easy to understand, put in busy places eg. Bus stops, railway stations, hospitals, health centres

   vii. Health Museums & Exhibitions

     Attract a large number of people. Increases awareness. Personal communication through workers who explain the exhibits.

   (ix) Folk Media

     Keerthan, katha, folk songs, dances, dramas, puppet shows, "Yaksha Gana", ghazals, Quawali can be used to create Health Awareness eg. AIDS Awareness

Planning & Management

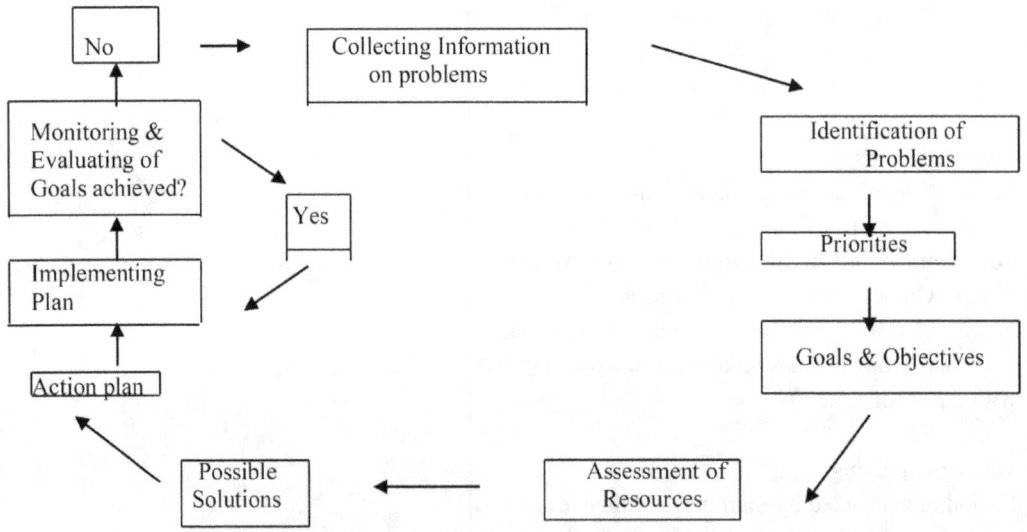

Health Education requires continuous evaluation to measure effectiveness of health education activities in achieving objectives, changes in KAP (Behaviour Change).

CHAPTER 11

ENVIRONMENT & HEALTH

Environment

   i.   Physical – Water, air, soil, housing, waste, radiation
  ii.   Biological – Plants, animals, bacteria, viruses, fungi, insects, rodents
 iii.   Social – Customs, culture, religion, habits, education, occupation, income

Sanitation

Sanitation is a way of life. It is the quality of living that is expressed in a clean home, farm, business, neighborhood and community.

Being a way of life, it must come from within the people; it is nourished by knowledge and grows as an obligation and an ideal in human relations.

Environmental Sanitation

Control of all those factors in a man's Physical Environment which exercises a deleterious effect on his physical development, health and survival. These factors include water, air, ventilation, lighting, noise, radiation, meteorology, housing, waste disposal.

Water

Safe & wholesome water

Water that is
(a)   Free from Pathogenic Agents
(b)   Free from harmful Chemical Substances
(c)   Pleasant to taste ie. free from colour, odour
(d)   Usable for domestic purposes

Water requirement

150 – 200 litres per capita per day per person.

Uses

Domestic – Cooking, drinking, bathing, ablution, gardening
Public – Swimming pools, fountains, ponds, tanks, public gardens
Industry
Agriculture
Electricity Production

Sources

Rain Water – Pure
Surface Water – Reservoirs, rivers, streams, tanks, ponds, lakes
Ground Water – Shallow wells, deep wells, springs

Sanitary Well

Location - More than 15m from sources of contamination
Lining - Cement lining with bricks
Parapet - Wall of 70-75 cm above the ground
Platform - Cement 1m around the well
Drain - To carry off spilled water to a Public Drain or a Soakage Pit constructed well beyond the cone of filtration.
Covering - Cement concrete
Hand Pump - For lifting the water
Consumer Responsibility - To keep it clean

Water Pollution

Pollution of water can be through:
(a) Sewage – Pathogenic Organisms
(b) Industrial and Trade Waste – Metals, Organic Chemicals
(c) Agricultural Pollutants – Pesticides, Insecticides
(d) Physical Pollutants – Heat, Radioactive Substances

Water Borne Diseases

Bacterial – Typhoid, Paratyphoid Fever, Cholera, Bacillary Dysentery, E Coli Diarrhoea
Viral – Rota Virus, Hepatitis A & E, Poliomyelitis
Protozoal – Amebiasis, Giardiasis
Helminths – Roundworm, Threadworm, Hydatid Disease
Leptospiral – Weil's Disease
Those due to Aquatic Host:
 i.   Snail – Schistosomiasis
 ii. Cyclops – Guinea Worm Disease, Fish Tape Worm

Water Quality Standards

Safe Water Criteria

1.   Physical Quality

Turbidity - Free from turbidity, < 5NTU units as measured by Nephelometric Turbidometer

Acceptable colour, taste, odour

Gross Alpha Radioactivity < 3 Picocurie/l

Gross Beta Activity < 30 Picocurie/l

2.   Chemical Quality

Free & Saline Ammonia	0.05mg/l or less
Albuminoidal Ammonia	0.1 mg/l or less
Nitrites	Nil
Nitrates	10mg/l or less
Chlorides	200 mg/l or less for Surface Water
	600 mg/l or less for Ground Water
Hardness	2mEq/l (100mg $CaCO_3$/l or less)
Total Solids	500 mg/l
Oxygen absorbed in 4-hours at 37° C	1mg/l
Arsenic & Lead	0.01 mg/l
Manganese	0.5 mg/l or less
Cadmium	0.005 mg/l or less
Selenium	0.01 mg/l or less
Mercury & Phenolic Substances	0.001 mg/l or less

3.   Bacteriological Quality

Presumptive Coliform Tests in a year:

No sample should show > 10 Coliforms/100 ml

95% of the samples during the year should show no Coliforms

No two consecutive samples should show 1–9 Coliforms/100ml

No sample should show E Coli.

Purification of Water on a Small Scale

1.   Household purification of water
2.   Disinfection of wells

1.   Household purification of water

   i.   Boiling

   5-10 mins of Rolling Boil kills Bacteria, Spores, Cysts, Ova

   Removes temporary hardness

   Must be kept in the same container after boiling

ii. Chemical Disinfection

    (a) Bleaching Powder - White Amorphous Powder, 33% available Chlorine

       Principle of Chlorination - To ensure free residual chlorine of 0.5mg/L after 1 hour of contact period

    (b) Chlorine Tab – 0.5g per 20L of water

    (c) Lime – Cheap, helpful in Gross Contamination

    (d) Iodine – High cost and Thyroid activity do not permit. Only accepted as emergency water purification

    (e) $KMnO_4$ – Oxidizing Agent, kills Vibrio Cholera; Drawback – Colour, smell, taste

iii. Filtration

        Pasteur Chamberland (Porcelaine)

Berkefeld (Infusorial Earth)

Katadyn (Silver Coated)

Filters Bacteria but not Viruses therefore, cannot prevent Polio, Hepatitis, Rotavirus

2.   Well Disinfection

Step 1 – Volume of water determined

Formula = $\Pi r^2 h$ X 1000 (1 cu m = 1000 litres)

Step 2 – Amount of Bleaching Powder required

Chlorine demand estimated by Horrock's Test

If 3rd cup of blue colour, then 3x2=6g required for 455 litres of water

(Roughly 2.5g Bleaching Powder for 1000 liters)

Step 3

Dissolve Bleaching Powder in water

Required quantity of Bleaching Powder prepared to a paste initially and later into a solution.

Contents stirred, allowed to sediment for 10 mins.

Supernatant Solution transferred to another bucket.

Step 4

Delivery of Chlorine Solution into the well

Bucket with Chlorine Solution lowered into the well, some distance below water surface, agitated vertically and horizontally

Step 5

Contact Period 1hour

Step 6

Orthotolidine Arsenite Test

Residual Chlorine estimated using OTA Test

It should be 0.5 mg/litre

Double Pot Method
It is a NEERI Device
Mixture of Bleaching Powder and Sand (1:2) in an Inner Pot which is kept in an Outer Pot.

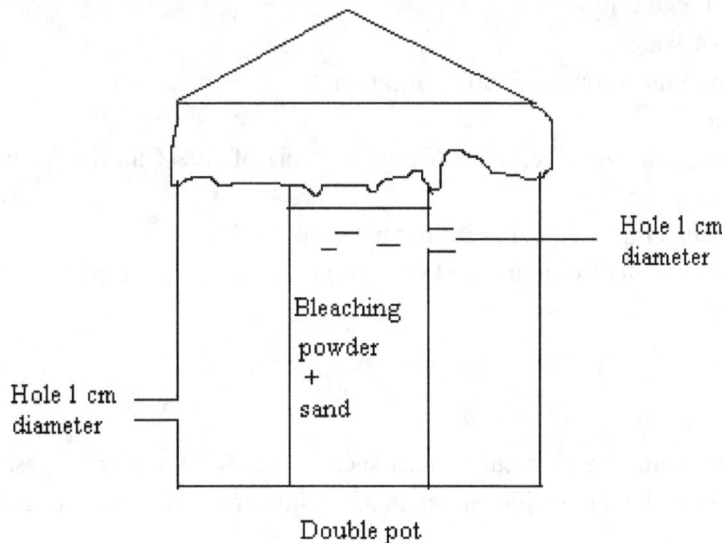

Double pot

Immersed in the well, effective for 4-weeks in Household Wells

Swimming Pool Sanitation

Contamination of swimming pool water due to:
(a)   Faecal Contamination
(b)   Urine
(c)   Organisms from skin, nasopharynx, eyes, ears

Diseases
   i.   Fungal and Viral infections of skin e.g. Epidermophyton, Trichophyton causing Athlete's Foot
  ii.   Infections of eyes, ears
 iii.   Infections of Upper Respiratory Tract
  iv.   Intestinal Infections
   v.   Accidents

Sanitation Measures

1.   Recommended Area - 2.2 sq m (24 sq ft) per swimmer
2.   Surveillance – Rules and regulations for those using swimming pool
     Persons with skin disease, sore eyes, cold, nasal or ear discharge or other communicable diseases should not be allowed to swim
     All swimmers to empty their Bladder and use toilet before entering the Swimming Pool

A Cleansing Shower with soap and water to be taken before entering the pool

Spitting, spouting of water, blowing nose prohibited in the pool

Swimming pool environment - Shower rooms, walkways and pool decks should be disinfected regularly

3. Filtration of Water

    Rapid Sand Filters for continuous filtration

4. Chlorination

    Widely used for Disinfection. 1.0 mg/l (1ppm) of free Chlorine provides residual protection against

    Bacterial and Viral agents. PH is kept between 7.4-7.8

5. Bacteriological quality should be kept close to drinking water quality.

Air pollution

Definition

Presence in the atmosphere of substances such as gases, mixtures of gases, particulate matter generated by human activities which affect human health, animals and plants.

Sources

(a) Automobiles

(b) Industries

(c) Domestic Sources

(d) Miscellaneous – Burning Refuse, Insecticides, Pesticides Spraying, Natural Sources (Dust, Fungi, Moulds, Bacteria)

Meteorological Factors

*   Air movement, climate affected air pollution
*   Winds help in dispersal and dilution of Air Pollutants
*   Topography (Mountains, tall buildings) weaken the winds
*   Temperature Inversion – Rapid cooling of lower layers of air causes little vertical motion and pollutants remain trapped leading to "Smog"

Air pollutants

Carbon Monoxide, Carbon Dioxide, Sulphur Dioxide, Lead, Hydrogen Sulphide, Hydrocarbons, Cadmium, PAH (Polynuclear Aromatic Hydrocarbons), Particulate Matter

Indoor Air pollution

It leads to ARI in young children, Chronic Lung Disease, Cancer, Stillbirths

Sources – Cigarette smoking, fuel smoke

Monitoring of Air Pollution

(a) Sulphur Dioxide – Major contaminant in urban, industrial areas and its concentration is estimated
(b) Smoke or Soiling Index – A known volume of air is filtered through White Filter Paper and measured by Photoelectric Meter
(c) Grit & Dust Measurement – Grit, dust, solids are collected and analysed monthly
(d) Coefficient of Haze – The amount of Smoke or Aerosol in the air is assessed
(e) Air Pollution Index – Arbitrary Index which includes one or more pollutants

Effects of Air pollution

1. Health Aspects

Immediate: Respiratory System (RS) – Acute Bronchitis, death by suffocation if air pollution is severe

Delayed: Chronic Bronchitis, Lung Cancer, Bronchial Asthma, Emphysema, Respiratory Allergies

Lead poisoning leading to decreased Neuropsychological Development

2. Social and Economic aspects

Destruction of plant life

Destruction of animal life, corrosion of metals, damage to buildings, cost of cleaning, maintenance, repairs, aesthetic nuisance

Prevention and Control

(a) Containment – Enclosure, ventilation and air cleaning
(b) Replacement – Electricity, natural gas instead of coal; Unleaded petrol
(c) Dilution – Green belts between industrial and residential areas
(d) Legislation – Air (Prevention & Control of Pollution) Act 1981, by GOI
(e) International Action – WHO established an international network of laboratories in London, Washington, Moscow, Nagpur, Tokyo

Noise

Definition

Wrong sound in the wrong place at the wrong time.

Sources

Automobiles
Factories
Industries
Aircrafts
Horns
Loudspeakers
Radios
TVs
Music Systems

Properties

Loudness > 85 dB can damage hearing

Frequency – Human ear can hear between 20-20,000 Hz

Effects of Noise Exposure

Auditory Effects	Non-Auditory effects
a) Auditory Fatigue appears at 90 dB & is greatest at 4000 Hz, may be associated with Whistling, Buzzing	a) Interference with speech
	(b) Annoyance
(b) Deafness Temporary – Results from exposure to noise but disappears after 24-hours Permanent - Repeated or Continuous Exposure to noise of 100 dB may lead to Permanent Hearing Loss by destruction of organs of Corti, Rupture of Tympanic Membrane may result from noise > 160 dB	(c) Efficiency reduced
	(d) Physiological changes - Increased BP, increased Heart Rate, increased Intracranial Pressure, giddiness, nausea, fatigue interferes with sleep, visual disturbance

Prevention and Control

1. Careful Planning of Cities
   (a) Separation of areas with industry and transport
   (b) Green Belts to separate residential areas from main streets
   (c) Widening of main streets
2. Control of Vehicles
   Vehicular traffic to be reduced in residential areas
   Prohibition of indiscriminate blowing of horn
3. Improve Acoustic Insulation of buildings
   Sound proofing of buildings
   Detached buildings instead of a single large building
4. Industries & Railways
   Industries – Control of noise at source
   Special areas, outside residential areas for industries, railways
   Green Belts to be created
5. Protection of Exposed Persons
   Ear plugs, ear muffs, Periodical Audiogram for workers exposed to noise > 85 dB in Frequency >150 Hz
   Regular rotation of workers
6. Legislation
   Hearing loss is compensable under legislation
7. Education
   Health Education on noise and prevention of ill effects will help in peoples' participation

Radiation

Sources

Natural	Man–made
1. Cosmic Rays 2. Environmental (a) Terrestrial (b) Atmospheric 3. Internal Potassium 40 Carbon 14	1. Medical & Dental X-rays, Radio Isotopes 2. Occupational X-rays 3. Nuclear – Radioactive fallout 4. Miscellaneous – TV, radioactive dial watches, luminous markers, isotope tagged products

Types

1. Electromagnetic Radiations – X-rays, Gamma Rays
2. Corpuscular Radiations – Alpha particles, Beta particles, Protons

Radiation Units

Potency of radiations measured as:
1. Roentgen - The unit of Exposure (Coulomb/kg)
2. Rad - The unit of Absorbed Dose (Gray)
3. Rem - Product of Absorbed Dose and Modifying Factors (Sievert)

Biological Effects

1. Somatic Effects

   Immediate
   i. Radiation Sickness
   ii. Acute Radiation Syndrome

   Delayed
   i. Acute Leukemia
   ii. Carcinogenesis
   iii. Foetal Developmental Abnormalities
   iv. Shortening of Life

2. Genetic
   i. Chromosome Mutations
   ii. Point Mutations

Prevention & Control

Radiation Protection

1. Unnecessary X-rays to be avoided
2. Protective Measures – Lead Shields & Lead Aprons
3. Periodical Medical Examination - Wearing Film Badge
4. Regular working hours
5. Recreation, holidays
6. Legislation   – ICRP – International Commission on Radiological Protection
   IAEA – International Atomic Energy Agency
   WHO – World Health Organisation
   These have been active in Radiation Protection

Heat Stress Indices

Indices:
(a) Equatorial Comfort Index – Temperature of still and saturated air
(b) Heat Stress Index – Represents % of Heat Storage Capacity of an average man
(c) Predicted Four Hour Sweat Rate (P4SR) – 4.5L/4-hours is the upper limit of tolerance (2.5L/4-hours optimal)

Effects of Heat Stress

1. Heat stroke – Temperature110°F (43°C), delirium, convulsions, loss of consciousness, dry and hot skin, sweating absent or decreased, often fatal Treatment – Rapid cooling in ice water bath, supportive treatment
2. Heat Hyperpyrexia – Temperature > 106°F, may lead to Heat Stroke
3. Heat Exhaustion   – Due to inadequate replacement of water and salts, temperature N or increased but not > 102°F (38°C), dizziness, weakness, fatigue
   Treatment – Normalizing fluid and Electrolyte balance
4. Heat Cramps   – Painful, spasmodic contractions of Skeletal Muscles in those doing heavy muscular work at high temperature, humidity due to loss of Na and Cl
5. Heat Syncope   – When patient stands for long time under the sun, becomes pale, BP falls and collapses due to pooling of blood in the lower limbs therefore, decrease flow of blood to the Heart and Brain

Global Warming

Emission of Green House gases into the atmosphere increasing from the beginning of the Industrial Revolution. Fossil Fuels emit CO_2.

Effects

Increase of 3°C in Global Surface Temperature by 2030
Rise in Sea Level 0.1–0.3m by 2050
Cyclones
Heatwaves
Droughts
Fresh Water Supplies
Agriculture
Forests
Industry
Transport
Human Health all may be affected
Change in Vegetation
Change in Insect Vectors
Cities warmer than rural areas

Housing

Housing Standards

Site	– Elevated, access to a street, away from breeding places of mosquitoes & flies, away from nuisances eg. Dust, smoke, smell, noise, traffic; soil dry, safe for foundation, subsoil water should be below 10 feet
Setback	– Open space all around the house In rural areas the built-up should not be > ⅓ of the total area In urban areas the built-up should be up to ⅔ of the total area There should be no obstruction of lighting and ventilation
Floor	– Pucca, impermeable, easily washable, free from cracks and crevices
Walls	– Strong, should not absorb heat and conduct heat, weather resistant, unsuitable for rats and vermin, not easily damaged, smooth, no cracks or crevices
Roof	– Low heat transmittance coefficient, height not < 10 ft.
Rooms	– Not < 2, one should be closed
Floor Area	– Not < 50 sq ft per person (optimum 100 sq ft)
Cubic Space	– 500 cu ft per capita (optimum 1000 cu ft)
Windows	– 2 windows per room, window area 1/5 of the floor area
Lighting	– Daylight should exceed 1% over half the floor area
Kitchen	– Separate, protected against dust, smoke, adequate lighting, provision for storing food, fuel, provisions, water supply, provision for washing vessels, floor impervious, adequate ventilation
Privy	– Sanitary privy is a must

Garbage & Refuse	– Storage facility and disposed daily in a sanitary manner
Bathing & Washing	– Facilities for bathing and washing to be available
Water Supply	– Safe and adequate
Cattle Shed	– Should be 25 ft from the dwelling

Over Crowding

1. Persons per room

1 room	2 persons
2 rooms	3 persons
3 rooms	5 persons
4 rooms	7 persons
5 rooms	10 persons

2. Floor Space – 110 sq ft for 2 persons
3. Sex Separation – Overcrowding if 2 persons > 9 years of age, not husband and wife, of opposite sex are obliged to sleep in the same room

Solid Waste Disposal

Solid Waste includes garbage (food waste), rubbish (paper, plastics, wood, metal, containers, glass), demolition products (bricks, masonry, pipes), sewage treatment residue (sludge-solids from coarse screening), dead animals, manure and other discarded items. It should not contain Night Soil.

Amount

0.25 – 2.5 kg per capita

Public Health Importance

If Solid Waste is allowed to accumulate:
(a) It decomposes, favours fly breeding
(b) Attracts rodents & vermin
(c) Pathogens may be conveyed back to man's food through flies & dust
(d) Possibility of water and soil pollution
(e) Unsightly appearance and bad odour

Sources

1. Street Refuse
2. Market Refuse

3. Stable Litter
4. Industrial Refuse
5. Domestic Refuse

Storage

Dust bins, paper sacks, public bins

Collection

Daily house to house collection, public bins cleared regularly.

Methods of disposal

3 Rs - **R**educe, **R**euse, **R**ecycle; Segregation of waste
(a) Dumping
(b) Controlled Tipping or Sanitary Landfill
(c) Incineration
(d) Composting
(e) Manure Pit
(f) Burial

(a) Dumping

To be done in low areas eg. Kolkata
Drawbacks – Refuse is exposed to flies, rodents; dispersed by wind; pollution of surface and groundwater, bad smell, unsightly appearance

(b) Controlled Tipping

i. Trench Method – On level ground, trench dug, refuse compacted & covered
ii. Ramp Method – Sloping terrain, excavation, refuse compacted & covered
iii. Area Method – Filling land depressions, disused quarries, clay pits
    Disadvantage – Requires supplemental earth from outside

Chemical, Bacteriological and Physical changes occur, Temperature > 60°C kills Pathogens and hastens decomposition, 4-6 months needed for complete decomposition

(c) Incineration

Burning of refuse at high temperature
Disadvantage – Loss to the community in terms of manure

(d) Composting

Combined disposal of Refuse and Night Soil

i. Bangalore Method (Hot Fermentation Method):
   Indian Council of Agricultural Research at IISc, Bangalore developed this method.

Trench – 90 cm deep, 1.5–2.5 m broad, 4.5–10 m long, first layer of refuse 15 cm; then Night Soil of 5 cm; alternate layers of Refuse & Night Soil till heap rises 30 cm above ground level, top layer Refuse, covered with excavated earth.

Temperature > 60°C within 1 week, decomposes Refuse and Night Soil, in 6 months decomposition is complete and it becomes Innocuous Manure.

Mechanical Composting (Aerobic Method)

Refuse is cleared of salvageable material like rags, bones, metal, glass. It is then pulverized and mixed with sewage in a rotating machine and incubated.

Composting is complete within 4–6 weeks.

(e) **Manure Pits**

In rural areas, garbage, cattle dung, straws, leaves are dumped into Manure Pits and covered daily with earth. Two such pits are created, when one is closed the other is used. In 4–6 months the compost converts into Manure.

(f) **Burial**

This is suitable for small camps. A Trench is dug, refuse is dumped daily into it and is covered with earth.

Compost to manure takes 4 – 6 months.

Public Education

Public Education helps to build awareness and maintain a clean environment.

Sullage Disposal

Definition

Sullage is waste water from bathrooms and kitchen which is devoid of excreta.

Soakage Pit

In rural areas Sullage is disposed by letting it into a Soakage Pit.

This is a trench, 3-m long, 3-m deep, 1-m broad. It is filled with irregularly shaped stones, bigger ones along the sides of the trench and smaller ones in the middle. It is covered with a Gunny Cloth as Tarred Mat so that the loose soil does not slip into the trench and block it.

Sullage from the houses is carried to the Soakage Pit with the help of submerged pipes. Before discharging it into the trench it is passed through an earthen pot filled with straw and provided with perforated bottom, so as to remove solid wastes, grease and detergents.

Bacteria and other organisms that grow around the stone particles act upon the Sullage as it sinks into the pit and converts it into harmless Inorganic Substances. The purified Sullage leaves the Soakage Pit and gets absorbed into the surrounding earth.

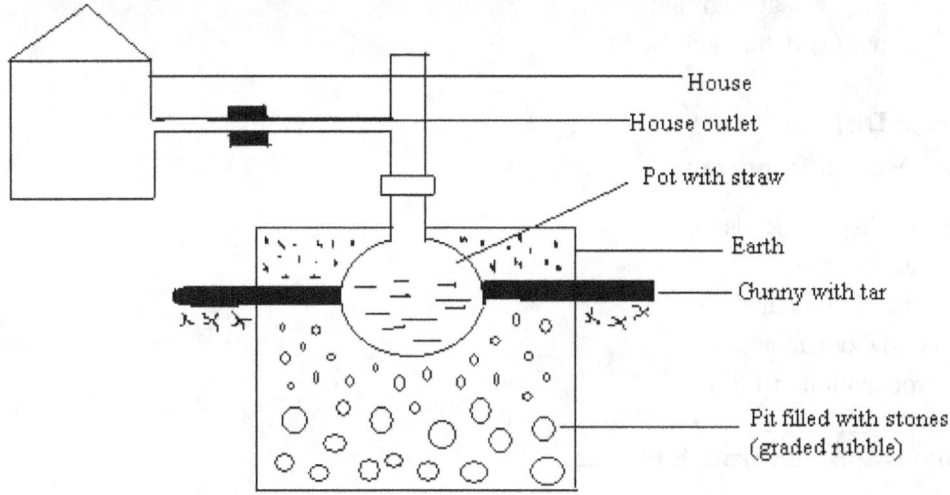

Methods of Excreta Disposal

I.   Unsewered Areas

1.   Service Type
Night Soil is collected by humans and disposed by Burying/Composting

2.   Non Service Type
(a) Bore Hole Latrine
(b) Pit Latrine
(c) Water Seal Latrines – PRAI, RCA, Sulabh Shauchalaya
(d) Septic Tank
(e) Aqua Privy

3.   Latrines for Camps & Temporary Use
(a) Shallow Trench Latrine
(b) Deep Trench Latrine
(c) Bore Hole Latrine
(d) Pit Latrine

II.   Sewered Areas
Water carriage system & sewage treatment

(a) Primary Treatment
Screening
Grit Removal
Plain Sedimentation

(b) Secondary Treatment
Trickling Filters
Activated Sludge Process

   (c) Other Methods
       i.   Sea Outfall
       ii. River Outfall
       iii. Sewage Farming
       iv. Oxidation Ponds

Excreta Disposal
Public Health Importance

Improper disposal leads to:
(a) Soil Pollution
(b) Water Pollution
(c) Food Contamination
(d) Propagation of Flies

Diseases spread through Faeces

(a) Typhoid
(b) Paratyphoid
(c) Cholera
(d) Diarrhea
(e) Dysenteries
(f) Viral Hepatitis
(g) Hookworm, Ascariasis, Amoebiasis

Transmission of Faecal-Borne Diseases

Sanitation Barrier to Transmission of Faecal-borne Disease:

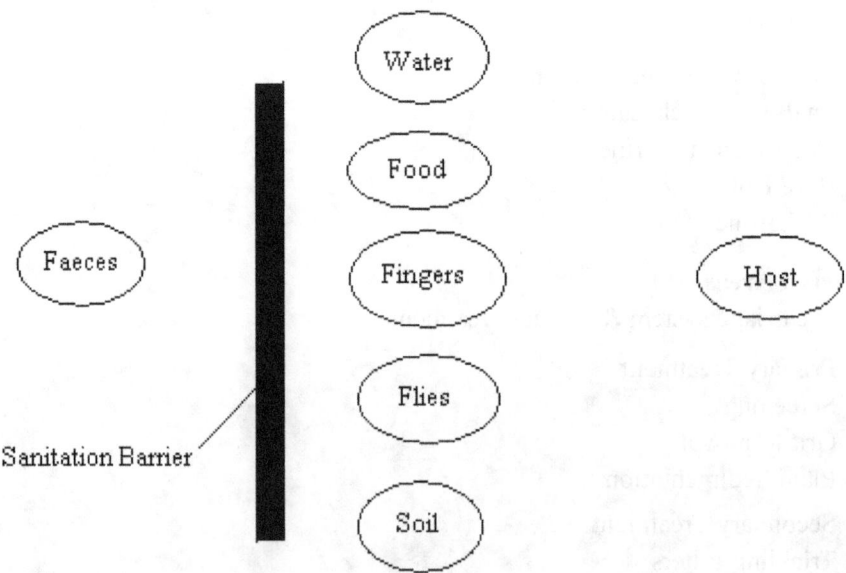

Bore-Hole Latrine

- It is a product of Rockefeller Foundation
- An Auger is required to Bore a hole
- Anaerobic Digestion
- Not very much in use today
- Serves for 1-year

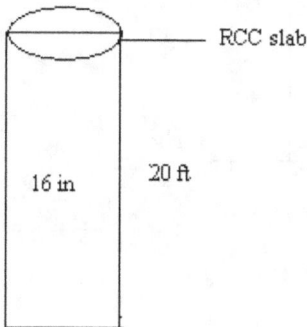

Pit Latrine

- It is a product of Singur Study
- Anaerobic Digestion
- Easy to Construct
- Good Longevity
- Serves 5 years for a family

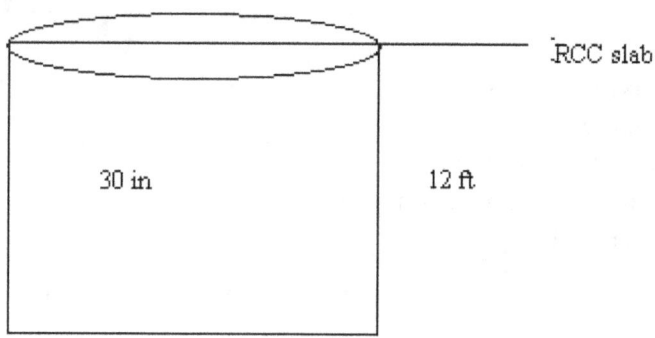

Septic Tanks

- Capacity 500 gallons
- Retention Period 24-hours
- Anaerobic Digestion

- Scum (Effluent) is let to the subsoil to undergo Aerobic Digestion
- Digested Sludge is bailed out once a year

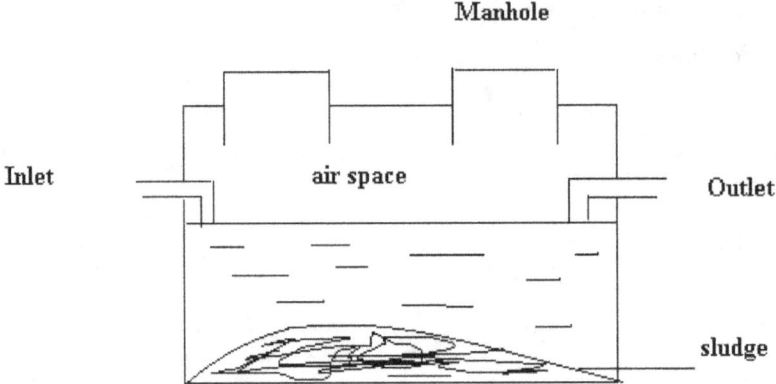

Water Seal Latrines

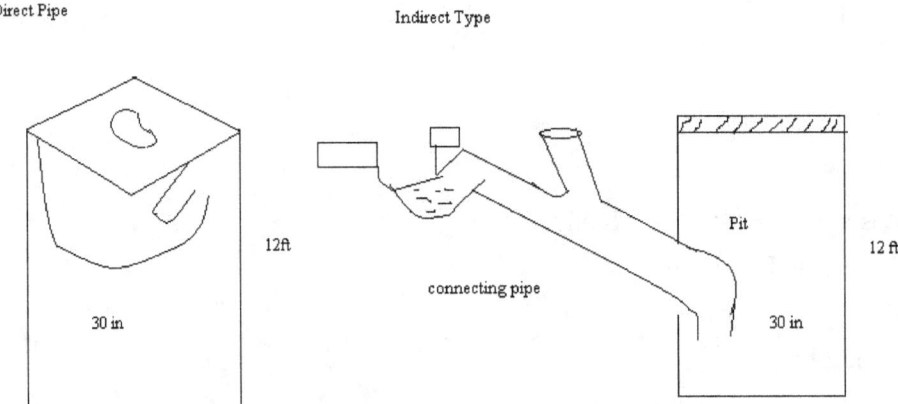

Aqua Privy

- It functions like a Septic Tank
- Anaerobic Digestion
- Treatment by Subsoil Irrigation
- Sludge to be removed at regular intervals
- 6 years for a small family

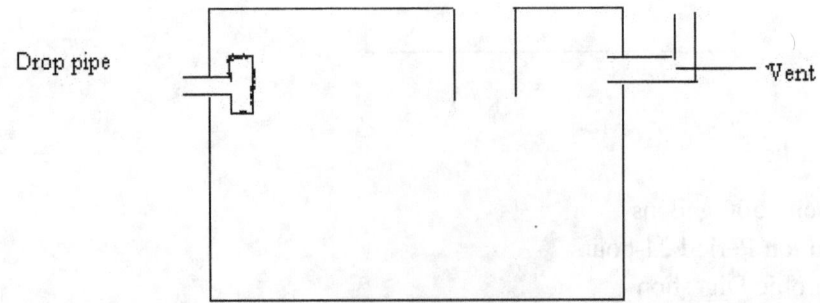

Shallow Trench Latrine

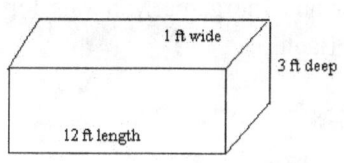

Deep Trench Latrine

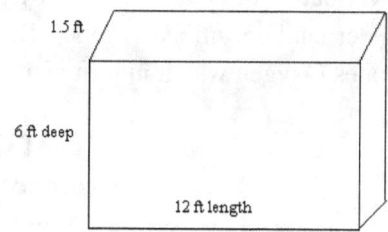

Intended for camps of short duration
Faeces should be covered with mud each time
When filled, it should be covered with earth
and compacted

Intended for Camps of long duration

Modern Sewage Treatment

Based on the Principles of Anaerobic and Aerobic Digestion:

(a) Sludge
  Sewage of 1 million gallons gives 20 tons of Sludge
  Sewage treatment (Anaerobic Autodigestion which yields Sludge)

  Sludge –
  (a) Digestion
  (b) Sea Disposal
  (c) Land Composting

(b) Effluent
  - Disposal by dilution in rivers, streams
  - Disposal on land for irrigation

(c) Other methods of Sewage Disposal
  (a) Sea Outfall
  (b) River Outfall
  (c) Land Treatment (Sewage Farming)
  (d) Oxidation Ponds
  (e) Oxidation Ditches

Oxidation Ponds

Other Names: Waste Stabilization Pond, Redox Pond, Sewage Lagoons
Useful for small communities of 100,000 population; Open shallow pool 1-1.5m deep.

Requirements for Oxidation Ponds:
  i. Algae
  ii. Bacteria which feeds on Decaying Organic Matter
  iii. Sunlight

Method of function:

Aerobic Oxidation of Organic Matter by Bacteria to Carbon Dioxide, Ammonia and Water Algae under sunlight utilizes Carbon Dioxide, Water and Inorganic Minerals for growth and liberates Oxygen which in turn is utilized by the Bacteria.

ENTOMOLOGY

Arthropod Borne Diseases

	Arthropod	Diseases Transmitted
1.	Mosquito	Malaria, Filaria, Viral Encephalitis (JE), Viral fevers (Dengue), Viral Hemorrhagic fevers (Yellow Fever, Dengue Hemorrhagic Fever)
2.	Housefly	Typhoid, Paratyphoid, Diarrhea, Dysentery, Cholera, Gastroenteritis, Amoebiasis, Helminthiasis, Poliomyelitis, Conjunctivitis, Trachoma, Anthrax, Yaws
3.	Sandfly	Kala Azar, Oriental Sore, Sandfly Fever, Oraya Fever
4.	Tsetse Fly	Sleeping Sickness
5.	Louse	Epidemic Typhus, Relapsing Fever, Trench Fever, Pediculosis
6.	Ratflea	Bubonic Plague, Endemic Typhus, Chiggerosis, Hymenolepis Diminuta
7.	Blackfly	Onchocerciasis
8.	Reduviid Bug	Chagas Disease
9.	Hard Tick	Tick Typhus, Viral Encephalitis, Viral fevers, Viral Hemorrhagic Fever (KFD), Tularemia, Tick Paralysis, Human Babesiosis
10.	Soft Tick	Q Fever, Relapsing Fever
11.	Trombiculid Mite	Scrub Typhus, Rickettsial Pox
12.	Itch Mite	Scabies
13.	Cyclops	Guinea Worm Disease, Fish Tapeworm
14.	Cockroaches	Enteric Pathogens

Mosquito

Anopheles Eggs

Habitat – Clean water, wells, tanks, streams
Identification – Found singly, both ends tapering, boat shaped, float and frill on either side

Anopheles Larva

Consists of a head
Segmented body covered with hair
Lies parallel, just below surface of water
Respiratory opening on the Dorsum of 8th segment
Siphon Tube absent
Palmate hair on abdomen

Anopheles Adult male

Palpi as long as Proboscis, clubbed end
Antennae long, feathery
Proboscis not adapted for piercing and sucking blood
Wings spotted

Public Health Importance - Nil

While resting – Proboscis, head, thorax and abdomen make an angle with the surface

Breeds in clear water and slow running streams

Anopheles Adult Female

Head has Proboscis and a pair of compound eyes, palpi and antennae
Proboscis specially adapted for piercing skin, sucking blood
Antennae hair short, scanty
Palpi as long as Proboscis
Wings spotted

While resting Proboscis, head, thorax and abdomen make an angle with the surface of water

Breeds in clean water, slow running streams

Public Health Importance - Vector of Malaria

Prevention

Antilarval and Anti-adult measures
Adult spraying with DDT, Pyrethrum
Mosquito Net
Antimosquito Cream - DEET

Culex Eggs

Habitat – Sullage water collections, sewage contaminated water drains, cesspools
Identification – Eggs cemented together in rafts, each raft has 200–300 eggs
Individual – Eggs cigar shaped
Control – Remove breeding places like drainage, oiling, fill up hollows

Culex Larva

Lies at an angle with the surface of the water
Has a head and segmented body
Conspicuous Siphon Tube
Long, slender body covered with hair

Culex Pupa

Comma shaped, large eyes
2 Breathing Trumpets, long and narrow

Culex Adult Male

Antennae feathery
Palpi long, tapering
Proboscis bent at an angle with body
Abdomen, head, thorax make an angle with the Proboscis which is parallel to surface

Breeds in dirty water eg. Cesspools, stagnant drains containing organic materials and polluted water

Public health importance – Nil

Culex Adult Female

Palpi shorter than proboscis - ⅓
Antennae short with some hair
Proboscis adapted for piercing skin and sucking blood
Abdomen, head, thorax make an angle with Proboscis which is parallel to the surface

Breeds in dirty water eg. Cesspools, stagnant drains containing organic materials and polluted water

Control

Adult – Pyrethrum spraying
     Mosquito net
     DEET Cream
Larva – Drainage, filling up ditches

Aedes

Eggs – Laid singly, cigar shaped

Larva – Lies at an angle with the surface of water
Has head and segmented body
Short and broad Siphon Tube

Pupa - Comma shaped
2 Breathing Trumpets, short and broad

Adult (Tiger Mosquito)

White stripes on black body

Breeds in artificial collections of fresh water
Eg. Inside the house - Flower vases, water coolers, refrigerator water;
Outside the house - Water in discarded tins, broken bottles, fire buckets, flower pots, earthen pots, tree holes, coconut shells, discarded tyres

Day time biters
Do not fly over long distances, usually < 100 m

Public Health Importance – Dengue, Chikungunya Fever, Filaria (Not in India), Yellow Fever (Not in India), Zika Virus Disease

Mansonia

Eggs - Laid under leaves – Pistia leaves, Water Hyacinth in clusters
One end conical and projecting

Larvae & Pupae – Attached to these plants by Siphon Tubes

Public Health Importance
Female Adults transmit Brugia Malayi

Control – Removal of water plants like Pistia and Water Hyacinth, Herbicides

Flies

Housefly
Eggs – 1-mm length
Resembles polished rice grains
Found in fresh manure or refuse collections

Housefly Larva

Length - ½ inch, hairless maggot, very active
Found in fresh manure, refuse, chronic wounds eg. Otitis Media in ears
Cylindrical anterior end, narrow, tapering

Adult

Large insect, dark colour, head, thorax, abdomen
Compound eyes – 1 pair
Mouth parts – Kept bent in a groove
1-pair of wings
3-pairs of legs, hairy

Public Health Importance – Diarrhea, Dysentery, Amoebiasis, Cholera, Poliomyelitis, Conjunctivitis

Control

Sanitation – Proper disposal of excreta and rubbish
Spraying – Pyrethrum, Fly traps, fly baits, screening

Sandfly

Eggs – 0.4 mm X 0.1 mm, torpedo shape, dark yellow

Larva – Head, neck, 12-body segments
Head highly chitinous, conspicuous
Body segments have hairy spines
Posterior end carries 2-pairs of very long Caudal hair
Yellow in colour and covered with fine hairs

Sandfly Male

Smaller than Mosquito
Whole body covered with profuse hair
Abdomen – Short, spindle shaped
Legs – Thin, long, hairy
Eyes – Very prominent
Proboscis – Starts from a projecting snout
Palpi longer than Proboscis and curved downwards
Wings kept vertical at rest
Posterior end of abdomen resembles the tail of an aeroplane because of external genitalia

Public Health Importance - Nil

Sandfly Female

Smaller than Mosquito

Whole body covered with profuse hair

Abdomen is short, spindle shaped

Legs – Thin, long, hairy

Eyes are very prominent

Proboscis starts from a projecting snout

Palpi longer than Proboscis and curved

Wings kept vertical at rest,

2nd Longitudinal vein branches twice, 1st branching taking place in the middle of the wing

Hopping – Sandflies hop about, do not fly

Public Health Importance – Kala Azar, Tropical Sore, Sandfly Fever

Control

1. Keep the area clean, especially cowsheds & surroundings
2. Spray DDT in the buildings, cowsheds
3. Sleep under net
4. Use Repellents
5. Cracks & Crevices to be plastered
6. Clear the vegetations & shrubs

Flea

Rat Flea – Xenopsylla Cheopis Female

Ectoparasites

Body flattened laterally, well segmented

Covered with bristles

No wings

Both sexes bite & suck blood

Females – Spermatheca well marked & semicircular

Males – Coiled structure, the penis

Public Health Importance – Plague, Endemic Typhus (Murine Typhus)

Flea Indices

1. General Flea Index – Average No. of all species per Rodent
2. Specific Flea Index – (X Cheopis Index, X Astia Index)

Average No. of Fleas of each species found per Rodent

3.   Percentage Incidence of Flea species – % of Fleas of each species found per Rodent
4.   Rodent Infestation Rate – % of Rodents infested with various Flea species

Importance – Flea Indices by themselves do not indicate an imminent Plague Epidemic but are useful indicators of the potential explosiveness of the situation should a Plague outbreak occur.

Blocked Flea

Fleas transmit infection by:
1.   Biting
2.   Mechanical Transmission
3.   Faeces

Biting – Chief method of transmission

Some Fleas become blocked due to multiplication of the Plague Bacilli in the Proventriculus or stomach. They are called Blocked Fleas.
Due to blockage the Flea is unable to obtain further blood meals.
Hunger causes it to bite more ferociously and makes it frantic to suck blood.

Every time it bites, instead of sucking blood it injects the Plague Bacilli into the wound.

Therefore, Blocked Fleas play a major role in the spread of the disease.
A partially Blocked Flea is more dangerous than a completely Blocked Flea.

Control

DDT, BHC, Malathion
Repellents
Rodent Control

Lice

Ectoparasites, dorsoventrally compressed
Both sexes transmit disease

Pediculus Human – Male

Wingless insect, lives on Mammalian Blood

Long narrow body, segmented abdomen

Conical Head – A Proboscis, a pair of jointed antennae, a pair of compound eyes, mouth parts adapted to suck blood

Males smaller than females

Claws on legs

Females larger than males
Deep notch at the apex of the last abdominal segment.
Deposits 300 eggs on hair or cloth

Public Health Importance – Typhus, Relapsing Fever, Trench Fever

Pubic Louse (Crab Louse)

Small size (square body)
Blunt & truncated head
Legs – strongly developed with claws at the end

Public Health Importance
Does not transmit disease but produces irritation.

Control

Apply Malathion Lotion or Permethrin Lotion after washing and drying hair.
Dust DDT in between skin and clothes and in between the layers of clothing.
T Ivermectin orally

Hard & Soft Ticks

Body compressed dorsoventrally
Head - Capitulum at anterior end in Hard Tick
In Soft Tick head on underside
Thorax & abdomen – Oval
Chitinous shield on dorsal surface of Hard Tick
Legs – 4 pairs

Public Health Importance
Hard Ticks – Tick Paralysis, Tick Typhus, Q Fever, Tularemia, Encephalitis, Hemorrhagic Fever (KFD)
Soft Ticks – Relapsing Fever, Q Fever, KFD

Control

Insecticidal – 5% DDT, 0.5% Lindane
Environmental – Cracks, crevices filled up, rodent control, dog control
Protection of workers – Protective, long clothing, pants, use tick repellents

Mites

Very small organisms, pin size head
Pass through life cycle of egg, larva, nymph, adult
Larva – 3-pairs legs,
Adult - 4-pairs legs

Sarcoptes Scabiei (Itch Mite)

Ectoparasites
Minute globular parasites visible to the naked eyes
4-pairs of legs

Lifecycle – Egg, larva, nymph, adult in 10 – 15 days

Public Health Importance
Scabies

Control

Treatment of all members of family, hostel
25% Benzyl Benzoate applied to all parts of body below chin and allowed to dry.
Repeat application after 12 hours; after another 12 hours, bath
All clothing and bed linen to be immersed in boiling water and washed with detergent powder.
Repeat application after 10 days.
10% Sulphur ointment
1% HCH (Lindane)
5% Tetmosol
Hygiene – Daily bath

Cyclops

Male and Female
Fresh water Crustacean
Pear shaped symmetrical body, forked tail
2-pairs antennae, 5-pairs legs and one eye
Lifespan 3-months

Female has a pair of egg sacs

Public Health Importance
Guinea Worm Disease, Diphyllobothrium Latum Disease (Fish Tape worm)

Control

Physical – Straining, boiling of water
Chemical – Chlorine 5 ppm, Lime, Abate
Biological – Barbel Fish, Gambusia Fish

Insecticides

Contact Poisons

Organochlorine Compounds

DDT – Dichlorodiphenyltrichloroethane

Residual insecticide, contact poison
Acts on the Nervous System of insects causing paralysis, convulsions & death

Application 100-200mg per sq ft area twice a year as 5% suspension; as 10% DDT Powder for control of Lice, Fleas, Ticks and Bugs

BHC – Benzene Hexachloride (Gammexane), Lindane

Residual Insecticide, contact poison
Dose 25-50 mg per sq ft

Applied 3 times per year

Organophosphorous Insecticides

Malathion

Dose 100 – 200 mg per sq foot every 3 months
Low toxicity
ULV spraying to prevent Dengue Hemorrhagic Fever, Mosquito Borne Encephalitis Epidemics

Abate – Temephos

Low toxicity
Dose 1 ppm used for control of A Stephensi in wells and domestic water containers

Natural compounds

Pyrethrum

Extract from Pyrethrum flowers
Active principles – Pyrethrins I & II, Cinerins I & II
Nerve poisons, contact poisons
Used as space spray

Mineral Oils

Eg. Kerosene, Crude Oil, Malariol
Used to kill Mosquito Larvae and Pupae
Oils suffocate the Larvae & Pupae
Cannot be used in drinking water or paddy fields

Stomach Poison

Paris Green

Composition – Copper Acetoarsenite, emerald green colour

Application – Applied as dust once a week on water surface as Anopheline Larvicide

Action - Stomach Poison

Rodents

Rattus Rattus, Rattus Norvegicus

Anti-Rodent Measures

1. Sanitation measures – Solid waste disposal, rat proof buildings, proper storage of foods, elimination of rat burrows
2. Trapping – Rat traps with baits
3. Rodenticides – Eg. Zinc Phosphide, Warfarin
4. Fumigation – Calcium Cyanide (Cynogas) for fumigation of rat burrows
5. Chemosterilants – A chemical that can cause temporary or permanent sterility in either sex or both. Rodent Chemosterilants are in the experimental stage.

Zoonoses

Definition – Diseases transmitted from vertebrate animals to man.

Bacterial

TB	Cattle, Goats
Brucellosis	Cattle, Goats, Pigs
Plague	Rats
Typhoid	Mammals, Birds
Leptospirosis	Rodents, Mammals

Viral

Rabies	Dog, Wolf
KFD	Monkeys, Cattle
Japanese Encephalitis	Wild Birds

Protozoan

Amoebiasis	Lower Primates
Leishmaniasis	Dogs
T Gondii	Mammals
Trypanosomiasis	Dogs

Helminthic

Hydatid	Dogs
Taenia	Cattle, Pigs
Trichinellosis	Pigs
Fasciolopsis	Dogs, Pigs
Ankylostomiasis	Dogs

Fungal

Dermatophytosis	Cats, Dogs, Horses
Ringworm	Poultry

Arthropod

Scabies	Domestic Animals

Rickettsial

Endemic Typhus	Rats
Rickettsial Pox	Mice
Scrub Typhus	Rodents
Q Fever	Cattle, Sheep

CHAPTER 12

HEALTH INFORMATION SYSTEM & HEALTH STATISTICS

Health Information System (HIS)

A mechanism for collecting, processing, analysing and transmission of information required for organizing and operating health services and also for research and training.

Components

HIS requires information and indicators about the following:
Vital Events
Demography
Health Status – Mortality, morbidity, disability, quality of life
Health Resources – Money, material, manpower, facilities
Health Service Utilization –Bed occupancy, OPD attendance
Health Service Outcome –Polio prevented, cure rate

Uses

Health status of community measured
Health care needs assessed
Health problems identified
Health status comparison at local, national, international levels
Planning, organizing, executing and evaluation are possible
Impact of health services is assessed
A tool for research activity

Sources of HIS

Registration of vital events
Notification of diseases
Census
Sample registration system
Hospital records

National registry of diseases
Survey Report
Screening Report
Surveillance Report

Recent Approaches

Local Area Network (LAN)
World Wide Web (www)
National library of medicine (Medline)
Environment and sick build (CDC)
Morbidity, mortality (CDC Wonder)

Health Statistics

Definition

Statistics – The science of collecting, processing, analysing and transformation of Data which is required for organizing and implementing health services.

Uses of Statistics

Helps in mapping health problems
Health care utilization
Comparison at local, national, international levels
Efficiency of programme is assessed
Helps in planning, organizing, implementing, evaluating health services

Measures of Central Tendency

Mean   – Arithmetic means widely used
           Summation of individual observations divided by the number of observations

Median – Data arranged in ascending or descending order of magnitude and then the middle observation is located

Mode   – The most commonly occurring value (fashionable) in a series of observations

Measures of Dispersion

Range – The difference between highest and lowest value or expressed from the lowest to highest value

Mean Deviation – Average of the deviations from arithmetic mean

$$MD = \frac{\sum (x - \overline{x})}{n}$$

Standard Deviation

Root Means – Square – Deviation

$$SD = \sqrt{\frac{\sum (x - \overline{x})^2}{n}}$$

Coefficient of Variation

$$CV = \frac{SD}{\overline{x}} \times 100$$

Normal Distribution

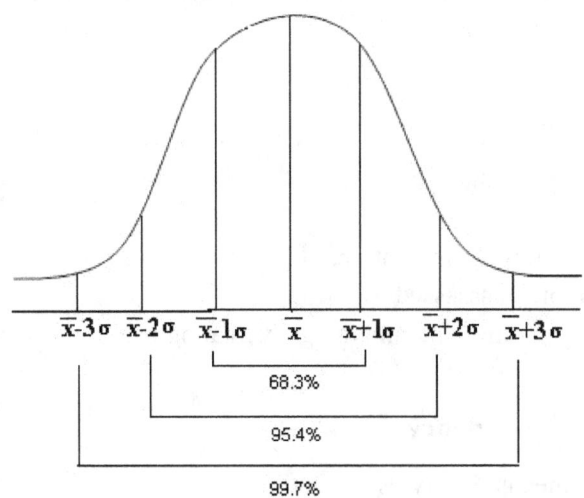

Smooth, bell-shaped symmetrical curve obtained by entering large number of observations.

Mean, Median, Mode all coincide

Total area of the curve is 1

Sampling

Definition – When a portion of a group is taken for a Study from a large group (universe).

Methods

Simple Random Sample

By random number or by lottery

Systematic Random Sample
Eg. Every 10th value taken

Stratified Random Sample
Stratification based on eg. Age, sex and to include each portion

Cluster Sampling
When a cluster is taken as in UIP

Significance Tests

Applied on qualitative or quantitative data
  i.   To find out the relationship or association, and
  ii. Whether the outcome of the study has occurred by chance or not

Common Significance Tests used:
(a) SE of the Mean
(b) SE of Proportion
(c) SE of Difference between 2 Means
(d) SE of Difference between 2 Proportions
(e) χ^2 test
(f) Z test
(g) T test

SE of the Mean $= S / \sqrt{n}$

SE of Proportion $= \sqrt{\dfrac{pq}{n}}$

SE of Difference between 2 Means

$$SE_{(\bar{x}_1 - \bar{x}_2)} = \sqrt{\frac{SD_1^2}{n_1} + \frac{SD_2^2}{n_2}}$$

SE of Difference between 2 Proportions

$$= \sqrt{\frac{p_1 q_1}{n_1} + \frac{p_2 q_2}{n_2}}$$

Chi Square Test

Alternate method of testing the Significance of Difference between 2 Proportions

Step 1
Test the Null Hypothesis
H_0 – No difference between the 2 groups
H_1 – There is a difference between the 2 groups

Step 2
In the table expected values are calculated:

$$E = \frac{\text{Row total X column total}}{\text{Grand total}}$$

$$\chi^2 = \sum \frac{(O - E)^2}{E}$$

Step 3
Finding the Degree of Freedom
$$d.f = (c\text{-}1)\,(r\text{-}1)$$

Step 4
Probability Tables
Published probability tables show that
For one degree of freedom the value of χ^2 for a probability of 0.05 (5% level of significance) is 3.84 and for a probability of 0.01 (1% level of significance) is 6.64.
If our value is > 3.84 it means that there is significant difference at 5% level.

Correlation & Regression

Correlation

To find out the linear relation between 2 variables eg. Height and weight, temperature and pulse, age and vital capacity, the Coefficient of Correlation is calculated.

$$r = \frac{\sum (x - \bar{x})\,(y - \bar{y})}{\sqrt{\sum (x - \bar{x})^2 \; \sum (y - \bar{y})^2}}$$

r tends to lie between -1 and +1
If r is near +1 it indicates a strong positive association between x and y.

A value near -1 indicates a strong negative association eg. When x increases, y decreases r = 0 indicates no association

Regression

To find out the value of one variable, knowing the value of the other, the Regression Coefficient is calculated.

$$y = \bar{y} + b(x - \bar{x})$$

$$\bar{y} = \text{mean of } y_1, y_2, y_3 \dots\dots y_n$$

$$\bar{x} = \text{mean of } x_1, x_2, x_3 \dots\dots x_n$$

$$b = \frac{\sum (x - \bar{x})(y - \bar{y})}{\sum (x - \bar{x})^2}$$

It is the Regression Coefficient of y upon x

Similarly, we can obtain the Regression of x upon y

PART 2

PART 2

CHAPTER 13

FAMILY WELFARE

Definition

Family Planning – A way of thinking and living adopted voluntarily, upon the basis of knowledge, attitudes and responsible decisions by individuals and couples, in order to promote health and welfare of the family group and thus contribute effectively to the social development of a country.

Objectives

- To avoid unwanted births
- To bring about wanted births
- To regulate intervals between pregnancies
- To control time at which births occur in relation to age of parents
- To determine the number of children in a family

Scope of family Planning Services

Aim of Family Planning:

- Proper spacing and limitation of births
- Advice on sterility
- Education on parenthood
- Sex education
- Screening for pathological conditions related to the Reproductive System eg Cervical Cancer
- Premarital consultation & examination
- Marriage counseling
- Genetic counseling
- Carrying out pregnancy tests
- Preparation of couples for arrival of first child
- Services for unmarried mothers

- Adoption services
- Teaching home economics & nutrition

Need for FP for Effective Family Welfare

Population problems are associated with:

1. ***Effects on Nation*** - Even if all resources are tapped to feed the added mouths, it is not sufficient.
   There will be low standard of living, unemployment, overcrowding
2. ***Effects on Family*** - Family income in India is low. If the number of people in a family increases parents will not be able to provide even the basic needs eg. Food, clothing, education
3. ***Effects on Mother*** - With increasing number of pregnancies a mother's health gets impaired; Problems of Anemia will make her more prone to infections, PPH and even death.
4. ***Effects on Child*** - The child gets little attention if pregnancies occur too frequently; Problems of Malnutrition (Kwashiorkor, Marasmus) and maternal deprivation occur.

According to John D Rockefeller, who was Chairman of the Population Council of USA, the objective of FP "is not the restriction of human life but rather its enrichment".

Health Aspects of Family Planning

Women's Health

Maternal mortality and morbidity decreases
Nutritional status is improved
Prevents complications of pregnancy & abortion

Foetal Health

Foetal mortality, chromosomal abnormalities are decreased

Infant & Child Health

Neonatal, Infant & under 5 Mortality is decreased
Health of infants at birth (birth weight) improves

Family Welfare Concept

Family Planning is associated with sterilization and birth control.
However, Family Welfare Programmes aim at improving the quality of life of the people.

Eligible Couples (ECs)	Target Couples
Currently married wherein wife is in the reproductive age (15–49 years) 150–180 ECs/1000 population EC register is a basic document for organizing Family Planning Services	Couples who have had 2-3 living children & on whom Family Planning was concentrated Later even families with one child, or newly married couples were included Now only the term EC is used

Couple Protection Rate (CPR)

Couple Protection rate is the percent of ECs effectively protected against childbirth by one or other approved methods of Family Planning. Eg. Sterilization, IUCD, oral pills, condoms

It is an indicator of prevalence of contraceptive practice in the community.
To achieve the Goal of NRR = 1, CPR should be > 60%

Small Family Norm

Initially 3-children family was propagated, later it was 2-children family.

Current emphasis is on 3 themes:

1. Sons or daughters – 2 will do
2. Second child after 3 years
3. Universal Immunization

National Family Welfare Programme - Refer National Programmes

Demography

Definition

The study of human population focusing on size, composition, distribution.
It deals with 5 Demographic processes:

(a) Fertility

(b) Mortality

(c) Marriage

(d) Migration

(e) Social Mobility

Demographic Cycle

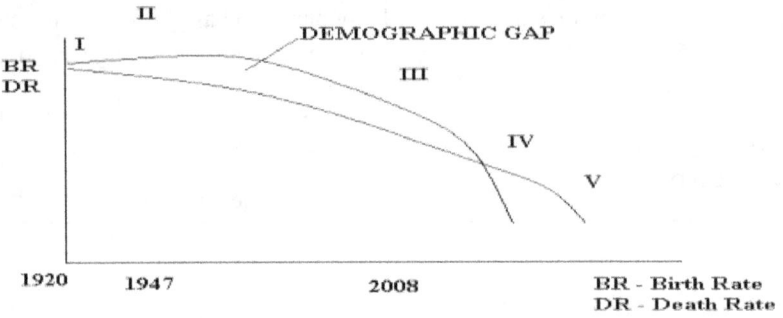

I **First Stage - High Stationary**
- High birth rate
- High death rate
- Population stationary eg. India till 1920

II **Second Stage - Early Expanding**
- Death rate begins to decline
- Birth rate remains unchanged
- Population growth eg. South Asia, Africa

III **Third Stage - Late Expanding**
- Death rate declines further
- Birth rate tends to fall
- Population growth because BR > DR eg. India, China, Singapore

IV **Fourth Stage - Low Stationary**
- Low birth rate
- Low death rate
- Population stationary – Zero population growth eg. Austria
- Growth Rate 0.1 eg. UK, Belgium, Denmark, Sweden

V **Fifth Stage - Declining**
- Birth rate < Death rate
- Population declines eg. Germany, Hungary

Demographic Gap

Difference between births & deaths
Indicates the rapid growth of population in a community.

Beginning of the Christian era the world population was 250 million to 7.7 billion (2019)

Age Sex Pyramid

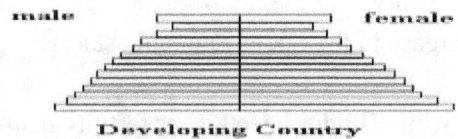

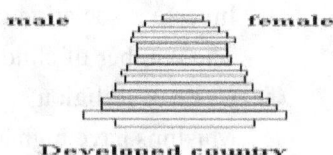

Developing Country	Developed Country
Broad base	Bulge in the middle
Tapering top	Narrower base
Eg. India	Eg. Sweden, Switzerland

Sex Ratio

Definition – No. of females per 1000 males

India – 940
Kerala – 957
Karnataka – 924

Population Density

382 people per sq km

Population Explosion

Causes

1. ***Increased Fertility***
   (a) Age at marriage
       According to Child Marriage Restraint Act, girls should be 18 years and boys 21 years to get married However, in BIMARU states (Bihar, Madhya Pradesh, Rajasthan, Uttar Pradesh), in villages & urban slums girls are getting married at 15 years of age.
   (b) Duration of Married Life
       Maximum births occur within 15 years of married life.
       Therefore, Family Planning should concentrate on this time period.
   (c) Spacing of Children
       Spacing children helps to decrease the fertility rate.
   (d) Education
       Inverse association between education & fertility
       Education is the best Family Planning method.
       The higher a person is educated, the less number of children he has.

(e) Economic Status

Inverse association of economic status & fertility.

The number of children decreases with increase in the Socio-economic status

(f) Caste & Religion

Muslims have higher fertility than Hindus while Hindus have higher fertility than Christians.

Lower castes have higher fertility than higher castes.

(g) Nutrition

Inverse relationship of nutritional status & fertility.

Well-fed societies have low fertility while poorly fed societies have high fertility

(h) Family Planning

Fertility decreases with Family Planning

(i) Others

Socio cultural factors – Wanting a male baby, value of children, place of women in the society, widow remarriage, urbanization, industrialization

(j) Universality of Marriage

Everyone gets married

2. *Decreased Mortality*

Due to

(a) Absence of natural checks eg. Famines, epidemics

(b) Mass control of diseases with National Programmes

(c) Better health facilities

(d) Advances in medical science eg. Chemotherapeutics, antibiotics, vaccines, insecticides

(e) Improvement in food supply

(f) Development of social consciousness in the community

(g) International Aid

3. *Increased Life Expectancy*

With advances in science, life expectancy has increased

Males 67 years, females 69 years.

Prevention & Control of Population Explosion

1. Family Planning – National Family Welfare Programme started in 1952

Spacing between 1st & 2nd delivery

Permanent method after 2nd child

2. Education

3. Improve Socio-economic status

4. Increase age of marriage & implement it

Fertility Related Statistics

1. ***Birth Rate***

    No. of births per 1000 estimated with mid-year population

    $$\text{Birth Rate} = \frac{\text{No. of live births during the year}}{\text{Estimated mid-year population}} \times 1000$$

2. ***General Fertility Rate (GFR)***

    No. of live births per 1000 women in the Reproductive Age Group (15-49) in a given year

    $$\text{GFR} = \frac{\text{No. of live births in an area during the year}}{\substack{\text{Mid-year female population of 15–49 years} \\ \text{in the same area same year}}} \times 1000$$

3. ***General Marital Fertility Rate (GMFR)***

    No. of live births per 1000 married women in the Reproductive Age Group of 15-49 years in a given year

    $$\text{GMFR} = \frac{\text{No. of live births in a year}}{\substack{\text{Mid-year married female population in the} \\ \text{age group of 15–49 years}}} \times 1000$$

4. ***Age Specific Fertility Rate (ASFR)***

    No. of live births in a year to 1000 women in any specified age group

    $$\text{ASFR} = \frac{\text{No. of live births in a particular age group}}{\text{Mid-year female population of the same age group}} \times 1000$$

5. ***Age Specific Marital Fertility Rate (ASMFR)***

    No. of live births in a year to 1000 married women in any specified age group

    $$\text{ASMFR} = \frac{\text{No. of live births in a particular age group}}{\substack{\text{Mid-year married female population of the} \\ \text{same age group}}} \times 1000$$

6. ***Total Fertility Rate (Completed Family Size) (TFR)***

    Average no. of children a woman would have if she were to pass through her reproductive years bearing children at the same rate as the women now in each age group.

    $$\text{TFR} = 5 \times \sum_{15\text{-}19}^{45\text{-}49} \text{ASFR}$$

7. **Total Marital Fertility Rate (TMFR)**

Average no. of children that would be born to a married woman if she experienced current fertility pattern throughout her reproductive span.

$$\text{TMFR} = 5 \times \sum_{15\text{-}19}^{45\text{-}49} \text{ASMFR}$$

8. **Gross Reproduction Rate (GRR)**

Average no. of girls that would be born to a woman if she experienced current fertility pattern throughout her reproductive span (15–49 years) assuming no mortality.

$$\text{GRR} = 5 \times \sum_{15\text{-}19}^{45\text{-}49} \text{ASFR, for female live births}$$

9. **Net Reproductive Rate (NRR)**

No. of daughters a newborn girl will bear during her lifetime assuming fixed age specific fertility & mortality rates.

This is a Demographic Indicator.

Goal is to achieve NRR = 1 (2-child norm); It can be achieved if at least 60% ECs practise FP.

10. **Child – Woman Ratio**

The no. of children 0–4 years per 1000 women of child bearing age of 15–49 yrs.

11. **Pregnancy Rate**

Ratio of no. of pregnancies in a year to married women in the age group of 15–49 years.

12. **Abortion Rate**

The no. of all types of abortions per 1000 women of child bearing age.

13. **Abortion Ratio**

Ratio of abortions performed during a particular time period by the no. of live births over the same period.

14. **Marriage Rate**

$$\text{Crude Marriage Rate} = \frac{\text{No. of marriages in a year}}{\text{Mid-Year population}} \times 1000$$

$$\text{Crude Marriage Rate} = \frac{\text{No. of marriages in the year}}{\text{No. of unmarried persons of 15-49 years}} \times 1000$$

Fertility Indicators

TFR   2.1
NRR   1
GRR   1
CPR   59.3%

Family Welfare Programme spent Rs.0.65 crore in the 1st plan to Rs 371,600 crore in the 12th plan.

Family Planning Methods

I   Spacing Methods
1.   Barrier Methods
     (a) Physical Methods
     (b) Chemical Methods
     (c) Combined Methods
2.   IUCD
3.   Hormonal Methods
4.   Post Conceptional Methods
5.   Miscellaneous

II.   Terminal Methods
Male sterilization
Female sterilization

Physical Methods

Condom

Most widely used barrier device by males
In India, it is known as NIRODH, a Sanskrit word meaning 'Prevention'.

Mode of Action – To prevent live sperms from meeting the ovum.

Method of use:
Fitted on the erect penis before intercourse.
Air must be expelled from the teat end to make room for ejaculate.
Condom must be held carefully when withdrawing from vagina to avoid spillage of seminal fluid into vagina.
A new condom must be used for each sexual act.
Should be properly disposed after tying a knot.

Failure Rate   – 2- > 20/100 women years; Most failures due to incorrect use.
            Effectiveness is increased by using with Spermicidal Jelly.

Advantages – Easily available, safe, inexpensive, easy to use, does not require medical supervision, no side effects, light, compact, easily disposable, prevents pregnancy and STDs/AIDS.

Disadvantages – May slip off or tear during coitus, interferes with sex sensation, many men do not use them regularly or correctly.

Brands Available –
  i.   Dry Nirodh - 3 pieces – 25p
  ii.   Deluxe Nirodh - 5pieces – Rs 2.00
  iii. Super Deluxe Nirodh - 4 pieces – Rs 3.00

Diaphragm

Is a Vaginal barrier
Description – Shallow cup made of synthetic rubber/plastic.
Size – 5-10 cms (2-4"), has a flexible rim made of spring or metal.
Important that a woman is fitted with a Diaphragm of appropriate size.

Hormonal Contraceptives

Introduction

It is the best spacing method between child births.
Over 65 million people in the world are estimated to be taking the Pill.
Approximately, 10 million in India use the Pill.

Classification

A. *Oral Pills*
    1. Combined Pill
    2. Progesterone only Pill
    3. Postcoital Pill
    4. Once a month Pill (Long acting)
    5. Male Pill

B. *Depot (Slow Release) Formulations*
    1. Injectables
    2. Subcutaneous Implants
    3. Vaginal Rings

1. **Combined Pill**
    A major spacing method of contraception.
    The original Pills in 1960s contained 100–200 mg of Synthetic Oestrogen & 10 mg of Progestogen.
    Today the Pill contains 30–35 mcg of Synthetic Oestrogen & 0.5–1 mg of Progestogen.

Method of Use

- To be taken orally for 21 days beginning on the 5th day of LMP followed by a break of 7 days during which menstruation occurs.
- Withdrawal bleeding occurs ie Uterine bleeding from an incompletely formed Endometrium caused by withdrawal of Exogenous Hormones.
- Loss of blood is half of that occurring in a woman having Ovulatory Cycle.
- If bleeding does not occur, the woman is instructed to start the second cycle one week after the preceding one. Ordinarily the woman menstruates after the second course of Pills.
- The Pill should be taken every day at a fixed time, eg. Before going to bed at night.
- If she forgets to take the pill, she should take it as soon as she remembers & take the next day's pill at the usual time.

Types of Pills

The Department of Family Welfare in the Ministry of Health & Family Welfare has made available 2 types of pills:

  i. Mala N   ii. Mala D

| Norgestrel | 0.3mg |
| Ethinyl Oestradiol | 0.03 mg |

Mala N is supplied free.
Mala D is in a package of 28 Pills (21 OCPs & 7 Ferrous Fumarate tabs) at Rs 2.00 per packet

Failure Rate – It is almost 100% effective
Annual Pregnancy rate < 1%

2. **POP (Progesterone only Pill)**
    Commonly called Minipill/Micropil
    Contains only Progesterone in small doses & is given throughout the cycle

    The commonly used Progestogens are:
    Norethisterone
    Levonorgestrel

    POP never gained widespread use because of:
    Poor cycle control
    Increased pregnancy rate

Advantages

Can be used in older women for whom Combined Pill is contraindicated because of Cardiovascular Risk.
May also be considered for young women with risk factors for Neoplasia.

3. **Post Coital Contraception**

Post Coital (or Morning After) contraception is recommended within 48 hours of unprotected intercourse, rape or contraceptive failure.

Two methods are available:

(a) IUCD

IUCD can be inserted, especially Cu T

(b) Hormonal

More often a hormonal method is preferable.

Double dose of the standard combined Pill where most Pills contain 50 mcg oestrogen

Take 2 Pills immediately, followed by 2 Pills after 12 hours.

Today's Pills contain 30–35 mg Oestrogen

So, 4 Pills to be taken immediately, followed by 4 Pills after 12 hrs.

Failure Rate

< 1%

If the method fails – MTP can be done

4. **Once a Month (Long Acting) Pill**

Experiments with once-a-month Pill have been disappointing.

Quinestrol – A long-acting Oestrogen + Short-acting Progestogen

Failure rate is too high

Bleeding is irregular

5. **Male Pill**

Experiments have been conducted since 1950 for male contraceptive.

The research has been along 4 main lines of approach:

Preventing Spermatogenesis

Interfering with sperm storage & maturation

Preventing sperm transport in the Vas

Affecting constituents of the Seminal Fluid.

A male pill made of Gossypol, a derivative of cotton seed oil, has been very much in the news.

It is effective in producing Azoospermia/Severe Oligospermia.

Disadvantage – 10% men may become permanently Azoospermic after taking it for 6 months.

Gossypol could be toxic.

Mode of Action of oral Pills

Combined Pills prevent release of ovum from ovary (Anovulatory Cycles) by blocking the Pituitary Secretion of Gonadotrophin which is necessary for ovulation.

POPs – (a) Render cervical mucous thick and scanty thereby, inhibiting sperm penetration
(b) Inhibit tubal motility thus, delay transport of the sperm & ovum to the uterine cavity.

Risks & Benefits

Risks	Benefits

(a) Cardiovascular Effects:
 - Myocardial Infarction, Cerebral Thrombosis, Deep Vein
   Thrombosis risk is increased with age & cigarette smoking
 - CVS complications are associated with Oestrogen content therefore, Oestrogen content has been decreased. Progestrogen has also been decreased because of untoward effects eg. Hypertension & Metabolic Effects
(b) Carcinogenesis
    No clear evidence of relationship with cancer
(c) Metabolic Effect
 - Positively related to Progesterone dose
 - High BP
 - Alteration in Serum Lipids (decrease high density Lipoproteins)
 - Increased Plasma Insulin
 	
These may also accelerate Atherogenesis leading to Myocardial Infarction & Stroke
(d) Others
- Liver disorders
- Hepatocellular Adenoma, Gall Bladder Disease (Cholestatic Jaundice)
- Subsequent Fertility – slight delay in conception
- Foetal Development –it might increase birth defects
- Ectopic Pregnancy – more likely in women taking POPs, but not in OCPs.
- Lactation – proportion containing high Oestrogen affects the quantity & constituents of Breast Milk
	- 100% effective in preventing pregnancy
	
	Non contraceptive benefits:
	- Protection against 6 diseases
	- Benign Breast Disorder eg. Fibrocystic Disease
	- Fibroadenoma
	- Ovarian Cysts
	- Ovarian Ca
	- Ectopic Pregnancy
	- PID (Pelvic Inflammatory Disease)
	- Iron Deficiency Anemia

Contraindications

Absolute:

Cancer of the Breasts & Genitals
Cardiac abnormalities
H/o Thromboembolism
Hyperlipidemia
Undiagnosed abnormal uterine bleeding
Liver Diseases

Special problems requiring medical surveillance:

Age > 40 years
Smoking & age > 35 years
Mild Hypertension
Chronic Renal Disease
Migraine
Epilepsy
DM
Gall Bladder Disease
H/o Infrequent Bleeding/Amenorrhea
Nursing mothers within 6 months

Combined Injectable Contraceptives

1. *Progestogen & Oestrogen monthly ± 3 days*

Mode of Action
(a) Suppression of ovulation
(b) Progestogen Effect on Cervical Mucus
(c) Progestogen Effect on Endometrium

In clinical trials – Cyclofem/Cycloprovera/Mesigyna have been found highly effective.

Failure rates 0.2 – 0.4%

Contraindications:
Confirmed/Suspected Pregnancy
Ca Breast/Ca Genitals
Past History or present CVS/Thromboembolic Disorder/DVT
DM
Migraine/Epilepsy
Not suitable within 6 months post-partum
Irregular Bleeding/Amenorrhoea

2. *Sub Dermal Implants*

Known as Norplant

Consist of 6 Silastic (Silicone Rubber) capsules containing 35 mg each of Levonorgestrel

Norplast (R)-2 consists of 2 small rods of Levonorgestrel.

The Silastic capsules/rods are implanted beneath the skin of the forearm/upper arm.

Contraceptive Effect is reversible on removal of capsules/rods.

Failure Rate – 0.7%

Disadvantages – Menstrual Irregularities

Surgical procedure necessary to insert/remove the implants

3. *Vaginal Rings*

- Contain Levonorgestrel
- Ring worn in vagina for 3 weeks of cycle & removed in the 4th week
- Hormone slowly absorbed through Vaginal Mucosa
- Lower dose used

Pill should mainly be used in younger women < 35 years for spacing pregnancies.

Females > 35 years should opt for other forms of contraception.

Pill should not be prescribed/continued for females > 40 years.

Medical supervision

Annual medical examination is required

B. Depot Formulations

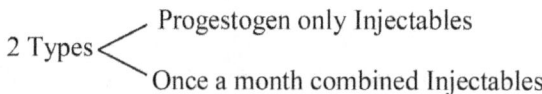

2 Types — Progestogen only Injectables

Once a month combined Injectables

DMPA (Depot Medroxyprogesterone Acetate) 150 mg to be taken every 3-months, IM	NET – EN (Norethisterone Enanthate)
Effectiveness – 99% women are protected from pregnancy for 3 months	200 mg to be taken every 2-months
Mode of Action – Suppression of ovulation, indirect effect on Endometrium, Fallopian Tubes & Cervical Mucus	Slightly increased Pregnancy Rate than DMPA
Advantage – Safe, effective, acceptable, minimum motivation required, can be used during lactation and women > 35 years	Suppression of Ovulation
Disadvantage – Side effects such as weight gain, irregular menstrual bleeding, prolonged infertility after use	Action on Cervical Mucus

Contraindications

Ca Breast
Genital Cancers
Suspected Malignancy
Undiagnosed Abnormal Bleeding

Intrauterine Devices

Definition

The most widely used Spacing method for Birth Control.

Types

(a) Non-medicated   I   Generation – Lippes Loop
                     II Generation – CuT
(b) Medicated   III Generation – Progestasert; Releases Hormone Progesterone
                                      or Levonorgestrel

Mechanism of Action

A foreign body reaction in the Uterus which causes cellular & biochemical changes in the Endometrium and Uterine Fluids thus, decreasing the viability of Gamete and decreasing Fertilization.

Progesterone IUDs – Local effect on Uterine lining, Cervical Mucus thickens and on Sperms.

Cu – Enhances cellular response in the Endometrium, alters biochemical composition of Cervical Mucus, may affect Sperm motility, survival.

Effectiveness

Failure Rate 0.5–3%

Contraindications

Absolute:

Pregnancy
Previous Ectopic pregnancy
Pelvic Inflammatory Disease
Vaginal Bleeding
Cancer Cervix, Uterus, Adnexia

Relative:

       Anaemia

       Menorrhagia

       Post PID

       Cervical discharge purulent

       Congenital malformation of Uterus

       Unmotivated person

Time of Insertion

Interval Period – Within 1st ten days of Menses

Post Abortal – After abortion

Post Puerperal Insertion - 6 weeks after Delivery

Follow Up

IUD wearer to be examined after 1st & 3rd Menstrual Period. Self-examination of threads/tail to be done regularly.

Side Effects & Complications

1. Bleeding
    Increased Vaginal Bleeding, Menorrhagia, Metrorrhagia
2. Pelvic Infection
    Pelvic Inflammatory Disease (PID). More risk for those having multiple partners; may lead to Tubal Block, Ectopic Pregnancy, Infertility
3. Pain
    Pain in lower abdomen, back pain
    Severe pain may indicate Uterine perforation.
4. Uterine Perforation
    Perforation more common if inserted immediate of Postpartum, < 6 weeks after Delivery.
    May be discovered incidentally in X–ray.
5. Pregnancy
    Failure rate of IUDs 0.5–3%
    Pregnancy can either be continued or removal of IUD or MTP.
6. Ectopic Pregnancy
    Prevention of Ectopic Pregnancy by not using IUD if past H/O PID, Ectopic Pregnancy. Signs of Ectopic Pregnancy taught to the user – Lower abdominal pain, scanty Vaginal Bleeding, Amenorrhoea
7. Expulsion
    More in those with Postpartum insertions
    Side effects – Pregnancy

8. Cancer & Teratogenesis

   No evidence of Cancer or Teratogenesis

9. Mortality

   Rare due to the complications eg. Septic spontaneous abortion/Ectopic Pregnancy

10. Fertility After Removal

    Not impaired provided there is no PID

Post Conceptional Methods

Menstrual Regulation (MR)

Aspiration of Uterine contents 6–14 days of missed Period, before pregnancy tests can determine pregnancy.

Cervical Dilation is indicated ——— in Nullipara or

Apprehensive subjects

Complications: Immediate – Perforation of Uterus

Bleeding

Late complications

Tendency of Abortion/Premature Labour

Infertility

Menstrual Disorders

Increased Ectopic Pregnancy

Rh Immunization

MR differs from abortion in 3 aspects:

Lack of certainty of pregnancy

Lack of legal restrictions

Increased safety of early procedures

MTP (Medical Termination of Pregnancy)

Definition

Abortion is the termination of Pregnancy before the Foetus becomes viable (capable of living independently).

ie. < 28 weeks, when the Foetus weighs approximately 1000 g.

World Wide: 30-55 million abortions take place in a year.

In India: 6 million ⟨ 4 million Induced
2 million Spontaneous

MTP Act 1971

The MTP Act was passed by the Indian Parliament in 1971 & came into force in 1972.

MTP Act 1971:

1. Conditions in which Pregnancy can be terminated
    (a) Medical – Where continuation of pregnancy might endanger the life of mother or cause grave injury to her physical or mental health.

    (b) Eugenic – Where there is substantial risk of the child being born with serious handicaps due to physical or mental abnormalities.

    (c) Humanitarian – Where pregnancy results from rape.

    (d) Socio-economic – Where there is risk of injury to the health of mother.

    (e) Failure of Contraceptive Devices – Unwanted pregnancy. This allows abortion on request, in view of difficulty in proving that pregnancy was not caused by failure of contraception.

The written consent of the guardian is necessary before performing an abortion in women < 18 years & lunatics, even if they are > 18 years.

2. Person/persons who can perform an Abortion
Only Registered Medical Practitioners having experience in OBG can perform an Abortion where

Pregnancy is < 12 weeks.

Where pregnancy is > 12 weeks & not > 20 weeks, the opinion of two Registered Medical Practitioners is necessary.

3. Where can an Abortion be done
A Government Hospital

A place approved by the Government

MTP Rules (1975)

Rules & regulations framed initially were altered in 1975.

1. Approval by Board
Under the new rules the CMO (Chief Medical Officer) of the district is empowered to certify that a Doctor has the necessary training in OBG to do Abortions.

2. Qualification to do Abortions
Registered Medical Practitioners can qualify through on-the-spot training.

If he has assisted a Registered Medical Practitioner in performance of at least 25 cases of MTP in a Government approved Institution.

The Doctor may also qualify if he has one or more of the following qualifications:

6 months Houseman-ship in OBG

A PG Qualification in OBG

Practice in OBG 3-years for those Doctors registered before the 1971 MTP Act

One year practice in OBG for those Doctors registered on or after the date of commencement of the Act.

3. **Place where an Abortion can be performed**

    Non-governmental Institutions may take up abortions provided they obtain a license from the CMO of the district.

Early Complications	Late Complications
Hemorrhage, Shock	Infertility
Sepsis	Spontaneous Abortions
Perforation of Uterus	Pre-term Labour
Cervical Injury	Low Birth Weight
Thromboembolism	Ectopic Pregnancy
Anaesthetic &	
Psychiatric Complications	

Miscellaneous

1. **Abstinence**

    The only method which is completely effective is Sexual Abstinence.

    It is sound in theory but difficult in practice.

2. **Coitus Interruptus**

    The oldest method of Voluntary Fertility Control which is widely practiced.

    Advantage – No cost, no appliances.

Method – The male withdraws before ejaculation, thereby preventing deposition of Semen into the Vagina.

Drawback – Precoital secretion of the male may contain Sperms & even a drop of Semen is sufficient to cause pregnancy.

The slightest mistake in timing of the withdrawal may lead to deposition of certain amount of Semen.

Failure Rate – 25%

3. **Safe Period (Rhythm Method)**

    It is also called the "Calendar Method" described by Ogino in 1930.

    Method – It is based on the fact that ovulation occurs 12–16 days from the LMP.

    A week before & a week after the Menses is considered a Safe Period (about 14 days).

Days on which conception is likely to occur are calculated as follows:

Shortest cycle – 18 days   Longest cycle – 10 days
(gives 1ˢᵗ day of Fertile Period)   (gives last day of Fertile Period)
Eg. Cycles of 26–31 days
26 – 18 = 8   31 – 10 = 21

Fertile Period during which the woman should not have intercourse would be 8–21 day of the Menstrual Cycle.

Drawbacks

Women's Menstrual Cycles are not always regular.
Only educated & responsible couples with high degree of motivation & cooperation can use this method
Compulsory Abstinence of Sexual Intercourse (SI) for one half of every month – what may be called Programmed Sex.
This method is not applicable during Postnatal Period.

High failure rate – 21/100 women years

Complications – Ectopic pregnancies, Embryonic abnormalities

4. **Natural Family Planning Methods**
    There are 3 Natural Family Planning Methods:

    (a) BBT Method
    (b) Cervical Mucus Method
    (c) Symptothermic Method

Couples abstain from SI during the Fertile Phase of the Menstrual Cycle.
They totally desist from using drugs/contraceptive devices.
The woman employs self-recognition of certain physiological signs & symptoms associated with Ovulation to ascertain the Fertile Period.

(a) BBT (Basal Body Temperature) Method:

Identification of rise of BBT at the time of Ovulation due to increase in production of Progesterone.
Temperature increases by 0.3–0.5°C up to the beginning of Menstruation.
Temperature is measured before getting out of bed in the morning.
Intercourse is restricted to the Post Ovulatory Phase.

Drawback – Abstinence is necessary for the entire pre-ovulatory period.

(b) Cervical Mucus Method

It is also known as the Billing's Method/Ovulation Method.

Observation of changes in characteristics of Cervical Mucus.

During Ovulation the Cervical Mucus is watery, clear, resembling a raw egg white, smooth, slippery and profuse.

After Ovulation (because of the Progesterone effect), the Cervical Mucus thickens & lessens in quantity.

Drawbacks – Requires a high degree of motivation & education.

(c) Symptothermic Method

Combines BBT, Cervical Mucus & Calendar Methods for identifying the Fertile Period.

NFP methods have little application in developing countries.

Male Sterilization (Vasectomy)

Male Sterilization is simple, safe, cheap when compared to Female Sterilization.

It can be performed in PHCs by trained Doctors under LA.

Method – A piece of Vas (1 cm) is removed after clamping.

The ends are ligated & folded back on themselves decreasing the risk of Re-canalisation at a later date.

Note - Acceptor is not immediately sterile after the operation, usually until 30 ejaculations. During this period another method of contraception must be used.

Failure Rate – 0.15 per 100 person years

Complications:

(a) Operation – Pain, Scrotal Hematoma, local infection.
Good Hemostasis, antibiotics will decrease the risk of these complications.

(b) Sperm Granules – Caused by accumulation of Sperms.
Appear 10–14 days after the operation.
Symptoms – Pain, swelling.
Signs – Hard mass, size 7mm.

Drawback – Sperm Granules may provide a medium through which Re-anastomosis of Vas can occur.
Sperm Granules eventually subside.
Use of metal clips to close the Vas may decrease/eliminate this problem.

(c) Spontaneous Re-canalization

Vas may re-canalise after damage

Incidence of re-canalization is 0-6%

Surgeon should explain this possibility to every acceptor prior to the operation & have a written consent.

5. Breast Feeding

Lactational Amenorrhoea provides some degree of protection against pregnancy.

5-10% women conceive during Lactational Amenorrhoea.

However, once Menstruation returns, continued Lactation no longer offers any protection against Pregnancy.

By 6 months of childbirth, 20–50% women are menstruating & in need of contraception.

6. Birth Control Vaccine

Research on Birth Control Vaccines is going on. Most advanced research involves immunization with a vaccine prepared from Beta Subunit of HCG (Human Chronic Gonadotrophin).

(Female Sterilization)

Female Sterilization – Accounts for 85%
Male Sterilization – Accounts for 10–15% } of all sterilizations

Advantages of Sterilization

It is a one-time method

It does not require sustained motivation

It provides most effective protection against pregnancy

The risk of complications is very less

It is the most cost-effective method

Conditions for Sterilization

Age of husband should not be < 25 years or > 50 years.

Age of wife should not be < 20 years or > 45 years.

If the couple has 3 or more living children, the lower limit of age of husband or wife may be relaxed.

The couple must have 2 living children at the time of the operation.

(d) *Autoimmune Response*

Vasectomy is said to cause an autoimmune response to the Sperms.

Blocking of the Vas causes reabsorption of Spermatozoa & subsequent development of antibodies against the Sperm.

(e) *Psychological*
Diminution of Sexual Vigour
Impotence
Headache
Fatigue

Causes of failure

(a) Some other structure instead of Vas ligated eg. Thrombosed vein, thickened Lymphatic. (Histological confirmation recommended in some countries/microscopic examination of smear by gently squeezing the Vas).
(b) Re-canalisation
(c) More than one Vas
(d) Sexual Intercourse before disappearance of Sperms from the Reproductive Tract

Post Operation Advice

Patient should rest for at least 2-hours post operation. During this period, he should be kept under observation for signs of shock. Before he leaves, the dressing should be examined for any untoward bleeding.

The patient should be told he is not sterile immediately after the operation; at least 30 ejaculations may be necessary before the Seminal Examination is negative.

Use contraceptives until Aspermia has been established.

Avoid taking bath for 24-hours after the operation & not wet the dressing.

Wear T Bandage/Scrotal support (Langot) for 15 days & keep the site clean & dry.

Avoid cycling/lifting weights for 15 days.

No need for complete bed rest.

No Scalpel Vasectomy (NSV)
It is a new technique
It is safe, convenient & acceptable
NSV project is being funded by UNFPA (United Nations Fund for Population Activities)

Female Sterilization

Female Sterilization can be done as an interval procedure, postpartum or post-abortal.

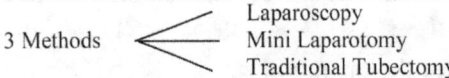

3 Methods
- Laparoscopy
- Mini Laparotomy
- Traditional Tubectomy

Laparoscopy

The technique of Female Sterilization through Abdominal Approach.
A special instrument is used - Laparoscope

Process

The Abdomen is inflated with gas (CO_2, Nitrous Oxide or air) & the instrument is introduced into the Abdominal Cavity to visualize the tubes.
Falope Rings (or clips) are applied to occlude the tubes.
OBG specialist trained in Laparoscopic Sterilization does the procedure.
It is not suitable for postpartum patients for 6 weeks.

Advantages

(a) Short operating time
(b) Short stay in hospital
(c) Small scar
(d) Falope Rings offer better scope for reversing tubal occlusion later, if necessary.

Follow up – By HWF & LHV, 7-10 days and then 12-18 months after the operation.

Complications – Uncommon
Eg. Puncture of large blood vessels and other viscera

Minilap Operation

Modification of Abdominal Tubectomy.
Simple procedure, small incision, 2.5-3 cms, under Local Anaesthesia.
Minilap/Pomeroy Technique, suitable procedure done at PHCs & in mass campaigns.
Suitable for Postpartum Tubal Sterilization

Traditional Tubectomy

Female Sterilization involves cutting & tying off the Fallopian Tubes (clamp, cut, ligate).
Postpartum Sterilization is done 1-3 days after Delivery.
Interval Sterilization is done at any time other than the following
Post-abortal – Eg. MTP or Tubectomy   Childbirth
                                                              Abortion

In Traditional Tubectomy – The abdominal operation is done in which a small piece of each Fallopian Tube is removed & ligated.
Anesthesia   General Anaesthesia
             Spinal

Hospitalization required for 1 week

Post OP – The woman can resume light household work after 10 days.
The woman should not carry heavy loads/do normal work for at least 3 weeks after the operation.
Sexual relations can be resumed 4 weeks after the operation.

Traditional Tubectomy is considered a major procedure.

CHAPTER 14

MATERNAL & CHILD HEALTH

Definition

Promotive, preventive, curative, rehabilitative health care for mothers and children which includes maternal health, family planning, child health, school health, health of handicapped children, children and adolescents.

Need for Specialized Services

1. Large Numbers: 20% mothers; 30% children < 15 years = 50% of population
2. High Risk Group: Mothers - Risk associated with childbearing
   Children - Risk associated with growth, development and survival
3. Preventable Problems: Mortality and Morbidity
4. Feasibility: MCH & FP are part of Primary Health Care

Mother and Child are one unit

1. Antenatal period Foetus is part of the mother.
2. Child Health is associated with Maternal Health. A healthy mother has a healthy baby.
3. Diseases of the mother during Pregnancy have effect on the baby.
   Eg Syphilis, German Measles, TORCHES Infections (Toxoplasma, Rubella, Cytomegalovirus, Herpes, Syphilis)
4. Drugs Taken by the mother have effect on the baby.
   Eg Tobacco, Alcohol, Medications
5. After birth, a child is dependent on mother Eg. Breastmilk.
6. During care of women, care of child is also required.
7. Mother is a child's first teacher
   Eg Socialization, Mental Development

Dr. Glen Doman researched on brain damaged children and found that when given appropriate stimulation they reached near normal development.

Therefore, normal children given sufficient stimulation can reach genius level.

Social Obstetrics

The study of interplay of social and environmental factors related to human reproduction and influence of these factors in the organization, delivery and utilization of obstetric services by the community eg, Age at marriage, child bearing, child spacing, family size, fertility patterns, education, socio-economic status, customs and beliefs, role of women in society, hot/cold foods.

Social Pediatrics

The study of interplay of social and environmental factors related to child health and development, prevention of morbidity, mortality and influence of these factors in the organization, delivery and utilization of child health care services by the community.

Preventive Pediatrics

Prevention of disease and promotion of physical, mental and social well-being of children so that each child may be able to achieve his genetic potential.

MCH Problems

1. Malnutrition - Anemia may cause post-partum Hemorrhage, PET, low birth weight, malnutrition related Diabetes Mellitus, Hypertension, Coronary Heart Disease.
2. Infection - Syphilis, German Measles, TORCHES, TB, Tetanus, Polio.
3. Unregulated Fertility - May lead to maternal mortality, infant mortality and morbidity.

ANTENATAL CARE

Preventive and promotive care during pregnancy (Antenatal period)

Aim

To achieve a healthy mother and a healthy baby at the end of pregnancy.

Objectives

(a) Decrease maternal and infant mortality and morbidity
(b) Promote, protect, maintain the health of mother
(c) Detect high risk cases
(d) Early detection and management of complications
(e) Remove anxiety
(f) Mothercraft education on child care, nutrition, personal hygiene and sanitation
(g) Family planning advice
(h) Care for under-fives

Services for Safe Motherhood (3Es)

1. Essential Care for All
2. Early Detection and Management of Complications
3. Emergency Care for those with Obstetric Complications

1. Essential Care for All

Early Registration 12-16 weeks
Regular Antenatal check ups
Ideal: once a month for 7-months
Twice a month in the 8th month
Once a week in the 9th month

Minimum 4 Antenatal visits:
At 12 weeks or as soon as pregnancy is known
At 28-34 weeks
At 36 weeks
At Full term

First Visit

Register and Prepare the MCH Card
History: Age >30 years or < 20 years
Diseases
General Examination: Anemia, BP, Pedal Edema, weight
Systemic Examination: CVS, RS, CNS
Abdominal Examination: Uterus height, Bimanual Palpation

Investigations

  i. Hb
 ii. Urine albumin, sugar, microscopy
iii. Blood Group, Rh
 iv. VDRL
  v. HBsAg
 vi. HIV

Treatment

Tetanus Toxoid - 1st dose
Iron and Folic Acid tablets - For prevention of anemia - 1 tab OD for 180 days
For treatment of Anemia - 1 tab BD for 180 days
T Mebendazole/Albendazole - If h/o passing worms in 2nd and 3rd Trimester

Antenatal Advice: Diet - Extra cereals, pulses, milk, sugar, GLV, Calcium, Iron

Rest – 8 hours at night and 2 hours in the afternoon

Danger Signs:

(a) Headache, blurring vision, epigastric pain, Pedal Edema
(b) Bleeding per Vagina
(c) Discharge per Vagina
(d) Decreased Foetal movements

Second Visit

History:

GE - Anemia, BP, Pedal Edema, weight (> 3kg/month PET)

Treatment:

Inj. Tetanus Toxoid - Second dose

IFA Tabs

Advice:

Diet, Rest, Danger signs

Third Visit

Enquire about place of delivery. Motivate Institutional delivery.

Give Disposable Delivery Kit (DDK), if delivery to be at home.

Advise 7 Cleans

Breast Feeding Advice:

(a) Initiate within half hour of birth
(b) Exclusive breastfeeding for 6 months (180 days)
(c) Continued breastfeeding till 2 years

Fourth Visit

Similar to the third visit

Risk Approach

Is a managerial tool

1. Elderly primi/teenage pregnancy
2. Short stature <140 cm
3. Antepartum Hemorrhage, Threatened Abortion

4. Diseases - CVS, Kidney, Liver, TB, Diabetes Mellitus
5. Pre-eclampsia, Eclampsia
6. Anemia
7. Malpresentations - Breech, transverse lie, oblique lie
8. Twins, multiple pregnancy
9. Bad obstetric history - Abortions, stillbirths, intrauterine death, manual removal of placenta
10. Previous Caesarian Section, Forceps Delivery
11. Elderly Grandmultiparas
12. Prolonged Pregnancy

Prenatal Advice

3Ds - Diet
Drugs
Danger Signs
Child Care
Personal Hygiene - Cleanliness, rest, sleep, bowels, exercise, smoking/tobacco chewing, dental care, sexual intercourse

Specific Health Protection

Asymptomatic Bacteruria, UTI - Risk to mother and Foetus - Pyelonephritis, preterm birth, low birth weight, perinatal mortality therefore, needs to be treated
Gestational Diabetes - Complications to mother and Foetus - High BP, pre-eclampsia, miscarriage/stillbirth, birth defects, big baby (>4.5kg)
Anemia
Other Nutritional Deficiencies
Tetanus
Syphilis
HIV
German Measles
Pre-eclampsic Toxaemia
Rh Status
Prenatal Genetic Screening

Mental Preparation

Removing the mother's fears

Family Planning Advice

Spacing between the 1st and 2nd pregnancy; permanent method (Vasectomy/Tubectomy) after 2nd child

Pediatric Component

Care of children under-five accompanying the mothers.

2. **Early Detection and Management of Complications**
   Pre-eclampsic Toxemia, Hypertension, Diabetes, Heart, Liver, Kidney Diseases, Anemia, Infections eg. TORCHES, Antepartum Hemorrhage, Abortions diagnosed and treated early.

3. **Emergency Care**
   First Referral Unit (FRU) - Eg. Community Health Centres, General Hospitals are equipped for emergency care.
   Specialists - Obstetrician, Pediatrician, Surgeon, Physician, Anaesthetist are available at FRU.

Facilities - Operation Theatre, Blood Transfusion and Manual Removal of Placenta

INTRANATAL CARE

Care given during Delivery.

Objectives

(a) Asepsis
(b) Early diagnosis and treatment of complications (Prolonged labour, antepartum hemorrhage, convulsions, malpresentations)
(c) Delivery with minimum injury to mother and infant
(d) Care of baby at delivery - Resuscitation, care of cord, care of eyes

Danger Signals During Delivery

(a) Sluggish pains/no pains after rupture of membranes
(b) Poor progress even with good pains for 1-hour after rupture of membranes
(c) Meconium-Stained Liquor
(d) Foetal Bradycardia (<100/min) or Tachycardia (>140/min)
(e) Excess show/bleeding during Labour
(f) Collapse during Labour
(g) Postpartum Hemorrhage or collapse
(h) Placenta not separated within half hour after Delivery
(i) Temperature > 38° C

Complications

Complications	Average time from Onset to Death	Place to Refer
Hemorrhage-APH	12-hours	FRU
PPH	2-hours	FRU
Ruptured Uterus	1-day	FRU
Obstructed Labour	3-days	FRU
Severe Anemia, CCF	2-hours to 1-day	FRU/CHC
Severe Toxaemia	2-days	PHC/CHC
Sepsis - After Abortion/ Delivery	6-days	PHC/CHC/FRU

7 Cleans During Delivery

1. Clean Hands
2. Clean Surface
3. Clean Razor Blade (New)
4. Clean Cord Tie
5. Clean Cord Stump (No Applicant)
6. Clean Vagina
7. Clean Perineum

Disposable Delivery Kit (DDK)

Plastic bag with following contents:

1. Soap
2. Razor Blade (New)
3. Cord Tie (Autoclaved)
4. Gauze (Autoclaved)

DDK is given to the mother if she wants a home delivery. Prevents complications eg. Sepsis, Tetanus, other infections.

Institutional Care

- Should be promoted
- 1% of Deliveries are abnormal; 4% of Deliveries are difficult.
- All high-risk cases require Institutional Services.
- Rest for 1-day, up and about from next day, discharge after 5-days of Delivery

Domiciliary Care

A Female Health Worker or Trained Dai conducts home Deliveries.

Advantages (a) Less fear because of familiar surroundings
(b) Less chances of cross infection
(c) Mother is able to keep an eye on her other children and domestic work

Disadvantages   (a)   Less medical and nursing care

                     (b)   Less rest

                     (c)   Diet may be neglected

Danger signals should be recognized early and referred to the right person, right place at the right time.

Rooming In

Definition

Keeping baby's crib by the side of mother's bed

Advantages

(a)   Breastfeeding better established

(b)   Mother can keep an eye on her baby

(c)   Better bonding between mother and baby

(d)   Mother can take care of the baby's needs

POSTNATAL CARE

Care given to the mother and baby after Delivery.

1.   Care of Mother

Objectives

(a)   To prevent complications

(b)   To restore mother to optimum health

(c)   Breastfeeding promotion

(d)   To provide Family Planning services

(e)   To provide Health Education

(a)   To Prevent Complications

    i.   Hemorrhage

       Primary Hemorrhage (within 6-hours after delivery) due to Cervical Tear, Vaginal Tear, Atonic Uterus

       Secondary Hemorrhage (6-hours to 6-weeks) due to retained products of conception, placenta or membranes

    ii.   Sepsis

       Puerperal Sepsis - Infection of the Genital Tract; symptoms and signs of temperature increase, pulse increase, abdominal pain and tenderness, foul smelling Lochia.

    iii.   Urinary Tract Infection - Burning and frequent micturition, fever with chills

    iv.   Breast engorgement, mastitis, breast abscess

    v.   Thrombophlebitis and Phlebothrombosis

Infection in the veins of legs. Leg tender, pale, swollen, Homan's sign positive; risk of Pulmonary Embolism and death

(b) **Restoration of Mother to Optimum Health**
   i.   Physical
     (a) Postnatal Check-ups - Ideal twice a day in the first 3 days, once a day till 1ˢᵗ week, once per month for the first 6-months, 2-3 per month till 1-year. Minimum at least 3 Postnatal Check-ups.
     (b) Postnatal Exercises - To tone up the Abdominal and Pelvic muscles
     (c) Anemia - Hb to be checked and iron supplementation, iron rich food advised
     (d) Nutrition – Healthy nutrition is necessary to regain strength
   ii. Psychological - Mother's fears should be addressed. Postpartum psychosis requires psychiatric referral and counseling.
   iii. Social – The infant should be taught to socialize

(c) **Breastfeeding**
Breastfeeding should be promoted from Antenatal period. It should be initiated within half hour after delivery, exclusive breastfeeding for 6-months and continued breastfeeding up to 2 years.
Feeding bottle should be avoided. It leads to Diarrhoeal diseases and Marasmus.

(d) **Family Planning**
FP should be promoted during Antenatal, Intra-natal, Postnatal periods.
All India Hospital Post-Partum Programme - Tubal Sterilizations carried out on the second or third day after Delivery.
Laparoscopic Tubal Operation should be done after Postnatal period of 6-weeks.
Spacing methods to be promoted between 1ˢᵗ and 2ⁿᵈ baby with IUD or conventional contraceptives (CC).
Oral contraceptives should not be used during Postnatal period as Oestrogen suppresses lactation.

(e) **Health Education**
   i.   Regular Health Check-ups
   ii. Birth Registration
   iii. Mothercraft Education should be given regarding nutrition, personal hygiene and environment, child-bearing, effective parenting, family planning, family budgeting, cooking demonstration

2. Care of Baby

Objectives

(a) Establishment and Maintenance of Cardiorespiratory Functions
(b) Maintenance of Body Temperature

(c) Avoidance of Infections

(d) Establishment of Feeding

(e) Early Detection and Treatment of Congenital and Acquired Disorders & Infections

(a) Establishment and Maintenance of Cardiorespiratory Functions

Clearing the Airway

To establish breathing – Keep the baby in the head down position, suction with rubber catheter/plastic catheter from the mouth and nostrils, Endotracheal Intubation and suction, oxygen to be given, if needed.

APGAR (Appearance, Pulse, Grimace, Activity, Respiration) Score

Sign	Score		
	0	**1**	**2**
Appearance	Blue, pale	Body pink, Extremities blue	Pink
Pulse, Heart Rate	Absent	Slow (<100)	>100
Grimace	No Response	Grimace	Cry
Activity	Flaccid	Some flexion of extremities	Active movements
Respiratory Effort	Absent	Slow, Irregular	Good cry
Total Score = 10	Severe Depression 0-3	Mild Depression 4-7	No Depression 7-10

Care of Cord

Cord should be cut after pulsation stops; baby gets extra 10ml blood. Sterilized instruments, cord ties and no applicant on cord to prevent Tetanus and other infections.

Care of Eyes

Eyes should be cleaned with sterile wet swabs, one for each eye from medial to lateral side. Ophthalmia Neonatorum can lead to blindness, should be prevented with Silver Nitrate/ Neomycin/Tetracycline eye drops. Causes include N Gonorrhoea, C Trachomatis, Staphylococci, Streptococci, Candida Albicans

Care of Skin

Bathe baby with soap and warm water to remove Vernix, Meconium, blood. Warm oil can be applied before bath.

(b) Maintenance of Body Temperature

N= 36.5-37.5°C.

Baby to be dried immediately after birth, wrapped in cloth and blanket over head and body with only face exposed and given to mother for skin-to-skin contact (Kangaroo mother). Baby should not be placed on cold surfaces eg Metallic tray, rubber sheet, weighing scale. Baby should be kept away from cold walls, open windows, draughts of air.

(c) Avoidance of Infections

Congenital infections with TORCHES cause high mortality.

It can be prevented by giving Rubella vaccine to teenage girls.

Penicillin injections should be given to mothers who are VDRL positive.

Persons with Respiratory Infections and GI Infections should not handle Neonates.

(d) Establishment of Feeding

Breastfeeding should be initiated within half hour of birth.

Colostrum should be given and demand feeding to be done.

Exclusive breastfeeding for 6-months (180 days) and complementary foods to be started after 6 months.

Cup and spoon or local measures eg. Palade/Olle can be used.

Avoid feeding bottles

(e) Early Detection and Treatment of Congenital & Acquired Disorders and Infections

i.   First Examination
To be checked for injuries, malformations, maturity assessed, cyanosis, breathing difficulty, imperforate anus, cerebral irritation (vomiting, bulging anterior fontanelle, convulsions, neck rigidity).

ii. Second Examination
Detailed examination within 24 hours - Body size, temperature, skin, CVS, RS, CNS, ABD, Spine, External Genitalia

iii.   Infections - Tetanus, Syphilis, HBV, HIV

iv. At Risk Infants:
Low birth weight
Twins
Birth Order ≥ 5
Weight < 70% of expected
Failure to gain weight during three consecutive months
Children with PEM
Children with Diarrhea
Artificial Feeding
Working Mother
Single Parent

v.   Neonatal Screening
PKU, Hypothyroidism, Coomb's Test, Sickle Cell Anemia, Hemoglobinopathies, Congenital Dislocation of Hips

BREASTFEEDING

B	-	Best for baby
R	-	Reduces incidence of allergies
E	-	Economical
A	-	Antibodies, greater immunity to infections
S	-	Stool inoffensive, never constipated
T	-	Temperature always correct and constant
F	-	Fresh milk - Never goes sour in the breast
E	-	Emotional bonding
E	-	Easy once established
D	-	Digested easily within 2-3 hours
I	-	Immediately available
N	-	Nutritionally balanced
G	-	Gastroenteritis greatly reduced

BABY FRIENDLY HOSPITAL INITIATIVE (BFHI)

1. Have a written Breastfeeding **policy** that is routinely communicated to all health care staff.
2. **Train** all health care staff in the skills necessary to implement this policy.
3. **Inform** all pregnant women about the benefits and management of Breastfeeding.
4. Help mothers to **initiate** Breastfeeding within half hour of birth.
5. **Show** mothers how to breastfeed and maintain lactation even if they are separated from their infants.
6. Give newborn infants **no food or drink** other than breastmilk unless medically indicated.
7. Practice **rooming in** - Allow mothers and infants to remain together 24-hours a day.
8. Encourage Breastfeeding on **demand.**
9. Give **no artificial teats or pacifiers** to Breastfeeding infants.
10. Foster the establishment of **Breastfeeding support groups** and refer mothers to them on discharge from the hospital or clinic.

LOW BIRTH WEIGHT

Definition

Birth weight < 2.5 kg

Causes

Preterm Babies	Small for Dates Babies
Multiple Births Acute Infections PET Cause not known	Maternal factors - Malnutrition, Anemia, Malaria, Toxaemia, Hypertension, heavy physical work, smoking/tobacco chewing, short stature, very young age, high parity, close birth intervals, low education, low SES Placental factors - Placental Insufficiency, Placental Abnormalities Foetal factors - Foetal Abnormalities, Intrauterine Infections, Chromosomal Abnormality, Multiple Gestation

Public Health Importance

Low birth weight babies have:
i.   High risk of dying - Perinatal, neonatal, infant mortality increases
ii. High morbidity - Diarrhoea, Pneumonia
iii. High risk of developing PEM

Global Strategy for Health For All

Indicator No.8 under Global Strategy for HFA by 2000,
Low birth weight should be < 10% among total live births

$$\text{Low birth weight \%} = \frac{\text{Live born babies with birth weight} <2.5 \text{ kg}}{\text{Total No. of live births}} \times 100$$

Global Scenario

Country	Low birth weight %
India	28
China	9
USA	7
UK	7
Sweden	5
Switzerland	5

Prevention

	Direct Interventions		Indirect Interventions
i.	Increasing Food Intake - Supplementary feeding in ICDS Centres, IFA Tabs, food fortification, enrichment for mothers	i.	Family Planning
		ii.	Avoidance of smoking/tobacco chewing
ii.	Controlling Infections - TORCHES, Malaria, UTI	iii.	Improve health and nutrition of young girls
		iv.	Maternity leave with full pay
iii.	Early Diagnosis and Treatment of Medical Disorders - Hypertension, PET, Diabetes Mellitus	v.	Improve SES
		vi.	Improve sanitation
		vii.	Improve Health & Social Services

Treatment of Low Birth Weight

< 2kg	> 2kg
NICU	Intensive care for 1-2 days
Feeding through nasal catheter	Breastmilk if suckling is good
Prevention of Infections eg Respiratory Infections, Septicaemia	Prevention of Infections

Causes of Deaths

(a)   Atelectasis

(b)   Congenital Malformation

(c)   Pulmonary Hemorrhage

(d)   Intracerebral Hemorrhage - Secondary to Anoxia, birth trauma

(e)   Pneumonia

(f)   Other infections

GROWTH & DEVELOPMENT

Definition

Growth - Increase in physical size.

Development - Increase in skills and function, intellectual, emotional and social aspects.

Factors Affecting Growth and Development

1.   Nutrition
2.   Exercise
3.   Genetic - Height, weight, mental development, IQ
4.   Environment - Sunshine, lighting, ventilation, good housing
5.   Freedom from infections eg. DD, ARI, parasites
6.   Mental Stimulation - Interactions of mother and child
7.   Psychological Factors - Love, tender care, effective parenting
8.   Age - Maximum growth during Foetal life, 1st year and puberty
9.   Sex - Growth spurt for girls is at 10-11 years while for boys it is at 12-13 years (Puberty)
10.   SES - Higher socio-economic status better weight and height
11.   Birth Order - 2nd and 3rd higher birth weight than 1st
12.   Family Planning – Birth spacing and small family

Methods of Assessment

1.   Weight for Age

Growth Chart:

Birth weight: 2.8-3.2 kg

Doubles by 5-months

Triples by 1-year

Quadruples by 2-years

1st year increases by 7-kg

2nd year increases by 2.5 kg

Thereafter 2-kg per year till puberty

At puberty - Boys 20 kg, girls 16 kg

2.   Height for Age

Length at birth 50cm

1st year 25 cm increase

2nd year 12 cm increase

Thereafter 5-cm per year till puberty

At puberty boys 20 cm, girls 16cm

3. Weight for Height - Nutritional wasting - low weight for height (Acute Malnutrition)
4. Head Circumference - At birth 34cm, CC 32cm; By 9-months it is equal.

   Indian children CC>HC at 2 years.
5. Chest Circumference - As above
6. Mid-Arm Circumference:

   N > 13.5 cm

   Mild to moderate malnutrition: 12.5-13.5cm;

   Severe Malnutrition < 12.5cm

Reference Values

(a) Harvard Standards
(b) WHO Standards based on NCHS (National Centre for Health Statistics)
(c) Indian Standards (ICMR)

Milestones of Development

Age in mths	Motor Development	Language Development	Adaptive Development	Sociopersonal Development
6-8wks				Looks at mother and smiles
3mths	Holds head erect			
4-5mths		Listening	Begins to reach out for objects	Recognizes mother Enjoys hide and seek
6-8mths	Sits without support	Experiments with noises	Transfers objects hand to hand	Suspicious of strangers
9-10mths	Crawling	Increasing range of sounds	Releases objects	
10-11mths	Stands with support	First words		
12-14mths	Walks wide base		Builds	
18-21mths	Walks narrow base	Joining words	Begins to explore	
24mths	Runs	Short sentences		Dry by day

GROWTH CHART- ROAD TO HEALTH CHART

- Road to Health Chart was designed by David Morley, modified by WHO.
- It is a visible display of a child's physical growth and development and is used for growth monitoring.
- Periodic weighing every month from birth to 60 months (5-years).
- Direction of growth curve is important - Flattening or falling indicates growth failure, a sensitive sign of Protein Energy Malnutrition (PEM).
- Space provided for general information - Name, registration, birth date, birth weight, H/O sibling health, immunization, introduction of complementary foods, family planning, reasons for special care.

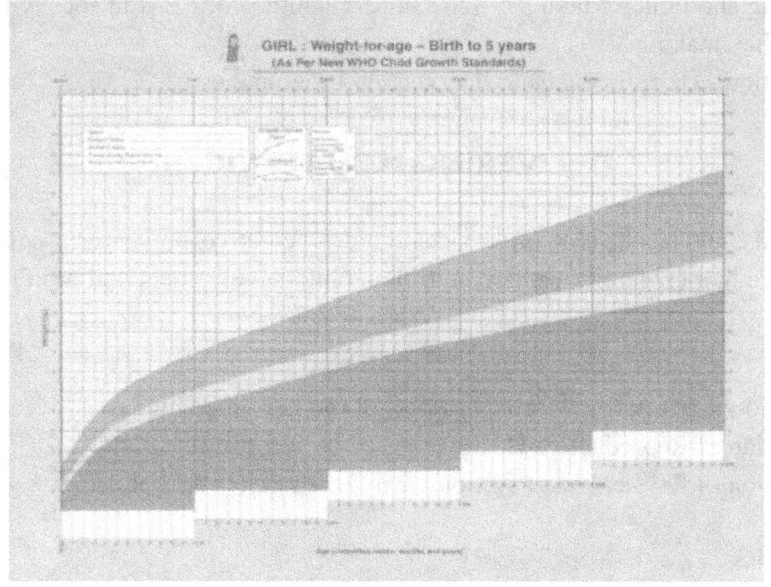

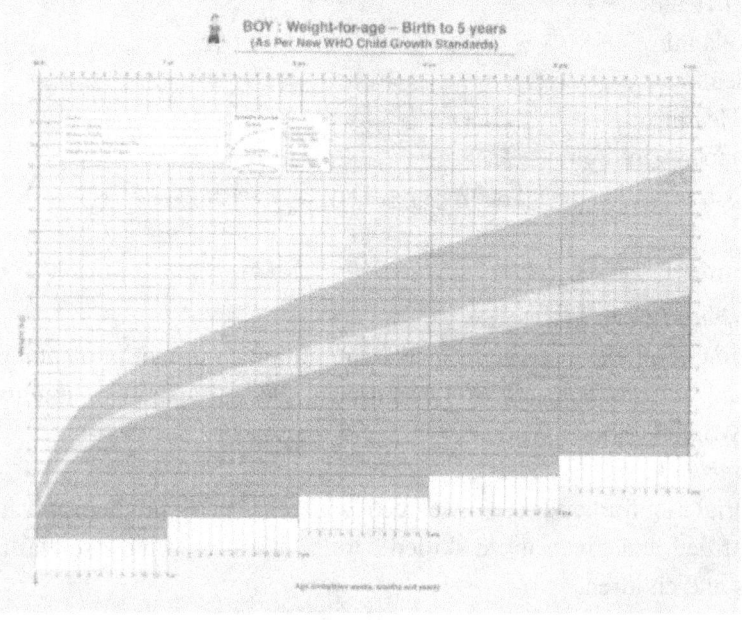

Growth charts should be maintained for all under 5 children in Anganwadis.

Uses of Growth Chart

1. For Growth Monitoring
2. Diagnostic Tool for early diagnosis and treatment of Protein Energy Malnutrition.
3. Tool for Action - Grade III Malnutrition in children should be referred to a hospital; Grade II should receive double food from Anganwadis.
4. Educational Tool – It is a visual of the child's growth, mothers can see how their children are growing and receive Nutrition Education.
5. Tool for Teaching about deleterious effects of illness eg. Diarrhea, ARI and importance of feeding adequately.
6. Planning and Policy Making – Shows the magnitude of PEM in society for planning and policy making.
7. Evaluation - Helps to evaluate Intervention Programmes

DELIVERING MCH SERVICES

Maternal and Child Health (MCH) services comprise curative, preventive, social aspects of Obstetrics, Pediatrics, family welfare, nutrition, child development and health education.

Objectives

1. Reduction in Mortality, Morbidity Rates of mothers and children
2. Promotion of Reproductive Health
3. Promotion of Physical and Psychological Development of a child

Components

(a) Maternal Health
(b) Family Planning
(c) Child Health
(d) School Health
(e) Handicapped Children
(f) Care of Children in special settings eg. Day care settings

Recent Trends

1. *Integration of Care*
   Integration of antenatal care, postnatal care, infant care, family planning.
   Personnel - Team consists of Obstetrician, Pediatrician, Community Physicians, Health Workers, Social Workers
2. *Risk Approach*
   Managerial tool for better use of scarce resources. At risk mothers and at-risk children are identified and given more skilled care, while providing essential care for other mothers and children.

3. *Manpower Changes*
   Wide range of workers:
   i.   Professionals - Specialists
   ii. Field Workers – Female Health Workers, Health Assistants, Dais, Anganwadi Workers, ASHAs
   iii. Voluntary Workers - Members of Women's Organizations
   iv. Primary Health Care

Essential Health Care is made universally accessible to individuals and acceptable to them through their full participation and at a cost the community and country can afford.

Its components of health education, promotion of food supply and proper nutrition, adequate supply of safe water and basic sanitation, MCH including FP, immunization, prevention of locally endemic diseases, treatment of common diseases and injuries and provision of essential drugs helps to improve the health of mothers and children.

Organization of MCH and FP Services

In Rural Areas

District Hospitals - All Specialists
CHC/FRU - Obs, Paeds, Surgeons, Physicians
PHC - Medical Officer
Subcentre – Female Health Workers
Village Level - Anganwadi Workers, Dais, ASHAs

In Urban Areas

Maternity Hospitals
Maternity Homes
Municipal Corporation Hospitals
Voluntary Organizations
Private Hospitals

INDICATORS OF MCH CARE

Maternal and Child Health status is assessed through measurements of
(a) Mortality
(b) Morbidity
(c) Growth and Development

MCH Indicators and Status:

Mortality Indicators	Current Status
Maternal Mortality Ratio/100,000 LB	113
Perinatal Mortality Rate/1000 LB	22
Neonatal Mortality Rate/1000 LB	23
Post-neonatal Mortality Rate	09
Infant Mortality Rate/1000LB	32
Under 5 Mortality Rate/1000 LB	36
Child Survival Rate %	96.3

MATERNAL MORTALITY RATIO

Definition

Maternal Death - Death of a woman while pregnant or within 42 days of termination of pregnancy, irrespective of duration and site of pregnancy, from any cause related to or aggravated by pregnancy or its management but not from accidental or incidental causes.

Maternal Mortality Ratio

Total No. of female deaths due to complications of pregnancy, childbirth, or within
<u>42 days of Delivery from Puerperal causes in an area during a given year</u> X100,000
Total live births in the same area and year

MMR in the world - 400/100,000 live births
MMR in India - 113/100,000 live births

Causes of MMR

Medical Causes	Social Causes
Obstetric Causes	Age at childbirth
Hemorrhage	Parity
Sepsis	Too close pregnancies
Abortions	Too many pregnancies
Toxaemias	Family size
Obstructed Labour	Poverty
Ruptured Uterus	Illiteracy, Ignorance, Prejudices
Non-Obstetric Causes	Malnutrition
Anaemia	Lack of Maternity Services
Associated Diseases - Cardiac, Renal, Hepatic,	Shortage of Health Manpower
Metabolic, Infectious Diseases	Delivery by Untrained Dais
Malignancy	Poor Environmental Sanitation
Accidents	Poor Communication, Transport
	Social Customs

Risk Approach

Elderly Primigravidae, Short Stature, Malpresentation, Antepartum Hemorrhage, Threatened Abortion, Bad Obstetric History (Previous stillbirth, intrauterine death, manual removal of placenta), Pre-eclampsia and Eclampsia, Twins, Hydramnios, Elderly Grand Multipara, Anemia, Prolonged Pregnancy, Previous Caesarian Section or Instrumental Delivery, Pregnancy associated with General Diseases (CVS, Kidney, Liver, TB, Diabetes)

Preventive and Social Measures

1. Early Registration of pregnancy
2. Minimum Antenatal Check-ups - 4
3. Tetanus Immunization
4. IFA Tablets Supplementation
5. Dietary Supplementation and Iron rich foods
6. Prevention of Complications eg. Eclampsia, malpresentation, ruptured uterus
7. Treatment of Infections during Pregnancy eg. Malaria, TORCHES
8. Training of Dais, Female Health Workers on Safe Delivery Practices, Infant Resuscitation
9. Clean Delivery Practices - 7 Cleans
10. Prevention of Infections and Hemorrhage during Puerperium
11. Institutional Deliveries
12. Promotion of Family Planning – 2-Child norm, Spacing of Pregnancy
13. Health Education to remove social and cultural factors which are negative to maternal health eg. Increasing age at marriage, Female Foeticide
14. Mortality Meetings - To identify cause of every maternal death

INFANT AND CHILD MORTALITY INDICATORS

Perinatal Mortality Rate

Definition

$$\frac{\text{Late Foetal Deaths} + \text{Early Neonatal Deaths in one Year}}{\text{Total Live Births in the same year}} \times 1000$$

or

$$\frac{\text{Late Foetal Deaths} + \text{Early Neonatal Deaths weight} > 1000g \text{ in one Year}}{\text{Total Live Births weight} > 1000g \text{ at birth in the same year}} \times 1000$$

=22/1000 Live Births

Causes

Antenatal Causes

*   Maternal Diseases - Hypertension, Diabetes, Cardiovascular, TB, Anemia
*   Toxaemia of Pregnancy
*   Malnutrition
*   Pelvic Diseases - Uterine Myomas, Ovarian Tumours, Endometriosis
*   Anatomical Defects - Uterine Anomalies, Incompetent Cervix

- Endocrine Imbalance and Inadequate uterine preparation
- Blood Incompatibilities
- Antepartum Hemorrhage
- Advanced Maternal Age >35 years or Teenage pregnancy < 18 years
- Maternal Height < 140 cm
- Bad Obstetric History
- Congenital Defects

Intranatal Causes

- Birth Injuries
- Asphyxia
- Prolonged Effort Time
- Obstetric Complications

Postnatal Causes

- Prematurity
- Respiratory Distress Syndrome
- Respiratory Infections
- Alimentary Infections
- Congenital Anomalies
- Multiple Pregnancies

Unknown Causes

Some cases, no causes

Social Causes

- Low socioeconomic status
- Illiteracy
- High parity
- Smoking/tobacco chewing

Infant Mortality Rate

Definition

Number of infant deaths per thousand live births in the same year.

$$\frac{\text{No. of infant deaths in a given year}}{\text{Total No. of Live Births in the same year}} \times 1000$$

= 32/1000 Live Births

Causes

Biological Factors

- Birth weight
- Birth order
- Birth spacing
- Family size
- High fertility
- Multiple births
- Age of mother

Economic Factors

Low Socio-economic Status

Cultural and Social Factors

Breastfeeding, Religion, Caste, Early marriages, Sex of child, Illegitimacy, Broken family, Maternal education, Quality of Mothering, Brutal Habits, Customs, Quality of health care, Indigenous Dai, Poor environmental sanitation

Neonatal Mortality Rate

Definition

$$\frac{\text{No. of deaths during Neonatal period (0-28 days) in a year}}{\text{Total Live Births in the same year}} \times 1000$$

= 23/1000 Live Births

Causes

Endogenous Factors

Prematurity, Intrauterine Growth Retardation
Twins
Congenital Anomalies
Birth injuries
Birth Asphyxia
Diarrhea
Acute Respiratory Infections
Tetanus
Syphilis
Sepsis

Hemolytic disease of newborn
Conditions of placenta and cord

Post-neonatal Mortality

Definition

$$\frac{\text{Total No. of deaths within 28 days to 1-year in a given year}}{\text{Total Live Births in the same year}} \text{ X 1000}$$

= 9/1000 Live Births

Causes

Exogenous Factors

* Environmental
* Social factors
* Diarrhea
* Acute Respiratory Infections
* Malnutrition
* Accidents
* Congenital Anomalies
* Large families
* F>M

1-4 Year Mortality Rate (Child Death Rate)

Definition

$$\frac{\text{No. of deaths of children 1-4 years during a year}}{\text{Total No. of children 1- 4 years in the middle of the year in that area}} \text{ X1000}$$

Causes

Infectious Disease - TB, DPT, Polio, Measles, Diarrhea, ARI, Other Febrile Diseases, Malnutrition, Accidents

Developing Countries	Developed Countries
Diarrhoeal Diseases	Accidents
ARI	Congenital Anomalies
Malnutrition	Malignant Neoplasms
Infectious diseases - (TB, DPT, Polio, Measles)	Influenza
	Pneumonia
Other Febrile Diseases	
Accidents and Injuries	

Under Five Mortality Rate - U5MR (Child Mortality Rate)

Definition

$$\frac{\text{No. of deaths of children} < 5 \text{ years in a given year}}{\text{Total Live Births in the same year}} \times 1000$$

$= 36$

Causes

- ARI
- Diarrhoea
- Malaria
- Measles
- HIV/AIDS
- Neonatal conditions - Preterm births, birth asphyxia, infections, injuries

Child Survival Index

Definition

A Child Survival Rate per 1000 births is calculated by subtracting U5MR from 1000, dividing by 10, shows % of those who survive up to the age of 5 years

$$= \frac{1000\text{-U5MR}}{10}$$

$= 96.3\%$

Preventive and Social Measures

1. **Prenatal Nutrition**
    Nutrition of the girl child and maternal nutrition helps to prevent low birth weight and its complications. ICDS helps with food supplementation during the Antenatal and Postnatal periods.

2. **GOBI FFF**
    Growth Monitoring
    Growth charts maintained for all under 5 children. They identify PEM early and treatment is given accordingly.

3. **Oral Rehydration Therapy (ORT)**
    ORT can decrease Diarrhoeal deaths due to dehydration.

4. **Breastfeeding**

Initiation of breastfeeding within half hour of birth, exclusive breastfeeding for 6-months, continued breastfeeding up to 2 years prevents Gastrointestinal, Respiratory infections and PEM.

5. **Immunization**

TB, DPT, Polio, Influenza, Hepatitis B Measles, Rubella is prevented through Immunization.

6. **Fertility Control**

Family Planning - Spacing 3-years between 1st and 2nd child; permanent method after 2 children.

7. **Female Literacy**

Educated women get married at later age, do not have early pregnancies, space their pregnancies, have less number of children, have better access to information, personal hygiene and child care and utilize health services.

8. **Feeding**

Breastfeeding and complementary feeding with locally available low-cost food at the right age.

9. **Provision of Primary Health Care**
   - Team approaches to provide MCH & FP services.
   - Early registration, early diagnosis and management of complications and emergency services in First Referral Unit (FRU)
   - Special Neonatal care for preterm IUGR Babies and training of Dais on the "7 Cleans".

10. **Sanitation**

Exposure to infections may be through contaminated food, polluted water, lack of hygiene, flies, poor housing and these need to be addressed to prevent child deaths.

11. **Socio-economic development**

Overall social and economic development of a community which includes education, improved nutrition, safe water, sanitation, improvement of housing condition, growth of agriculture and industry, availability of commerce and communication.

CHILD HEALTH PROBLEMS

1. Low birth weight
2. Malnutrition - PEM, Iron deficiency Anemia, Vit A deficiency, Iodine deficiency
3. Infections - Diarrhea, ARI, TB, Diphtheria, Pertussis, Tetanus (DPT), Measles, Rubella, Malaria, HIV/AIDS

4. Parasitosis - Ascariasis, Hookworm, Amoebiasis, Giardiasis
5. Accidents - Trauma, burns, falls, Road Traffic Accidents
6. Poisoning - Medicines, Pesticides
7. Behavioural Problems - Delinquents, social, psychological problems
8. Other Factors affecting health of children - Maternal health, family, socio-economic status (education, occupation, income), environment, social support and health care

Rights of the Child

As per the Indian Constitution:

i. Article 24 prohibits employment of children below 14 years in factories
ii. Article 39 prevents abuse of children of tender age
iii. Article 45 provides for free and compulsory education for all children until they complete 14 years of age

UN Declaration of the Rights of the Child

1. Right to develop in an atmosphere of affection and security and wherever possible in the care and under the responsibility of his/her parents
2. Right to enjoy the benefits of social security, including nutrition, housing and medical care
3. Right to free education
4. Right to full opportunity for play and recreation
5. Right to a name and nationality
6. Right to special care, if handicapped
7. Right to be among the first to receive protection and relief in times of disaster
8. Right to learn to be a useful member of society and to develop in a healthy and normal manner and in conditions of freedom and dignity
9. Right to be brought up in a spirit of understanding, tolerance, friendship among people, peace and universal brotherhood
10. Right to enjoy these rights regardless of race, colour, sex, religion, national or social origin

14th Nov is the Universal Children's Day

National Policy for Children

"It shall be the policy of the State to provide adequate services to children, both before and after birth and through the period of growth, to ensure their full physical, mental and social development. The State shall progressively increase the scope of such services so that, within a reasonable time, all children in the country enjoy optimum conditions for their balanced growth."

UNDER FIVE'S CLINIC

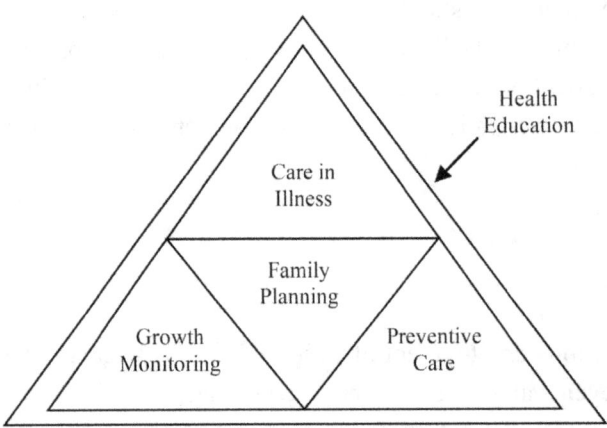

1. **Care in Illness**
   Care and treatment of sick children comprising diagnosis, treatment of acute illness, chronic illness (physical, mental, congenital and acquired abnormalities), disorders of growth and development.
   X-ray, lab services and referral services to be made available.

2. **Preventive Care**

Immunization - World's greatest public health tool against TB, DPT, Polio, Hepatitis, Influenza, Measles, Rubella.

Nutritional surveillance - To detect and treat PEM, Anemia, Nutritional Blindness.
ICDS provides supplementary feeding for under five children.
Health check-up of Anganwadi children every 3 months by Medical Officer of PHC.

Oral Rehydration Therapy - Diarrhoeal episodes, 3 per year in under 5 children.
Diarrhoea can lead to dehydration and death or malnutrition.
Oral Rehydration prevents deaths due to dehydration.

Iodised Salt - Should be used to prevent Iodine Deficiency Disorders.

3. **Growth Monitoring**
   Anganwadi workers maintain growth charts of under five children. Appropriate action should be taken according to nutritional status.

4. **Family Planning**
   For health and welfare of preschool children, Family Planning is most important.
   Spacing of 3 years between 1st and 2nd child and permanent method after 2 children.

5. **Health Education**

   Health Education on Infant and Young Child Feeding (IYCF), keeping the child clean, immunization, environmental sanitation, safe water, home management of Diarrhea, Acute Respiratory Infections.

CONGENITAL MALFORMATION

Definition

Diseases which are determined before or during birth are known as Congenital Malformation.

Causes

1. Genetic Factors

   Chromosomal Abnormalities - Down's, Klinefelter's, Turner's Syndromes
   Inborn Errors of Metabolism - Phenylketonuria, Tay-Sachs Disease, Galactosemia
   Others - Huntington's Chorea, Thalassemia, Sickle Cell Disease, Hemophilia
   Conditions with possible Genetic Etiology - Congenital Dislocation of Hip, Neural Tube Defects, Club Foot

2. Environmental Factors

   Infections - TORCHES
   Drugs - Thalidomide, Stilboesterol, Anticonvulsants, Anaesthetic, Antithyroid Drugs, Alcohol
   Irradiation
   Maternal Diseases - Diabetes, Cardiac Failure
   Dietary Factors - Folic Acid Deficiency

Risk Factors

Maternal Age - > 30 years
Consanguinity - First cousin, uncle-niece marriages

Investigations

  i.   Alphafoetoprotein - Neural Tube Defects
 ii.   Ultrasound - Anencephaly
iii.   Amniocentesis – Down's Syndrome, Neural Tube Defects
 iv.   Chorionic Villi Sampling - Chromosomal Anomaly, Sex

Prevention

1. Discourage reproduction after birth of malformed baby.
2. Avoidance of pregnancy where malformations are likely eg. Advanced maternal age.

3. Identification and removal of Teratogens - Drugs (Thalidomide), Steroid Hormones, Folate Antagonists, Anticonvulsants, Infective Agents (TORCHES), Physical Agents (X-rays, Irradiation).
4. Avoidance of drugs in pregnancy except where absolutely necessary.

India MCH Goals and Current Level

INDICATOR	CURRENT Level	NHP 2017
Family Planning Indicators		
CBR	20.0	21
TFR	2.2	2.1
CPR	67.0	Meet all needs
Mortality Indicators/1000		
IMR	32	28
Neonatal Mortality Rate	23	16
U5MR	36	23
MMR	113	100
Services (% Coverage)		
Infants immunized for:		
BCG	92	
DPT3	89	
Polio3	89	
HepB3	89	
Hib3	89	
Measles2	80	
Rotavirus	35	
PCV3	6	
Pregnancy women TT	87	
ANC 4X	51.0	
Institutional delivery	79	
Delivery by trained personnel	81	
Low birth weight babies	28	

SCHOOL HEALTH PROGRAMME

Definition

Comprehensive care of health and well-being of children throughout their school years.

Objectives

1. Promotion of positive health
2. Prevention of diseases
3. Early diagnosis, treatment and follow-up of defects

4. Awakening of health consciousness in children
5. Provision of healthful environment

Aspects

i. Health appraisal of school children and school personnel
ii. Remedial measures and follow-up
iii. Prevention of Communicable Diseases
iv. Healthful school environment
v. Nutritional Services
vi. First Aid and Emergency Care
vii. Mental Health
viii. Dental Health
ix. Eye Health
x. Health Education
xi. Education of Handicapped Children
xii. School Health Records

i. Health Appraisal

Health appraisal of students, teachers and other school personnel is done annually.
Periodic Medical Examination of school children - History, Physical Examination, height, weight, vision, hearing, dental screening.
Medical Examination.
Daily morning inspection by teacher - Flushed face, fever, rash, coughing/sneezing, sore throat, red watery eyes, headache, Diarrhea, body pain, disinclination to play, listlessness or sleepiness, Pediculosis, Scabies, Ringworm, finger nails.
Referral to School Medical Officer if there are any symptoms or signs of illness

ii. Remedial Measures and Follow-up

After Medical Examination, treatment and follow-ups are important

iii. Prevention of Communicable Diseases

Immunization programme – DPT at school entry, TT at 10 years and 16 years.
Hepatitis injection, if not given earlier.

iv. Healthful School Environment

(a) Location - Centrally situated, away from busy places, cinema houses, factories, railway tracks, market places
(b) Site - Elevated ground
(c) Structure - Single storey, heat resistant walls
(d) Class Rooms - Verandahs, not > 40 students per classroom
(e) Furniture - Single desk and chair, minus type desk
(f) Doors and windows - Broad windows, combined door and windows area at least 25% of floor space, cross ventilation
(g) Colour - White inside the classrooms

(h) Lighting - Natural light

(i) Water supply - Safe and potable water

(j) Eating Facilities - Canteen and approved vendors

(k) Lavatory - 1 urinal per 60 students; 1 latrine per 100 students

v. **Nutritional Services**

Mid-day meals - Should provide one-third calories and half protein required by children.

Applied Nutrition Programme with assistance from UNICEF.

Specific Nutrients should be given if required.

vi. **First Aid and Emergency Care**

Teachers trained during Teachers Training Programmes to give first aid and emergency care in case of accidents and injury, Gastroenteritis, Colic, Fits, Fainting.

vii. **Mental Health**

School teacher has a positive and preventive role in Mental Health.

Relaxation should be planned for in the curriculum.

Psychologist and vocational counselors required in schools.

viii. **Dental Health**

Dental Caries and Periodontal Diseases are common.

Dentists and Dental Hygienists should attend to dental problems and teach Dental Hygiene.

ix. **Eye Health**

Screening and treatment of Refractive Error, Squint, Amblyopia, Eye Infections, Trachoma and Vit A Administration

x. **Health Education**

(a) Personal hygiene - Skin, hair, teeth, clothing

(b) Environmental Health

(c) Family life education

In Child-to-Child Programmes, the children who get educated, educate other children, their parents and community.

In high schools WHO's 10 life skills education includes:

1. Problem Solving
2. Decision Making
3. Creative Thinking
4. Critical Thinking
5. Communication Skills
6. Interpersonal Relationships
7. Self Awareness
8. Empathy
9. Dealing with Stress
10. Dealing with Emotions

Age-Appropriate Health Promotion

Primary School	Middle School	High School
Health, growth, development Personal hygiene Personal safety Nutrition, Exercise Prevention of diseases - Malaria, Dengue, TB, Diarrhoea, Worm Infestation	Pubertal changes Eye care Oral hygiene Nutrition, Exercise HIV/AIDS Prevention Yoga, Meditation Substance abuse prevention Mental health Bullying prevention Internet safety, Media Literacy	Sexual & reproductive health Substance abuse prevention Violence prevention Unintentional injury treatment Road safety Nutrition, Exercise Yoga, Meditation

xi. Education of Handicapped Children

Handicapped children should be educated to reach their maximum potential and be economically independent in later life.

INSPIRE:
The Seven Strategies for ending violence against children:

- **I** - Implementation and enforcement of laws
- **N** - Norms and values
- **S** - Safe environment
- **P** - Parent and care giver support
- **I** - Income and Economic strengthening
- **R** - Response and support services
- **E** - Education & Life Skills

xii. School Health Records
Cumulative Health Record of each student should be maintained.

School Health Administration

(a) Primary Health Centres
Medical Officer of Primary Health Centre is in charge of School Health Programmes in that area.

(b) School Health Committees
Recommended to form School Health Committees at village, block, district, state and national levels to help mobilize resources and make School Health Programmes self-supporting and sustainable.

JUVENILE DELINQUENCY

Definitions

Delinquent – A child who has committed an offence.

Juvenile – A boy/girl below 18 years of age

Causes

Biological Causes

Hereditary Defects, Chromosomal Anomaly (XYY), feeble mindedness, physical defects, Glandular Imbalance

Social Causes

Broken Homes - Death of parents, separation, step mother

Disturbed Conditions - Poverty, alcoholism, parental neglect, ignorance about childcare, too many children

Other Causes

Absence of recreational facilities, cheap recreation, sex thrillers, urbanization, industrialization, cinemas, television, slum dwelling

Features of Delinquent Behaviour

Juvenile crime, incorrigible, ungovernable, habitually disobedient, desert their homes and mix with immoral people, behaviour problems, antisocial practices

Preventive Measures

1. *Improvement of Family Life*
    Parents should be educated on Effective Parenting.
2. *Schooling*
    Healthy teacher-pupil relationship.
    Early diagnosis and psychotherapy for behaviour problems.
3. *Social Welfare Services*
    Parent counseling, child guidance, educational facilities, general health services, recreation facilities.

CHILD GUIDANCE CLINIC

Objective

To prevent children from becoming Neurotics and Psychotics in later life.

Criteria

Children with Juvenile Delinquency.

Children and adolescents who are not fully adjusted to their environment.

Team Work

Comprising Psychiatrists, Clinical Psychologists, Educational Psychologists, Psychiatrics, Social Workers, Public Health Nurses, Pediatricians, Neurologists, Speech Therapists, Occupational Therapists.

Services

Psychiatrists helped by others for correct diagnosis and treatment.
Pediatrician takes care of physical health.

Psychotherapy - To restore positive feelings of security.
Methods Used - Play therapy, counseling, easing parental tensions, reconstruction of parental attitudes, change in physical environment.

If sound foundations of Mental Health are laid in childhood and adolescence, the same will continue into adulthood.

CHILD PLACEMENT

1. *Orphanages*
   For children who have no home or could not be cared for by parents.
   However, mass care is undesirable because children lack warmth of family life to develop emotional security and participate in activities to enable them to become good citizens.

2. *Foster Homes*
   Rearing children in Foster Homes provides the child with security, love and affection.

3. *Adoption*
   Children are legally adopted.
   It confers upon the child and adoptive parents the rights and responsibilities similar to natural parents.

4. *Borstals*
   Boys over 16 years of age who are difficult to be handled by a Certified School or have misbehaved are sent to a Borstal. This institution falls in a category between a Certified School and an Adult Prison.

5. *Remand Homes*
   The child is placed under the care of Doctors, Psychiatrists and other trained personnel.
   Mental and physical well-being is improved.
   Elementary schooling, arts and crafts, games and other recreational activities are taken care of.

HANDICAPPED CHILDREN

Definition

Handicap - A disadvantage for an individual resulting from an impairment/disability that prevents the fulfillment of a role that is normal (Depending on age, sex, social and cultural practice) for that individual.

Impairment - Any loss or abnormality of psychological, physiological or anatomical structure or function.

Disability – A lack of ability to perform an activity in a manner/within the range considered normal for a human being.

Causes

Physically Handicapped	Mentally Handicapped	Socially Handicapped
Birth Defects: Hare Lip, Cleft Palate, Talipes, Cerebral Palsy, Congenital Heart Disease Infections: Polio Accidents: Burns, Injuries	Genetic Conditions: Chromosomal Abnormality, Down's Syndrome, Turner's Syndrome, Klinefelter's Syndrome, PKU, Tay-Sachs Disease, Galactosaemia, Microcephaly, Congenital Hypothyroidism Antenatal Factors: Neural Tube Defects, Rh Incompatibility, Infections (TORCHES), Drugs, Irradiation Perinatal Factors: Birth Injuries, Hypoxia, Cerebral Palsy Postnatal Factors Head Injuries, Accidents, Encephalitis, Physical and Chemical agents eg. Lead, Mercury Poisoning Miscellaneous: Maternal Malnutrition, PEM, IDD, Consanguineous Marriages, Pregnancy > 40 years	A Child whose opportunities for healthy personality development and full unfolding of potentialities is hampered by certain elements in the social environment eg. Parental Inadequacy, Environmental Deprivation, Emotional Disturbances eg. Orphans, Neglected and Destitute Children

Prevention

Primary Prevention	Secondary Prevention	Tertiary Prevention
i. Genetic Counselling: Avoid pregnancy > 30 years, Avoid consanguineous marriages	i. Early Diagnosis: Parents should bring child to pediatrician for evaluation	i. Disability Limitation
ii. At-Risk Approach: Identify people with Chromosomal and Sex-linked diseases and advise iii. Immunization: Polio, Rubella iv. Nutrition: Maternal Nutrition v. Others Health care during prenatal, natal and postnatal periods, avoidance of infections, drugs, X-rays	ii. Treatment: Physical medicine and Rehabilitation, Physiotherapy, Occupational Therapy, Speech Therapy, Music Therapy	ii. Rehabilitation: Medical, surgical, social, educational, vocational measures for training and re-training the individual to the highest possible level of functional ability

WHO ICF (International Classification of Functioning, Disability & Health)

Components of ICF

(a) Functioning & Disability
- Body Function and Structure - Anatomy, Physiology, Psychology of body
- Activity and Participation – Person's functional status, communication, mobility, interpersonal interactions, self-care, learning, applying knowledge

(b) Contextual Factors
- Environmental Factors
  Family, work, governmental agencies, laws, cultural beliefs
- Personal Factors
  Race, age, gender, educational level, coping styles

ADOLESCENT HEALTH PROBLEMS

Definition

Children within the ages of 10-19 years are known as Adolescents.

Problems

Communicable Diseases - STDs, HIV/AIDS
Others - Malaria, Dengue, TB, Diarrhoeal Diseases, Acute Respiratory Infections

Mental Diseases - Delinquency, Suicides, Depression, Anxiety
Substance Abuse - Drugs, Tobacco, Alcohol
Reproductive Health - Unwanted pregnancy, Abortion
Education - School or College drop-outs

Prevention

 i. ARSH Programme - Adolescent Reproductive & Sexual Health Programme
 ii. Life Skills education

CHAPTER 15

GERIATRICS

Definition

Geriatrics – The care of aged people.

Gerontology – The study of physical and psychological changes of old age.
In India 8% of the population is of people over 60 years of age.

Health Problems

1. Problems due to Aging
Eyes - Cataract, Glaucoma
Ear - Nerve Deafness
Failure of special senses
RS - Emphysema
Bones - Osteoporosis

2. Problems associated with Long Term Illness
CVS - Atherosclerosis of Heart and Blood Vessels (Multifactorial causes - Diet, physical inactivity, overweight, hereditary, stress) which leads to Coronary Heart Disease and Stroke

RS - Chronic Bronchitis, Asthma, Emphysema

Cancer
Females: Breast Cancer, Cervical Cancer
Males: Prostatic Cancer, Lung Cancer, Oropharyngeal Cancer especially among smokers

Accidents - Fracture neck of Femur, Colle's Fracture

Diseases of Locomotor System - Osteoarthritis, Rheumatoid Arthritis, Gout, Ankylosing Spondylitis, Fibrositis, Myositis, Neuritis

Endocrine System - Diabetes Mellitus, Hypothyroidism

Genitourinary System - Benign Prostatic Hypertrophy, Nocturia, Dysuria, Frequency and urgency of Micturition

3. *Psychological Problems*
   (a) *Mental Changes*
       Memory impaired, rigidity of outlook, dislike of change, irritability, decreased income, decreased standard of living

   (b) *Emotional Changes*
       Failure to accept aging leads to bitterness, inner withdrawal, depression, weariness of life, suicidal.

   (c) *Sexual Changes*
       At 40-50 years, cessation of reproduction in women and decreased sexual activity in men.

Prevention

Primary Prevention	Secondary Prevention	Tertiary Prevention
Healthy Habits:	Screening:	Rehabilitation:
No Smoking	Diabetes Mellitus	Physical Deficits
No Alcohol	Hypertension	Cognitive Deficits
Normal body weight	Coronary Heart Disease	Functional Deficits
Nutrition	Stroke	
Physical Activity	Breast Cancer	Caretaker Support
Sleep	Cervical Cancer	Introduction of Support
	Prostatic Cancer	Prevent loss of autonomy
CHD Risk Factors	Colorectal Cancer	
	Anemia	
Immunization	Urinary Incontinence	
Tetanus	Tuberculosis	
Pneumovax	Syphilis	
Influenza	Dental Caries	
Injury	Periodontal Diseases	
Osteoporosis	Medication side effects	
	Depression	
	Stress	

Social Welfare Measures
• National Assistance
• Pension Scheme
• Home Care Services
• Old Age Homes
• Counselling to Accept Old Age

Facilities for Elderly Citizens

- Travel Concession (Train, bus, air)
- Wheel chair facility at Railway Stations, Airports
- Battery operated car facility for disabled persons
- Lower berth reservation in Railways
- Income Tax Rebate
- Geriatric Clinics
- Medical Insurance Benefits at lower rates
- No waiting in bank, post office
- Meals on Wheels services
- Free facility for hearing aids
- Free facility for Presbyopic correction glasses

Chapter 16

COMMUNICABLE DISEASES

Smallpox

An acute infectious disease caused by Variola virus characterised by fever, headache, vomiting, sometimes convulsions and rash centrifugal distribution, passes through stages of macule, papule, vesicle, pustule, scab, scarring. Smallpox has been eradicated in 1980.

Smallpox Eradication Factors:

1. No animal reservoir
2. No carrier
3. Detection of cases is simple - characteristic rash on visible parts of body
4. Persons with subclinical infection do not transmit the disease
5. Lifelong immunity after recovery from the disease
6. Vaccine highly effective, easily administered, heat stable
7. International cooperation

Chickenpox

Magnitude of the Problem

World - 4.2 million severe complications
4,200 deaths
India - 66,963 cases
50 deaths (2018)

Clinical Features

(a) Pre-eruptive Stage
    Fever, shivering, malaise, back pain
    In children -1 day,
    In adults- 2-3 days

(b) Eruptive Stage

Differences between Smallpox and Chickenpox

	Smallpox	Chickenpox
Incubation	12 days	14 days
Prodromal Symptoms	Severe	Mild
Rash Distribution	Palms and soles, exterior surfaces and bony prominences (Axilla free)	Palms and soles seldom affected Axilla affected
Rash Characteristics	Deep seated Vesicles multi-locular, umbilicated, only one stage	Superficial Unilocular, dewdrop like Pleomorphic – different stages of rash at one time
Evolution of Rash	Slow, passes through stages of Macule, Papule, Vesicle, Pustule Scabs form 10-14 days after rash appears	Very rapid 4-7 days
Fever	Subsides with appearance of rash, may rise during Pustular stage	Temperature rises with each fresh crop of rash

Complications

Varicella Hemorrhagic, Pneumonia, Encephalitis, Acute Cerebellar Ataxia, Reye's Syndrome

Maternal Varicella causes Foetal wastage, birth defects eg. Cutaneous scars, atrophied limbs, microcephaly, low birth weight, varicella in newborn, oncogenicity

Laboratory Diagnosis

Vesicle fluid examination under electron microscope shows round particles (Brick shaped in Smallpox)

Scrapings of the floor of Vesicles show multi-loculated giant cells coloured by Giemsa Stain

Serology used in Epidemiological Surveys

Control

No specific treatment

Control measures - Notification, isolation for 6 days, disinfection of soiled articles from nose and throat discharges

Prevention

(a) VZIG: Varicella Zoster Immunoglobulin within 72 hours of exposure
Dose: 1.25 ml-5 ml IM

(b) Vaccine
Chickenpox vaccine 0.5 ml; one dose within 12 months -12 years
2 doses > 13 years 6-10 weeks apart

Measles (Rubeola)

Magnitude of the Problem

Global - 9.7 million >140, 000 deaths
India - 20,895 cases; 34 deaths (2018)

Definition

An acute, highly infectious disease of childhood caused by Myxovirus.

Epidemiology

Agent Factors

Agent - RNA Paramyxovirus

Source of Infection – Other cases of measles (Carriers not known)

Infective Material - Secretions from nose, throat, respiratory tract during Prodromal and early stages of the rash.

Communicability - Highly infectious during Prodromal and Eruption of rash (4 days before and 5 days after appearance of rash); Isolation of patient for 1 week from Eruption of rash.

Secondary Attack Rate - > 80% among susceptible household contacts

Host Factors

Age - Infancy, childhood

Sex - Equal

Immunity - Active immunity through measles infection, vaccination

- Passive immunity through maternal antibodies up to 9 months

Nutrition - Malnourished child, infection very severe, mortality high

Environmental Factors

Temperate Climate - In winters

India – During winters and early spring (Jan-Apr)

Overcrowding, poor ventilation, poor socio-economic status

Transmission - Droplet infection, droplet nuclei

Portal of entry - Respiratory Tract

Incubation Period - 14 days

Clinical Features

Fever, Upper respiratory infection (Coryza, cough), rash

1. Prodromal Stage - Fever, Coryza, sneezing, nasal discharge, cough, red eyes, lacrimation, photophobia.
2. Eruptive Stage - Koplik's Spots on Buccal Mucosa opposite 1st and 2nd upper molars, 1-2 days before rash.
    Rash Macular/Maculopapular, begins behind ears, then face, neck, down to lower extremities within 2-3 days, discrete or confluent, fades in the same order of appearance, leaves brownish discolouration
3. Postmeasles Stage - Malnutrition, growth retardation, chronic illness due to increased susceptibility to bacterial and viral infections, Diarrhea, Acute Respiratory Infections, Cancrum Oris, Pyogenic Infections, Candidosis, Reactivation of PTB

Complications:

Post measles diarrhea, Pneumonia, Otitis Media, SSPE (Subacute Sclerosing Panencephalitis)

Prevention of Measles

WHO Measles Elimination Strategy

Catch up – One-time nationwide vaccination campaign for children between 9months-14 years

Keep up - Routine services aimed at vaccinating > 95% of each successive birth cohort

Follow up - Subsequent nationwide vaccination campaign every 2-4 years for children

Measles Vaccine - Live attenuated vaccine, tissue culture vaccine (Chick embryo/Human diploid cell line), freeze dried, given at 9 months and one and half years, 0.5 ml SC.

Combined Vaccine - MMR Vaccine given at 15 months

Immunoglobulin
Immunoglobulin (Human) 0.25 ml/kg body weight given within 3-4 days of exposure
Live vaccine should be given 8-12 weeks later

Eradication of Measles

Measles can be eradicated because:

1. Good vaccine, heat stable
2. 2 Doses
3. Requires immunization coverage for 96% of children < 1 year
4. Cumulation in immunity gap should be prevented

Control Measures

1. Isolation for 7 days after onset of rash
2. Immunization of contacts within 2 days of exposure
3. Prompt immunization at the beginning of an epidemic
4. Surveillance

WHO Targets to be met by 2015 for Eradication

- Raise routine measles 1 coverage to > 90%, nationally
- Reduce annual measles incidence to < 5/million
- Reduce measles mortality by > 95% when compared with the year 2000

Rubella (German Measles)

Magnitude of the Problem
Globally - Yearly > 100,000 babies are affected with Congenital Rubella Syndrome

Definition
An acute childhood infection, mild, short duration (3 days), fever, Lymphadenopathy, Maculopapular Rash.
Infection in early pregnancy may result in serious congenital defects including death of Foetus.

Epidemiology
Agent Factors
Agent - RNA virus of Togavirus family

Source of Infection - Clinical or subclinical cases (No carrier state)

Period of Communicability - 1 week before symptoms to 1 week after rash appears

Host Factors

Age - Mainly childhood 3-10 years. Changing trend to ≥15 years after widespread immunization

Immunity – Life-long immunity after infection, infants of immune mothers protected upto 6 months, 40% of women of child bearing age are Rubella susceptible

Environmental Factors

Temperate countries – During winters and spring
Epidemics every 4-9 years

Transmission

Droplet infection, droplet nuclei
Crosses placental barrier (Vertical Transmission) and infects Foetus - Congenital Rubella Syndrome

Incubation Period

2 weeks

Clinical Features

Asymptomatic in majority (Subclinical) of cases

Case: (a) Prodromal - Coryza, sore throat, low grade fever
      (b) Lymphadenopathy - Postauricular, Posterior Cervical Lymphadenopathy
      (c) Rash - Face, trunk, extremities, minute, discrete, pinkish, macular rash (Not confluent), spreads rapidly, clears as rapidly within 3 days
      (d) Complications - Congenital Malformations

Congenital Rubella Syndrome - Infants born with defects secondary to intrauterine infection, implied by presence of IgM Rubella antibodies soon after birth or IgG antibodies persisting > 6 months.

- Rubella infection inhibits cell division, leading to congenital malformations and low birth weight, deafness, cataracts, cardiac malformations.
- Others eg. Glaucoma, Retinopathy, Microcephalus, Cerebral Palsy, IUGR, Hepatosplenomegaly, Mental Retardation and Motor Retardation.
- Infection during 1st trimester disastrous for Foetus. Serious infection may lead to spontaneous abortion, stillbirth or infant may develop a classical triad of Patent Ductus Arteriosus, cataract and deafness.
- Infection in 2nd trimester may cause deafness.
- Infection after 16 weeks causes no abnormalities.

Investigations

- HAI - Hemagglutination Inhibition Test - 2 samples taken wherein 1st is within 5 days of onset of illness, 2nd 2 weeks later
- ELISA Test
- Radioimmunoassay

Prevention

Single dose of Live attenuated vaccine, 0.5 ml SC
MMR combined vaccine given at 15 months

MUMPS

Magnitude of Problem

Annual incidence: 100-1000 cases/100,000 population
Peaks every 2-5 years

Definition

An acute infectious disease caused by Myxovirus with predilection for Glandular and Nervous tissues resulting in non-suppurative enlargement and tenderness of one or both Parotid Glands.

Epidemiology

Agent Factors

Agent - Myxovirus Parotiditis, RNA Virus

Source of Infection - Clinical and Subclinical cases

Period of Communicability - 1 week before symptoms to 1 week after

Secondary Attack Rate - 86%

Host Factors

Age - 5-15 years

Immunity - One attack clinical or subclinical induces lifelong immunity
Infants < 6 months are immune due to maternal antibodies

Environmental Factors

Cases occur throughout the year, peak in winters, spring

Overcrowding, poor ventilation

Mode of Transmission

Droplet infection

Incubation Period

2 weeks

Clinical Features

Subclinical in 30-40% of cases
Pain and swelling in one or both Parotid Glands

Others - Testes, Pancreas, CNS, Ovaries, Prostate may be affected
Fever, headache, constitutional symptoms 3-5 days in severe cases

Complications

- Orchitis, Oophoritis, Pancreatitis, Meningoencephalitis, Myocarditis
- Rarely Bilateral Orchitis leading to sterility
- Mumps leading to Diabetes has occurred in children

Prevention

(a) Vaccination - Live attenuated vaccine
    Combined vaccine - MMR 0.5 ml IM at 15 months of age

(b) Immunoglobulins
    Specific Immunoglobulin (Mig) is available

Control

- Isolation of cases
- Disinfection of articles used by patient
- Contacts kept under surveillance

INFLUENZA

Magnitude of Problem

Pandemic - Every 10-40 years
Epidemic of Influenza A - Every 2-3 years
                 Influenza B - Every 3-6 years
1918 - Spanish Influenza
1957 – Asian Influenza
1968 - Hong Kong Influenza
2009 - Swine Influenza
2012 - MERS
2019 – COVID-19

Definition

An Acute Respiratory Infection caused by Influenza virus Types A, B, C characterised by fever, chills, malaise, cough and muscular pains. Pandemics are caused by Type A. Epidemics all over world which last 6-8 weeks.

Epidemiology

Agent Factors

Agent - Orthomyxoviridae Type A, B, C.
Two distinct surface antigens - Haemagglutinin (H) and Neuraminidase (N)
H Antigen initiates infection, N Antigen responsible for release from infected cells

Antigenic Shift - Sudden complete or major change

Antigenic Drift - Antigenic change is gradual over a period of time

Reservoir of Infection - Animals and birds (Swine, horses, dogs, cats, poultry, wild birds)

Source of Infection - Case or subclinical cases

Period of Infectivity - 1-2 days before and 1-2 days after onset of symptoms

Host Factors

Age - All ages

Sex - Both sexes

Human Mobility - Important in spread of disease

Immunity - Subtype specific, Antibodies against HA and NA important in Immunity, no Cross Immunity

Environmental Factors

Season – During winter months in the Northern Hemisphere
During winters or rainy months in the Southern Hemisphere
India - In summers, overcrowding, poor ventilation

Mode of Transmission

Droplet infection/droplet nuclei from sneezing, coughing, talking

Portal of entry – Respiratory Tract

Incubation Period

18-72 hours

Clinical Features

Fever, chills, aches and pains, coughing, general weakness, secondary bacterial infection leading to Pneumonia

Investigations

1. Virus Isolation - Nasopharyngeal secretions by Indirect Fluorescent Antibody Technique and Egg Inoculation
2. Paired Sera - 2 Serum specimens one during acute phase and another 14 days later during convalescent stage - rising CF Antibodies

Prevention

(a) General - Good ventilation, avoidance of crowded places, hand washing, cough etiquette, masks
(b) Vaccines
   i. Killed Vaccines - Vaccine strains grown in Chick Embryo killed by formalin or betapropiolactone
      2 doses of 0.5 ml for adults
      > 3 years (0.25 ml within 6 months–3 years) at one month interval
   ii. Live attenuated vaccine - Administered as nose drops
   iii. Newer Vaccines - Split Virus Vaccine, Neuraminidase Specific Vaccine, Recombinant Vaccine
(c) Antiviral Drugs - Imantadine 100 mg BD for 3-5 days

Avian Influenza (H_5N_1)

Influenza virus which primarily affects birds, rarely affects pigs and humans

Swine Flu (H_1N_1)

Pandemic in 2009 which lasted 19 months

Definition

H_1N_1 Influenza virus can affect the Lower Respiratory Tract and cause rapidly progressive Pneumonia

Incubation Period

2-3 days upto 7 days

Suspected Case:

- Person with Acute Febrile Respiratory Illness (>38°C)
- Within 7 days of close contact with c/o Influenza A, or
- Within 7 days of travel to areas where there are ≥1 confirmed cases, or
- Resides in a community where there are ≥1 confirmed cases

Probable Case:

- Person with Acute Febrile Respiratory Illness
- Is positive for Influenza A but unsubtypable for H_1, H_3
- Is positive for Influenza A by Rapid Test/IFA & meets criteria for suspected case, or
- Individual with clinically compatible illness who died of an unexplained Acute Respiratory Illness epidemiologically linked to a probable/confirmed case

Confirmed Case:

- Person with Acute Febrile Respiratory Illness
- Laboratory confirmed Influenza A by ≥1 of the following tests - Real Time PCR, Viral Culture, 4-fold rise in H_1N_1 Antibodies

Transmission

Droplet infection

Clinical Features

- Uncomplicated Influenza
  - (a) Influenza like illness - Fever, cough, sore throat, Rhinorrhoea, headache, malaise, muscle pain
  - (b) GI illness - Diarrhea, vomiting

- Complicated/Severe Pneumonia
  Shortness of breath, Dysponea, Tachypnea, Hypoxia, &/or radiological signs of LRTI-Pneumonia; CNS-Encephalopathy, Encephalitis, Renal Failure, Multiorgan Failure, Septic Shock

Risk for Severe Disease

Infants, young children < 2 years
Pregnant women
Persons with COPD
Persons with Cardiac Disease
Persons with metabolic disorders (Diabetes Mellitus), Chronic Renal Disease, Chronic Hepatic Disease
Persons ≥ 65 years

Lab Diagnosis

RT-PCR
C/S

Control

Isolation - 7days + 24 hours after fever subsides
T Tamiflu (Oseltamivir) - 75mg/day X 10 days
Zanamivir for children

Vaccine - Inactivated vaccine, single dose, IM upper arm

COVID 19

COrona **VI**rus **D**isease-20**19**, caused by SARS-CoV-2
Started in Wuhan, China in Dec 2019
RNA virus with spike shaped protein, sensitive to UV rays, high temperature, lipid solvents eg. Ethanol, Chlorine
Led to Global Pandemic

Variants - Delta, Lambda, Omicron

Globally 11 crore cases; 24.5 lakh deaths (Feb 2021)
India - First case in Kerala, 30 Jan 2020
Maharashtra, Delhi, Kerala, Andhra Pradesh, Karnataka, Tamil Nadu worst hit states.

Mode of Transmission

Direct or indirect contact with infected persons
Droplet infection, airborne infection, fomite transmission

Period of Communicability

1-3 days before symptoms upto 1-2 weeks

Incubation Period

2-14 days

Clinical Spectrum

Asymptomatic to severe diseases

Acute Respiratory Infections (ARI)

Definition

Acute infection of the Respiratory Tract from nose to alveoli; Acute Upper Respiratory Infection (Common cold, Pharyngitis, Otitis Media) and Acute Lower Respiratory Tract Infection (Epiglottitis, Laryngitis, Laryngotracheitis, Bronchitis, Bronchiolitis, Pneumonia.

Pneumonia is a major cause of death.

Magnitude of the Problem

Global 0.2 million out of 5.83 million deaths in under-five year old children.
India – 6 Episodes/child/year which is a major cause of death.
Developing countries - Incidence of Pneumonia is 20-30%. About 5 episodes/child/year among < 5 years old children

Epidemiology

Agent Factors

Agent: Bacteria – Bordetella Pertusis, Corynebacterium Diphtheriae, Haemophilus Influenzae,
Klebsiella Pneumoniae, Legionella Pneumophilia, Staphylococcus Pyogenes, StreptococcusPenumoniae, Streptococcus Pyogenes
Virus – Adenovirus, Enteroviruses (ECHO, Coxackice), Influenza A, B, C, Parainfluenza, Measles, Respiratory Syncitial Virus, Rhinoviruses, Coronavirus
Others – Chlamydia, Coxiella Burnetti, Mycoplasma Pneumonia

Host Factors

Age – Usually infants & children or the elderly
Sex – M > F

Environmental Factors

- Climatic conditions
- Housing, overcrowding, poor ventilation, industrialization, indoor air pollution, smoking, low socio-economic status

Mode of Transmission

Airborne route – Droplet infection, droplet nuclei

Clinical features

History – Age, cough duration, whether child is able to drink, whether infant has stopped feeding well, antecedent illness (eg. Measles), fever, drowsy, convulsions, difficulty in breathing, blue, treatment history.

Physical Examination-

1. Count breaths in one minute – fast breathing
   If $\geq$ 60/min in child < 2 months
   $\geq$ 50/min   2 months – 12 months
   $\geq$ 40/min   12 months – 5 years
2. Look for chest indrawing
3. Look & listen for Stridor
4. Look for Wheezing
5. See if child is abnormally sleepy
6. Feel for fever or low body temperature
7. Check for severe malnutrition
8. Check for Cyanosis

Classification of Illness, treatment, home care and prevention – Refer ARI Control Programme.

Severe Acute Respiratory Syndrome (SARS)

Definition

A Viral disease caused by the Coronavirus.
Death in 10% of cases.

Magnitude of Problem

First case detected in 2002, a health worker in China. Spread to Hong Kong, Singapore, Vietnam, Taiwan, Toronto.

Incubation period

2 – 7 days

Mode of Transmission

Droplets or fomites

Epidemiology

Age – Mostly adults

Risk Groups – Health care workers exposed to severally ill patients.

Exit screening of passengers from International flights recommended by WHO.

Clinical Features

1. ***Suspect Case*** – High fever (>38^{0}C) and cough or breathing difficulty & close contact of suspect with probable case of SARS

H/o travel to SARS affected area

Residing in affected area

Person with unexplained Acute Respiratory Illness (ARS) resulting in death after 1st Nov 2002, but on whom no autopsy has been performed & one/more of following has been observed:

- Close contact with suspect/probable case of SARS
- History of travel to affected areas/Residing in affected area

2. ***Probable Case***
- Suspect case with radiographic evidence of infiltrates consistent with Pneumonia/ Respiratory Distress Syndrome.
- Suspect case with autopsy finding consistent with Respiratory Distress Syndrome

Exclusion Criteria

If there is an alternative diagnosis

Complications

Pulmonary Decompensation, ARDS, Nosocomial Infections, Tension Pneumothorax, Pulmonary Oedema

Treatment

- Ventilatory Support
- Ribavirin/Lopinavir/Ritonavir/Interferon
- IV Immunoglobulin
- Corticosteroids

Prevention

1. Surveillance & prompt identification of persons with SARS
2. Isolation
3. Protection of medical staff treating patients
4. Identification & Isolation of suspected cases
5. Exit screening of international travelers
6. Timely & accurate reporting & sharing information with authorities and Governments

Diphtheria

Definition

An acute infectious disease caused by Corynebacterium Diptheriae resulting in Anterior Nasal, Faucial, Laryngeal Diphtheria; skin, conjunctive, vulva may be affected.

Bacilli multiply locally in the throat, release powerful toxins which cause greyish membrane over tonsils, Pharynx or Larynx which cannot be wiped away; marked congestion, oedema or local tissue destruction.

Cervical Lymphadenopathy and neck may be swollen (Bull neck); signs and symptoms of Toxaemia (fever, headache, malaise, tiredness, prostration).

Fatality 10% in untreated and 5% in treated cases.

Magnitude of Problem

Developed countries - Rare
India - Endemic disease, declining trend. Incidence 4090 cases, 64 deaths (2013)

Agent factors

Agent – Corynebacterium Diphtheriae, Gram Positive non-motile organism.
It is of 3 types – Gravis, Mitis, Intermedius; Produces powerful Exotoxin.

Source of Infection

i. Case – Subclinical and clinical cases
ii. Carriers important in transmission
   Temporary or chronic carriers, nasal or throat carriers

Infective Material

Nasopharyngeal Secretions, discharge from skin lesions, contaminated fomites, possibly infected dust.

Period of Infectivity

- Unless treated, infective for 2–4 weeks from onset of disease
- Carriers infective for longer periods
- Case or carrier non-communicable when at least 2 cultures from nose and throat 24 hours apart are negative for Diphtheria Bacilli.

Host Factors

Age - 1-5 years; shift in age to school age in countries with widespread immunization.
Sex – Both equal

Immunity

Maternal Antibodies in first few months of life
Large proportion acquires Active Immunity through Inapparent Infection

Environmental Factors

All seasons
Increased during winters
Over-crowding, poor ventilation, poor socio-economic status

Mode of Transmission

- Droplet infection
- Fomites (cups, thermometers, toys, pencils) contaminated by Nasopharyngeal Secretions of the patient
- Direct transmission to susceptible host from Infected Cutaneous Lesions.

Portal of Entry

  i. Respiratory route – most common
 ii. Non-respiratory routes – Skin where cuts, wounds, ulcers may get infected with Diphtheria Bacilli; Umbilicus in newborn; eye; middle ear; genitalia

Incubation Period

2–6 days

Clinical Features

Respiratory Tract Forms

i.   Pharyngotonsillar Diphtheria

Sore throat, difficulty swallowing, fever. Throat – Erythema and grey membrane which may bleed if you try to remove it.

Oedema Submandibular area and Cervical Lymphadenopathy giving appearance of Bull Neck.

ii. Laryngotracheal

Hoarseness and croupy cough may extend into Bronchial Tree leading to severe disease

iii. Nasal Diphtheria

Mildest form, localized to Septum or Turbinates of one side of the nose, membrane may extend into Pharynx

Non-respiratory mucosal surface - Conjunctiva, genitals

iv. Cutaneous Diphtheria – Secondary infection of previous skin abrasion or infection Ulcer surrounded by Erythema and covered with membrane

Schick Test

Intradermal test for:

i.   Presence of Antitoxin therefore, Immunity Status, and

ii. Hypersensitivity to Diphtheria Toxin or other proteins of Diphtheria Cells

Method

0.2 ml (1/50 MLD) of Schick Test Toxin ID into forearm while into opposite arm the same toxin inactivated by heat (control)

Negative Reaction	Positive Reaction	Pseudo-positive Reaction	Combined Reaction
No reaction if patient is immune	Test arm: Circumscribed red flush 10-50 mm diameter in 24-36 hours maximum by 4-7th day, Slowly fades into brown patch & skin desquamates Control arm - No change Interpretation: Person susceptible to Diphtheria	Red flush equally in both arms, Less circumscribed than true positive, Fades quickly and disappears by 4th day Allergic reaction test - Negative	Test arm true positive, Control arm - Pseudo-positive Susceptible to Diphtheria Allergic to toxin, should be vaccinated with caution Doses of vaccine greatly reduced & no. of injections increased

Schick Test largely replaced by measurement of Serum Antitoxin Level by Haemagglutination Test.

Control of Diphtheria

1. *Cases & Carriers*

    Early detection – Active search for cases & carriers among family & school contacts; Swabs from nose, throat cultured

    Isolation - Cases, suspected cases, carriers isolated in hospital for 14 days. Discharged only after 2 consecutive nose, throat swabs taken 24 hours apart are negative.

    Treatment

    Cases – Diphtheria Antitoxin 10,000-80,000 IM/IV after test dose 0.2ml SC to detect Sensitisation to Horse Serum, Penicillin (2.5L every 6 hours) or Erythromycin (250 mg every 6 hours) for 6 days

    Carriers – Erythromycin orally for 10 days

    Immunity status upgraded

2. *Contacts*

    Throat swabbed & immunity status determined.

Primary Immunization or booster within previous 2 years	Primary Immunization or booster > 2 years before	Non immunized
No action	One booster Diphtheria Toxoid given	Prophylactic Penicillin/ Erythromycin Diphtheria Antitoxin 1000-2000 units Diphtheria Toxoid - Active Immunization

Surveillance of contacts

  i. Clinically, daily for 1 week
 ii. Bacteriologically, weekly for several weeks.

3. *Community*

    Pentavalent Vaccine – 6weeks, 10weeks, 14weeks

    DPT - 1½ years, 5 years 0.5ml deep IM

Whooping Cough (Pertussis)

Definition

An acute infectious disease of young children caused by B Pertussis resulting in fever, irritating cough with Whoop (loud crowing inspiration) called "Hundred Day Cough" by Chinese.

Magnitude of Problem

World - A significant cause of death in infants
India - Decline in disease; 18,006 cases; 8 deaths (2018)

Epidemiology

Agent factors

Agent – B. Pertussis (in <5% B Parapertussis)

Source of Infection – Case (Mild, missed, unrecognized cases usually)

Infective Material – Nasopharyngeal & Bronchial secretions; contaminated objects

Infective Period – A week after exposure to 3 weeks after onset of Paroxysmal Stage

Secondary Attack Rate – 90%

Host Factors

Age – Infants & Pre-school children

Sex – F > M

Immunity – Through Infection and Immunization

Environmental Factors

Throughout year but more during winters & spring
Overcrowding, poor ventilation, low socio-economic status

Mode of Transmission

Droplet infection
Direct contact
Freshly contaminated fomites

Incubation Period

7 – 14 days

Clinical Course

3 stages – i. Catarrhal stage lasting 10 days
ii. Paroxysmal stage 2-4 weeks
iii. Convalescent stage 1-2 weeks

Illness lasts 6 – 8 weeks

Complications

Bronchitis, Bronchopneumonia, Bronchiectasis, Paroxysms may precipitate Subconjunctival Hemorrhages, Epistaxis, Hemoptysis, Punctate Cerebral Hemorrhages leading to convulsions or coma

Control

1. ***Cases & Contacts***
   Cases – Early diagnosis, isolation, treatment, disinfection of nasal & throat discharges. Early diagnosis by Bacteriological Examination of nose & throat secretions by Naso-Pharyngeal swabs using Fluorescent Antibody technique
   Isolation till non-infectious

   Treatment with Erythromycin 30-50 mg/kg body weight in 4 divided doses for 10 days.

   Others – Ampicillin, Septran, Tetracycline (Antibiotics control secondary bacterial infections, do not reduce frequency, severity of spasms)

   Contacts Prophylactic Antibiotic (Erythromycin or Ampicillin) for 10 days.

2. ***Active Immunization***
   DPT 3 doses 0.5ml deep IM at 6weeks, 10weeks, 14weeks, 1½ years, 5years

Meningococcal Meningitis

Definition

Cerebrospinal Fever, acute communicable disease caused by N Meningitidis characterised by headache, vomiting, stiff neck progressing to coma.

Magnitude of Problem in the World

Outbreaks in Africa, Asia, America, Europe

Magnitude of Problem in India

Endemic in BIMARU states
3300 cases, 152 deaths (2018)

Epidemiology

Agent Factors

Agent – N Meningitidis, Gram –ve Diplococci
Source of infection – Carriers & Cases
Period of Communicability – Until nose & throat discharges do not contain Meningococci
Cases rapidly lose infectiousness within 24-hours of treatment

Host Factors

Age – Children & young adults
Sex – Both
Immunity – By subclinical infection, clinical infection
Vaccination
Infants receive passive immunity from mother

Environmental Factors

Cold months of the year
Overcrowding, poor ventilation, low socio-economic status, poor housing conditions

Mode of Transmission

Droplet infection

Portal of Entry

Nasopharynx

Incubation period

3 – 4 days

Prevention & Control

Cases – Antibiotics – Penicillin or Chloramphenicol, Ampicillin, Ceftriaxone

Carriers – Rifampicin to eradicate carrier state

Contacts – Chemoprophylaxis
Rifampicin 600 mg BD x 2 days, or
Sulfadiazine 1g BD x 2 days (if sensitive)

Mass Chemoprophylaxis – Rifampicin to total population in closed & medically supervised communities

Other drugs – Ciprofloxacin, Minocycline, Spiramycin, Ceftriaxone

Immunization – Vaccines from Gp A, C, Y or W135
Immunity for 3-years, booster every 3 years
High risk population identified & vaccinated

Environmental Measures:
Prevention of overcrowding
Improved housing

(Carriers seen in Meningitis, Diphtheria, Typhoid, Salmonellosis, Amoebiasis, Hepatitis B, AIDS, Gonorrhoea)

Tuberculosis

Definition

An Infectious disease caused by M Tuberculosis. Primarily, it affects the lungs causing Pulmonary TB. It may also affect the Intestines, Meninges, Bones & Joints, Lymph Glands, Skin & other tissues.

Magnitude of the Problem

World:

It is a public health problem
Annual risk of TB infection is 0.5-2%
One PTB patient can infect 10-15 persons per year
TB is one of the top 10 causes of death

India:

25% of world's TB is in India.
Incidence Rate is 167/100,000 population/year
Prevalence Rate of all forms of TB is 195/100,000 population/year
TB Death Rate is 17/100,000 population/year
MDR TB among new TB cases is 2.2%%
Problem of TB is likely to become aggravated because of AIDS

Diagnosis

Bacteriologically confirmed TB case - One from whom a biological specimen is positive by Smear Microscopy/culture/Xpert MTB or RIF.

Clinically diagnosed TB case - One who does not fulfil bacteriological confirmation but diagnosed with active TB by clinician/medical practitioner and decided to give full course of TB treatment.

Epidemiological Indices

1. Incidence of infection (Annual Infection Rate)
   Number of new TB cases and recurrent cases in a year.
2. Prevalence of Infection
   Number of TB cases at a given point in time.
3. Mortality from TB
   Number of deaths caused by TB in HIV negative people.
4. Case Fatality Rate
   Number of deaths due to TB/Number of cases.
5. Case Notification Rate
   Number of new and recurrent TB cases notified to WHO for a given year per 100,000 population
6. Case Detection Rate
   Number of notifications of new and recurrent cases in a year divided by the estimated incidence of such cases in the year
7. Prevalence of Drug Resistant Cases
   Prevalence of patients excreting TB Bacilli resistant to Anti-TB drugs

Classification of TB

Based on Anatomical Site	Based on Previous TB Treatment	Based on Drug Resistance	Based on HIV Status
PTB Extra PTB	New patients Previously treated patients: i. Relapse patients ii. Treatment after failure iii. Treatment after loss to follow up iv. Other previously treated patients v. Patients with unknown previous treatment history	i. Monoresistance ii. Polydrug resistance iii. Multidrug resistance iv. Extensive drug resistance v. Rifampicin resistance	i. HIV Positive TB ii. HIV Negative TB iii. HIV status unknown TB

Treatment Outcomes for TB Patients

Outcome	Definition
Cured	PTB patient with Bacteriologically confirmed TB at the beginning of treatment who was smear/culture negative in the last month of treatment and on at least one previous occasion
Treatment completed	TB patient who completed treatment without evidence of failure but with no record to show Sputum Smear/Culture results in last month of treatment and on one previous occasion were negative
Treatment failed	TB patient whose Sputum Smear/Culture is positive at $\geq$5months during treatment
Died	TB patient who dies before/during treatment
Lost to follow-up	TB patient who did not start treatment or treatment interrupted for $\geq$2mths
Treatment success	Sum of cured and treatment completed

Epidemiology

Agent Factors

Agent - M Tuberculosis – Facultative Intracellular Parasite

Human strain – Responsible for majority of cases
It is readily killed by sunlight, 2% Lysol, 25% Phenol for 1 hour. In dried Sputum it survives several days.

Bovine strain – In cattle (Killed by boiling milk)

Atypical Mycobacteriae –

   i.   Photochromogens
  ii.   Scotochromogens
 iii.   Non-photochromogens
  iv.   Rapid growers

Source of Infection

Human Source – Open cases of Pulmonary Tuberculosis

Bovine Source – Infected milk

Communicability

Patients are infective as long as they remain untreated.
Effective treatment reduces infectivity by 90% within 48 hours.

Host Factors

Age – All ages.
Increased from 1% in under 5 age group to 30% at 15 years.
Elderly also affected.

Sex – M > F

Heredity – Not a hereditary disease but susceptibility to the disease is hereditary.

Risk Factors

Smoking, Alcoholism, Diabetes, Malnutrition, AIDS, Fatigue, Mental Exertion

Immunity

Gained through natural infection, BCG Vaccination, Atypical Mycobacteria

Environmental Factors & Social Factors

- Poor housing (Small, ill ventilated), large families, overcrowding, poverty, illiteracy
- With improvement of living standards in developed countries, disease rate came down long before Antituberculosis drugs were discovered.
- Following customs help to spread TB – Indiscriminate spitting; open mouthed coughing, sneezing; smoking from common pipe

Clinical Features

Presumptive Pulmonary TB

 i. Cough > 2 weeks
 ii. Fever > 2 weeks
 iii. Significant weight loss
 iv. Haemoptysis and any abnormality in CXR

Investigations

Sputum Smear – 2 times
First is Spot Sputum when patient comes to the TB Centre, he is given a sputum container & asked to collect the next morning sputum & bring it to the centre; This is the second specimen.

Spot sputum is obtained by asking patient to stand, place his hands on his hips, take a deep breath, cough forcibly. He is then asked to collect the sputum in his mouth & spit it out gently into a waxed paper cup.

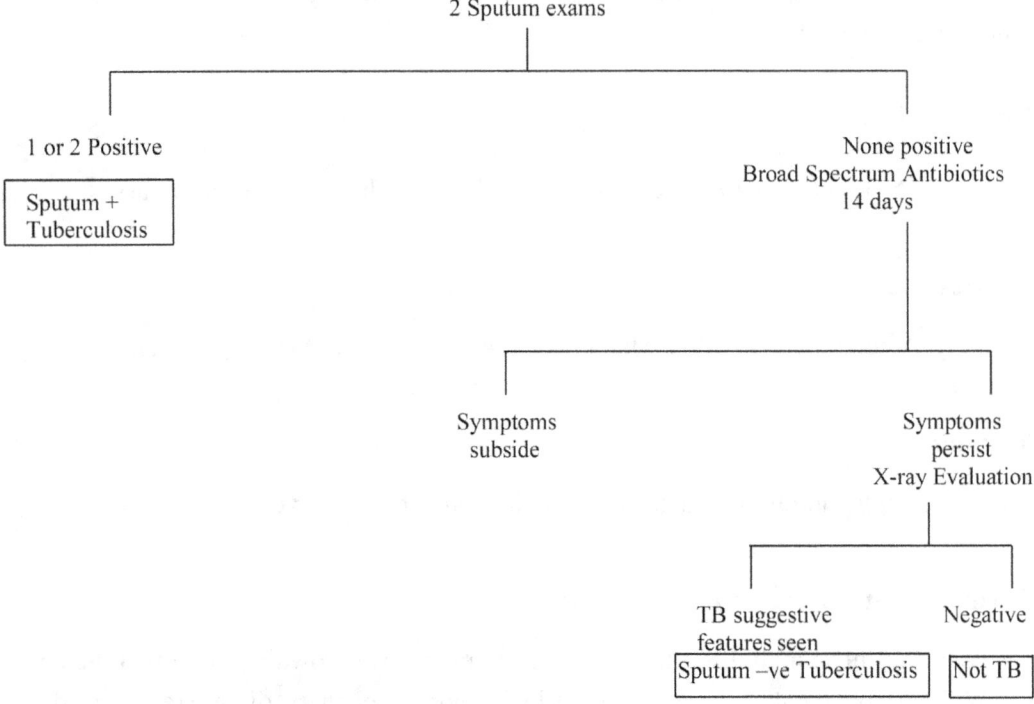

Ziehl Neelsen Staining

- Smear is stained with Z-N Staining.
- Carbol Fuchsin poured on slide & heated intermittently for 5 minutes to keep the dye steaming.
- Slide is washed with water.
- Slide covered with 20% Sulphuric Acid for 1-min and washed with water. This is repeated till the smear has faint pink colour.
- Slide is washed & placed in 95% Alcohol for 2-mins.
- Slide is washed and counter stained with Methylene Blue.
- The slide is washed & air dried.
- The stained slide is examined under oil immersion microscope.
- Slender rods against a blue background are AFBs.

Diagnosis of Infection

By Tuberculin Test or Mantoux Test.
Carried out by injecting intradermally on the surface of forearm 1TU of PPD 0.1 ml
(WHO advocates PPD-RT-23 with Tween 80)
Result of the test is read after 72 hours (3rd day)

Tuberculin reaction consists of Erythema & Induration:

Positive> 10 mm diameter

Doubtful 6 – 9 mm

Negative < 6 mm

Positive Tuberculin test means:

i. Person is infected with M Tuberculosis (does not mean he is suffering from the disease)

ii. Person has been successfully Immunized with BCG

iii. Person has been infected with one of Atypical Mycobacteria Photochromogens, Scotochromogens, Non-Photochromogens, Rapid Growers.

Primary Prevention

- BCG Vaccination
- Dust suppression and control measures in industries where there is risk of Silicosis
- Improve standards of living
- Improve literacy
- Health Education on:

   (a) TB not a hereditary disease

   (b) It is caused by germ that spreads through prolonged close contact

   (c) It is a curable disease but patient has to take continuous treatment for 6–9 months

   (d) Cardinal symptoms - Cough with expectoration, fever > 2weeks

   (e) One should cover one's mouth & nose while coughing or sneezing & not indiscriminately spit everywhere

   (f) AIDS predisposes to TB therefore avoid indiscriminate sex; use condoms in case of unprotected sex

Secondary Prevention

A. *Early Detection*

   (a) *Contact tracing & surveillance*

   Contacts of known case of TB - Family, school, occupation and neighbourhood are subjected to

   Clinical & Sputum Examination.

   (b) *Sputum Examination*

   Sputum of patients attending PHC or other health facility with cough > 2weeks examined for AFB.

   (c) *Symptomatic Surveys*

   Health workers identify individuals with cough, fever, chest pain, unexplained weight loss, obtain their sputum & send it to PHC for sputum microscopy.

   (d) *Special Surveys*

   Conducted on high-risk individuals eg. Hospital inpatients, nurses, slum dwellers, bus conductors; migrant labourers, school teachers, workers in dusty industries

Management

Treatment Regimen – Drug Sensitive TB

Type of TB	Intensive Phase	Continuation Phase
New Cat I	2HRZE	4HRE
Previously Treated Cat II	2HRZES+1HRZE	5HRE

FDC Dosage for Adult TB

Weight Category (kg)	No. of Tabs (FDCs mg) IP HRZE 75/150/400/275	CP HRE 75/150/275	Inj SM g
25-39	2	2	0.5
40-54	3	3	0.75
55-69	4	4	1
≥70	5	5	1

MDR/RR-TB (Cat IV)

IP (6-9 mths)	CP (18 mths)
Z Eto E Cs Lfx Km (PEECOK)	Eto E Cs Lfx (EECO)

XDR-TB

IP (6-12 mths)	CP(18 mths)
Cm, PAS, Mfx, High dose INH, Cfz, Lzd, Amx/Clv	PAS, Mfx, High dose INH, Cfz, Lzd, Amx/Clv

Pediatric PTB

Presumptive Pediatric TB

Persistent fever, cough >2weeks, loss of weight or no weight gain, H/O contact with infectious TB cases.

FDC Dosage for Pediatric TB

Wt. Category (kg)	IP HRZ 50/75/150	E 100	CP HRE 50/75/150	Inj. SM (mg)
4-7	1	1	1	100
8-11	2	2	2	150
12-15	3	3	3	200
16-24	4	4	4	300
25-29	3+1A	3	3+1A	400
30-39	2+2A	2	2+1A	500

Sputum collection, disinfection & disposal

Sputum is collected in paper cups, rags or coconut shells, mixed with saw dust & burnt or collected in old tins & put boiling water over it or use Spittoons filled with 2% Lysol or 25% Phenol, later buried in soil.

Health Education – Patients educated to cover nose & mouth during coughing & sneezing (Cough etiquette);
Not spit everywhere indiscriminately.

Attendants of open cases advised to wear masks while tending the patient.
Highly susceptible contacts are not allowed to go into the room where patient is or sent to a relative's place.

Bedaquiline Conditional Access Programme

Class of Drug - Diarylquinoline
Criteria - Adults >18years with MDR TB
Females should not be pregnant or using birth control methods
INH Preventive Therapy

For all HIV infected children
All TST positive children receiving Immunosuppression Therapy
Child born to mother with TB in pregnancy

Adults and adolescents – INH 300mg + Pyridoxine 50mg/day for 6-months
End TB Strategy (2015)

Vision   World free of TB: zero deaths, disease and suffering due to TB

Goal   End Global TB Epidemic

Indicators	Milestones		Targets	
	2020	2025	SDGs 2030	End TB 2025
Reduction in No. of TB deaths compared with 2015 (%)	25	75	90	95
Reduction in TB incidence rate compared with 2015 (%)	20	50	80	90 <10/100,000
TB affected families facing catastrophic costs due to TB (%)	zero	zero	zero	zero

Dracunculiasis

Definition

Guinea Worm Disease caused by Dracunculus Medinensis & transmitted by Vector Cyclops.

Epidemiology

Agent Factors

Agent – Dracunculus Medinensis
Reservoir – Infected person harbouring Gravid female

Host Factors

Susceptibility universal
Multiple, repeated infections may occur
Human Habit – Washing, bathing in surface water using Step Wells

Environmental Factors

Season – Dry season – March to May;
Contact between Guinea Worm cases & drinking water is greatest in places with Step Wells.
June – September in places where ponds are used.
Temperature – 25-30^0 C when Larvae develop the best (Tropical, Subtropical regions)

Mode of Transmission

Water Based Disease – Through Cyclops with infective stages of Guinea Worm

Eradication

Strategies:

   i.   Provision of safe drinking water (Piped water, hand pumps)
   ii. Control of Cyclops – Physical method (Straining, boiling)
        Chemical method (Chlorine, Lime, Abate)
        Biological method (Barbel fish, Gambusia fish)
   iii. Health Education - Eg. Boiling, sieving drinking water; preventing water contamination by infected people
   iv. Surveillance – Active search for new cases
   v.   Treatment of Cases – Niridazole, Mebendazole, Metronidazole

Food Poisoning

Definition

Acute Gastroenteritis caused by Bacteria, Toxins, Chemical Substances

Characterised by:
  i.   H/o Ingestion of common food
  ii. Many people affected at the same time
  iii. Same signs & symptoms

Salmonella	Staphylococcal	Botulism	Cl Perfringens	B Cereus
Common Agent – S Typhimurium, S Cholera Suis, S Enteritidis	Common Enterotoxins of Staphylococcus Aureus heat stable, resist boiling ≥ 30 mins	Botulus Sausage, rare, most serious, kills ⅔ of cases Exotoxin of Cl Botulinum Type A, B, E	Cl Perfringens (Welchii)	Bacillus Cereus Aerobic, Spore bearing, motile, gm +ve rod
Source: Farm animals, poultry through contaminated meat, millet, milk products, sausages, custards, eggs & egg products; rats & mice contaminate foodstuff by their urine, faeces	Ubiquitous in nature present on skin, nose, throat of men, animals, cows with mastitis, salads, custards, milk & milk products contaminated by Staphylococci	Soil, dust, animal's intestinal tract, enters food as spores present in home preserved foods – home canned vegetables, smoked or pickled fish, home-made cheese, low acid foods	Faeces of humans, animals Soil, water, air Foods - Meat, meat dishes, poultry food cooked ≥ 24hours before eating, cooled slowly at room temperature, reheated prior to eating.	Soil, raw, dried & processed foods, Spores can survive cooking & germinate in favourable temperature
Incubation period 12 – 24 hours	1 – 6 hours	12 - 36 hours	6 – 24 hours	1 – 6 hours Emetic type 12 – 24 hours Diarrhea type

Salmonella	Staphylococcal	Botulism	Cl Perfringens	B Cereus
Mechanism of Food poisoning: Organisms multiply in intestines leading to Enteritis & Colitis	Toxins preformed in food where Bacteria have grown	Toxin preformed in Anaerobic Conds, affects Parasympathetic Nervous System	Spores survive cooking, if cooked meat & poultry not cooled enough spores will germinate. Organisms multiply 30 – 50^{0}C produce toxins Alpha, Thetatoxin	2 Enterotoxins Emetic form Diarrhoeal form
Cl Features: Fever, chills, nausea, vomiting, diarrhea, convalescent carriers last several weeks	Vomiting, cramps, diarrhea, blood & mucus, Toxins affect Intestine & CNS	GI symptoms: Slight Dysphagia, Diplopia, Ptosis, Dysarthria, Blurring of Vision, muscle weakness, Quadriplegia, Fever absent, consciousness retained. Fatal – due to Respiratory or Cardiac failure. Toxin Thermolabile therefore heating food to 100° C for few mins makes food safe. Rx Antitoxin – 50,000–100,000 units IV Guanidine Hydro Chloride 15–40mg/kg orally. Medical & Nursing Care	Diarrhea, Abdominal cramps 8–24 hours after consumption of food. Fever, nausea, vomiting rare, illness short (24 hours), recovery rapid, no deaths. Prevention – cooking food just prior to consumption or if it is to be stored rapid, adequate cooling.	Emetic type – Upper GI Symptoms Diarrhea type – Lower GI Symptoms, abdominal pain, Diarrhea Toxins preformed Rx Symptomatic

Investigations

(a) Secure complete list of people & history

Questionnaire – Foods eaten, place of consumption, time of onset of symptoms, symptoms of illness (Abdominal pain, nausea, vomiting, Diarrhoea, fever, headache, prostration)

General Information: Name, age, sex, address, occupation

(b) Laboratory Investigations

Stool ⎤
Vomit ⎬ Culture and Sensitivity
Food ⎦

Stool samples of kitchen employees, food handlers to be tested.
Samples examined Aerobically, Anaerobically & Phage Typing.

(c) Animal Experiments

Food given to Rhesus monkeys
Mice injected with saline filtrate of foodstuff in Botulism

(d) Blood for Antibodies – Useful for Retrospective Diagnosis

(e) Environmental Study – Inspection of eating places, kitchen, questioning food handlers.

(f) Data Analysis – According to time, place, person distribution; food specific attack rates. Case control study can be done to find out association of illness with food.

Prevention & Control

(a) Food Sanitation

i. Meat Inspection – Examined by veterinary staff before & after slaughter.
ii. Personal Hygiene – Important among individuals in handling, preparing & cooling of food
iii. Food Handlers – Those with infected wounds, boils, diarrhoea, dysentery, throat infection should be excluded from handling food
iv. Food Handling Techniques - Bare hands should not be used for handling cooked food. Food must be thoroughly cooked. Cold storage preserves food. Pasteurisation of milk and milk products.
v. Sanitary Improvement – Sanitisation of work places, utensils, equipment. Food premises to be kept free from rats, mice, flies, dust.
vi. Health Education – For food handlers on clean habits, personal hygiene

(b) Refrigeration

Food to be kept in cold storage if not eaten immediately. Golden rule "cook & eat the same day".

(c) Surveillance

Food samples obtained from food establishments periodically, subjected to laboratory analysis.

Amoebiasis

A disease caused by the Entamoeba Histolytica, an Anaerobic Parasitic Amoebozoan.

Epidemiology

Agent Factors

Agent – E Histolytica

Trophozoites short lived outside human body, not important in disease transmission.
Cysts are infective to man, survive several days in faeces, sewage, water, soil; not affected by chlorine in usual dose; readily killed if dried, heated (55^0C) or frozen.

Reservoir
Man – Cases & carriers especially food handlers.

Source
Faeces containing cysts.

Period of Communicability
May be years, as long as cysts are excreted.

Host Factors

Age – All
Sex – Equal
Immunity – Cell medicated immunity prevents Invasive Amoebiasis

Environmental Factors

Rainy season
Poor sanitation, use of night soil in agriculture
Poor socio-economic status
Lack of safe water
Sewage seepage into water supply

Mode of Transmission

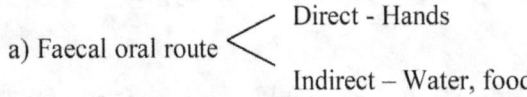

a) Faecal oral route
Direct - Hands
Indirect – Water, food

b)   Sexual Transmission – Oral Rectal contact among male homosexuals

c)   Vectors – Flies, cockroaches, rodents contaminate food & drink

Incubation Period

2 – 4 weeks

Clinical features
- Intestinal Amoebiasis – Abdominal discomfort, Diarrhoea, Dysentery
- Extra Intestinal Amoebiasis – Liver (Liver Abscess), lungs, brain, spleen, skin

Prevention & Control

1.   *Primary Prevention*
   (a)   Sanitation – Safe disposal of excreta
   (b)   Water supply – Water filtration, boiling kill cysts
   (c)   Hand Washing – After defaecation, after cleaning a child who has defaecated, before preparing food, before eating, before feeding a child.
   (d)   Food Hygiene – Fruits, vegetables thoroughly washed with detergents in running water. Uncooked fruits, vegetables disinfected with Acetic Acid (5%-10%) or Vinegar.
   Food handlers to be examined periodically, treated & educated on food hygiene practices eg. Hand washing.
   (e)   Health Education – Of the public.

2.   *Secondary Prevention*
   (a)   Early Diagnosis
   Clinical features & Investigations:
   Stool Microscopy for Trophozoites containing red cells
   Serological Test – Positive in extra Intestinal Amoebiasis - Indirect Haemagglutination Test (IHA)
   Counter Immunoelectrophoresis (CIE) & ELISA Test

   (b)   Treatment
   Symptomatic Cases:
   Metronidazole 30mg/kg body weight/day in 3 divided doses
   Tinidazole can also be used for 8–10 days. Secnidazole – A single dose.
   Liver Abscess – Referred to hospital

   Asymptomatic Cases:
   In endemic area, not to be treated except if they are food handlers. In non-endemic area they should be treated.
   Diiodohydroxyquin 650 mg TDS (Adults) or 30 – 40 mg/kg body weight per day for 20 days or
   Diloxanide Furoate 500 mg TDS for 10 days

Ascariasis and Hookworm Infections

Ascariasis	Hookworm Infection
Infection of Intestinal Tract	Infection of Intestinal Tract
	Endemic Index Chandler Index Average No. of Eggs per g of stools < 200 Hookworm infection is not of much significance 200 – 250 may be regarded as potential danger 250 – 300 minor public health problem > 300 Important Public health problem; used in epidemiological studies & impact of mass Rx
Epidemiology Agent Factors:	
Agent – Ascaris Lumbricoides	Agent – A Duodenale, N Americanus
Reservoir – Man	Reservoir – Man
Infective material – Faeces containing fertilized eggs	Faeces containing Ova of Hookworm Immediate source – Soil contaminated with Infective Larvae
Host Factors: Children Both sexes Contribute to malnutrition – Roundworms rob man of his food	All ages Both sexes Malnutrition is predisposing factor Host parasite balance Occupation – Farmers
Environmental Factors: Temperature – Low temperature inhibits the development of eggs Soil – Clay soil Human habits – Indiscriminate Defaecation	24 – 32°C Porous soil (sandy) Oxygen required for growth & development of Larvae
Period of Communicability – Until all fertile females are destroyed & stools negative	Moisture – Required for survival Rainfall - > 40inches & shade – protects Indiscriminate Defaecation; walking barefoot
Mode of Transmission Faecal oral route Direct – Fingers contaminated with soil Indirect – Infective eggs ingested with food (salads) drink	As long as person harbours the Parasite Enters body through feet by penetrating skin A Duodenale, also by oral route (contaminated vegetables, fruits)
Incubation period 2 months	N Americanus 7 weeks A Duodenale 5 weeks-9 months
Clinical Features Abdominal pain, nausea, cough (Tropical Pulmonary Eosinophilia), live worms passed in stool or vomited, Intestinal Obstruction	Effect of Disease: Individual – Anemia, growth retardation, Increase in morbidity, low birth weight, Abortion, Still-births Community – Impaired Lactation, low work output, economy, quality of life

Prevention & Control

1. Sanitary disposal of human excreta
2. Provision for safe drinking water
3. Food hygiene
4. Health Education – Use of sanitary latrine, personal hygiene, avoiding indiscriminate Defaecation

Secondary Prevention

Drugs – Albendazole, Mebendazole, Levamisole

Mass treatment – Periodic deworming every 6 months in children

In Hookworm Infection – Rx of Anaemia with Ferrous Sulphate for 3 months after Hb 12g%

Viral Hepatitis

Infection of Liver caused by half dozen viruses (Hepatitis A, B, C, D, E, G)

Hepatitis A	Hepatitis E
Epidemiology Agent Factors Agent – Hepatitis A Virus Enterovirus of Picornaviridae family	Hepatitis E Virus
Resistance-Fairly resistant to heat, chemicals, withstands heating to 60°C for 1-hour not affected by chlorine in usual doses sensitive to – UV rays, boiling 5-mins, autoclaving Reservoir of Infection-Human cases Asymptomatic to severe ones (children) Period of Infectivity 2 weeks before to 1week after onset of Jaundice Infective material – Man's faeces, Blood, serum, other fluids during brief stage of Viraemia Virus Excretion – In faeces 2 weeks before to 1 week after onset of jaundice May also be excreted in urine	Man's faeces
Host Factors Age – Children (by 10 years 90% are immune) Sex – Both equal	Young adults 15–40 years

Hepatitis A	Hepatitis E
Immunity – Immunity after infection for life	
In Endemic areas most people acquire	
immunity through Subclinical Infection	
Environmental Factors	
Season – Throughout the year,	
More during heavy rainfall periods	
Poor sanitation	Poor sanitation
Overcrowding	Overcrowding
Modes of Transmission	
i. Faecal – Oral Route	Faecal – Oral route
Major route	Water borne disease
Direct – Person to person contact through	
hands, eating utensils	
Indirect – Contaminated water, food, milk	
ii. Parenteral Route	Contaminated water, contaminated food
Rarely (By blood, blood products, skin	
penetration	
through contaminated needles)	
iii. Sexual Transmission	
Rare, in Homosexual through Oral – Anal	
contact	
Incubation Period	
15-45 days (2–6 weeks)	
Clinical features	2–9 weeks
Fever, chills, headache, fatigue, aches, pains,	
Anorexia, nausea, vomiting, dark urine,	Acute Viral Hepatitis,
jaundice, yellow conjunctiva, yellow skin	Self-limiting,
	Fulminating Hepatitis E,
	Particularly pregnant women,
	Intrauterine infection may cause abortions,
	intrauterine death, high perinatal morbidity,
	mortality
Lab – (i) HAV particles or Specific Viral	
Antigens in faeces	
ii. Rise in anti HAV Titre	
iii. Detection of IgM Antibody to HAV in	
Serum	
(Ig G indicates past infection & immunity)	
Prevention & Control	
(a)Control of Reservoir – Difficult because	
i. Faecal shedding of virus high during	No specific treatment
incubation period & early phase of	Supportive measures only
illness	

Hepatitis A	Hepatitis E

ii. Large no. of Subclinical cases
iii. Low socio-economic profile of population.
Control measures to be followed, notification, complete bed rest, disinfection of faeces, fomites with Sodium Hypochlorite 0.5%
(b) Control of Transmission – Personal & community hygiene
   i. Hand washing
   ii. Sanitary disposal of excreta
   iii. Safe water supply
   iv. Autoclaving of syringes, needles, equipment
(c) Control of susceptible population
Human Immunoglobulin
Family contacts – 0.02ml/kg body weight
Institutional Outbreaks - (3.2mg/kg body weight)
Travellers to developing countries
– 0.02-0.05ml/kg
body weight 3.2–8.0 mg/kg body weight every 4 months
Vaccines
Hepatitis A Vaccine – 2 doses 6–18 months apart
Combination Vaccine Hepatitis A & B; 0, 1, 6 months
	Sanitary disposal of excreta
	Safe water supply
	Food hygiene
	
	No immunoglobulin
	
	No vaccine available

Hepatitis B	Hepatitis C	Hepatitis D	Hepatitis G

Definition
Acute Systemic Infection mainly affecting the Liver
 	
Epidemiology
Agent Factors:
Agent – Hepatitis B Virus
3 morphological forms
  i. Small spherical particles
  ii. Tubules
  iii. Dane particles – Infectious
	Infection of liver caused by Hepatitis C virus
	
	Single stranded RNA virus
	A Flavivirus
	Genus
	Hapacivirus
		Infection due to Hepatitis D virus – Delta Hepatitis occurs in association with Hepatitis B (carrier state) not significant infection in India
		
		Agent – Hepatitis D virus
			Infection due to Hepatitis G virus.
			
			Discovered in 1996
			
			Hepatitis G virus – a Flavivirus

Hepatitis B	Hepatitis C	Hepatitis D	Hepatitis G
Reservoir Carriers (5 to 10% of patients) Cases (inapparent to symptomatic cases) Infective material Contaminated blood Others – Saliva, vaginal secretions, semen Resistance Quite stable – survives for days on environmental surfaces Sensitive to Sodium Hypochlorite, heat, Sterilization in Autoclave ½ - 1hour Period of Communicability 1 month before Jaundice & during acute phase of disease. In chronic carriers - Period of communicability several months – years, or until disappearance of HBsAg & appearance of surface antibody Host Factors Age 15-19 years Acute Hepatitis B infection in perinatal 1% 1-5 years 10% > 5 years 30% Chronic HBV infection Perinatally 95% 1–5 years 80% > 5 years 5–10 % High risk groups Surgeons, health care personnel, laboratory personnel, infants of HBV carrier mothers, Immuno compromised patients, homosexuals, prostitutes, percutaneous drug abusers	Adults Men > women		

Hepatitis B	Hepatitis C	Hepatitis D	Hepatitis G
Humoral & Cellular responses Hepatitis B virus has 3 Antigens – Stimulate antibodies Surf Antigen HBsAg Anti HBs Core Antigen HBcAg Anti HBc e Antigen HBeAg Anti HBe Modes of Transmission i. Parenteral Route Blood borne infection transmitted by infected blood & blood products - Blood transfusion, Dialysis, contaminated syringes, needles, skin pricks, handling infected blood, surgical, dental procedures, Immunization, tattooing, ear piercing, nose piercing, ritual circumcision, acupuncture, shared razors, tooth brushes Perinatal Transmission HBV carrier mother to Baby At birth leak of maternal blood to baby's circulation; ingestion or accidental inoculation of blood Usually Anicteric Diagnosis-HBsAg 60-120 days after birth Sexual transmission Sexually promiscuous; homosexuals Other Routes Child – Child Horizontal Transmission through physical contact. Cuts, grazes, scabies, impetigo. Blood sucking Arthropods (Mosquito, bedbugs) suspected	Parenteral route transfusion of contaminated blood or blood products IV drug users who share needles	Same as Hepatitis B	Blood transfusion

Hepatitis B	Hepatitis C	Hepatitis D	Hepatitis G
	Occupational hazard in health care workers therefore universal precautions to be taken. Traditional circumcision, tattooing, scarification with contaminated instruments can spread the disease		
Incubation Period 6weeks – 6 months	Minimal 6 weeks – 4 months		
Clinical features Viral Hepatitis may → Chronic carrier (5–10%) Chronic Active Hepatitis, Cirrhosis, Primary Liver Cancer HBsAg present	Mild, asymptomatic, insidious onset Chronicity in ≥ 50% Chronic active Hepatitis, Cirrhosis, Liver Cancer HbsAg absent	Same as Hepatitis B	
Prevention & Control i. Hepatitis B vaccine (a) Plasma derived vaccine Formalin inactivated subunit Viral vaccine of HBsAg (6) RDNA – Yeast derived vaccine, Recombinant DNA vaccine elaborated from cultures of Yeast cloned with HbsAg s-gene Dose – 20mcg Initially, 1 month, 6 months IM	Interferon treatment No vaccine	Immunization Ag Hepatitis B also protects against Delta Hepatitis	
Children < 10 years ½ dose Infants & children < 2 years Anterolateral aspect of thigh			
Indications Children, adolescents < 18 years,			

Hepatitis B	Hepatitis C	Hepatitis D	Hepatitis G

High risk population, high risk sexual behaviour, partners, household contacts of HbsAg positives, injecting drug users, persons requiring frequent blood/ blood products, recipients of Organ Transplantation, occupational risk eg. Health care workers, international travelers to HBV Endemic countries
  b. Hepatitis B Immunoglobulin
HBIG for immediate protection for people acutely exposed to HbsAg positive blood.
eg. surgeons, nurses, lab workers. Newborn infants of carrier mothers, sexual contacts of acute Hepatitis B patients.
2 Doses 0.05–0.07ml/kg at 1-month apart
  c. Passive – Active
     Immunization
HBIG & simultaneously Hepatitis B
Vaccine administered
  d. Other Measures
Blood donors screened
Voluntary blood donation encouraged.
Sterilization of all instruments, syringes, needles disposable, simple hygiene measures.
Carriers – Should not share razors, toothbrushes, should not donate blood, use
	No immunoglobin		

Typhoid Fever (Enteric Fever)

Definition

An acute communicable disease caused mainly by S Typhi resulting in continuous fever for 3–4weeks, relative Bradycardia, Lymphoid Tissue involvement, constitutional symptoms.

Epidemiology

Agent Factors

Agent – S Typhi in majority of the cases
S Para A, S Para B infrequently
S Typhi has O, H, V Antigens & number of Phage types
Readily killed by drying, pasteurization, disinfectants

Reservoir – Man - Cases – Mild, missed, severe
-       Carriers – Temporary – Incubatory, convalescent 6–8 weeks
        Chronic – Excrete Bacilli for > 1-year
        Organisms persist in Gall Bladder & Biliary Tract
        Typhoid Mary gave rise to 1300 cases
        Chronic urinary carriers associated with abnormality of Urinary Tract

Source – Faeces & urine of cases/carriers form primary source
Secondary sources – Contaminated water, foods, fingers, flies

Host Factors

Any age. Maximum 5–19 years
M > F but carriers more in females
Immunity – Antibody stimulated by Infection/Immunization.

S Typhi intracellular, cell mediated immunity
Local intestinal immunity contributes to resistance to infection.
Gastric acidity – Contributes to resistance to infection.

Environmental & Social Factors

Throughout year, but peaks in Jul–Sept (Rainy season) & increase fly population. Open defaecation, urination, poor sanitation, health ignorance, contaminated water, ice, ice creams, contaminated food, sewage farming.

Incubation period

10–14 days

Modes of Transmission

Faecal oral route

Urine oral route

Directly – Through soiled hands with faeces or urine of cases or carriers

Indirectly – By contaminated water, milk, food, flies

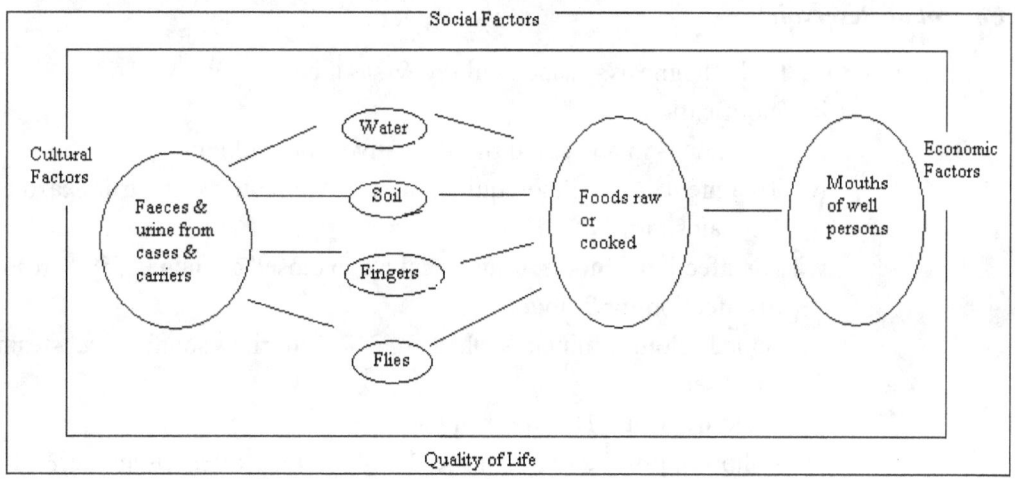

Dynamics of Typhoid Fever Transmission

Clinical Features

Fever with chills (fever step ladder pattern), headache, cough, sore throat, coated tongue, malaise,

abdominal pain, constipation or Pea Soup Diarrhea, abdominal distension

Relative Bradycardia

Rash (Rose spots) - 2nd week of disease

Complications – Intestinal Hemorrhage, Intestinal Perforation, Pneumonia, Myocarditis, Psychosis, Cholecystitis, Nephritis, Osteomyelitis

Blood – Leucopenia

Urine & stool culture positive for Salmonella

Splenomegaly, tenderness

Investigations

i. Microbiological Procedures
    Isolation of S Typhi from blood, bone marrow, stools, urine

ii. Serological Procedures
    Widal test measures agglutinating Antibody levels against O & H Antigens

iii. New Tests – IDL Tubex Test can detect Antibodies within mins.
    Typhidot takes 3-hours to perform.

Control of Typhoid

1. Control of Reservoir
2. Control of Sanitation
3. Immunization

1. Control of Reservoir

(a) Cases   i.   Early diagnosis – Blood culture & stool c/s

            ii.   Notification

            iii.   Isolation – In a hospital till 3 negative stool cultures

            iv.   Treatment – Fluoroquinolones, Ampicillin, Cotrimoxazole, Cephalosporin

            v.   Disinfection – Stools, urine, received in closed containers, 5% Cresol disinfection for 2-hours.
Soiled clothes, linen soaked – 2% Chlorine solution & steam sterilised.
Hand hygiene - Doctors & nurses

            vi.   Follow Up – Stools & urine 3 – 4 months after discharge & 12 months to identify carriers.

(b) Carriers

     i.   Identification – By cultural & Serological Examination
Duodenal drainage establishes presence of Salmonella in Biliary Tract carriers Vi Antibodies present in 80% of carriers

     ii.   Treatment – Ampicillin or Amoxycillin 4–6g/day & Probenecid (2g/day) for 6 weeks.

     iii.   Surgery – Cholecystectomy with Ampicillin Therapy highly successful
Nephrectomy in refractory cases when kidney damaged

     iv.   Surveillance – Carriers kept under surveillance, should be prevented from handling food, milk, water

     v.   Health Education – On hand washing with soap & water after defaecation or urination, before preparing food

2. Control of Sanitation

     i.   Safe water – Should be supplied to community after proper filtration & chlorination

     ii.   Sanitation – Construction & use of sanitary latrines

     iii.   Food Hygiene – Proper preparation & cooking of food

3. Immunization

     i.   Vi Vaccine – Contains Vi Polysaccharide single dose SC or IM. Protection after 7 days after
Injection & maximum by 1 month. Re-vaccination every 3 years.

ii. Typhoral (Oral Typhoid Vaccine)

Ty21a – Enteric coated capsule of Lyophilized Vaccine contains not less than 10^9 viable attenuated

Salmonella Typhi Strain Ty21a.

Immunization of adults & children > 6-years. One capsule on days 1, 3, 5 one hour before meal with cold or lukewarm milk or water.

Protection, 2-weeks after last capsule upto 3 years.

Booster every 3 years.

Poliomyelitis

Definition

An acute infection caused by RNA virus primarily affecting human Alimentary Tract but may infect

CNS in 1% of cases resulting in paralysis and possible death.

Endemic countries – Pakistan, Afghanistan

India - Polio eradicated by 2014

Epidemiology

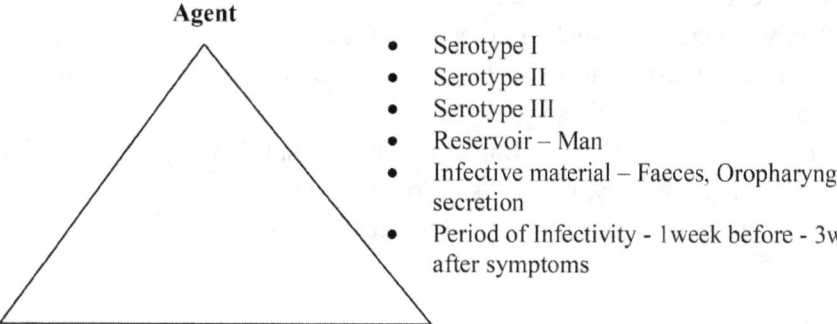

Agent
- Serotype I
- Serotype II
- Serotype III
- Reservoir – Man
- Infective material – Faeces, Oropharyngeal secretion
- Period of Infectivity - 1week before - 3weeks after symptoms

Environment
- Rainy Season
- Water contamination
- Poor Sanitation
- Overcrowding

Host
Infants mostly
Sex - M:F - 3:1
Risk – Fatigue, Trauma, Tonsillectomy, Injection
Immunity

Mode of Transmission

i. Faeco-Oral Directly – Contaminated fingers
   or
   Indirectly – Contaminated water, milk, foods, flies, articles of daily use
ii. Droplet Infection – During acute phase of disease when virus is in the throat

Incubation Period

7-14 days

Clinical Features

  i. Inapparent or Subclinical Infection
     91–96% of Poliovirus infection.
     No symptoms, recognition by virus isolation or rising Antibody Titres.
 ii. Abortive Polio or Minor Illness
     In 4–8% of infection causes mild, self-limiting illness, recovers quickly. Diagnosis cannot be made clinically, recognition only by virus isolation or rising Antibody Titre.
iii. Non-Paralytic Polio
     In 1% of infections.
     Disease synonymous with Aseptic Meningitis, stiffness & pain in neck & back for 2–10 days, recovery rapid.
 iv. Paralytic Polio
     In < 1% of infections.
     Virus invades CNS & causes Paralysis. Acute Flaccid Paralysis – Acute onset of fever, constitutional symptoms (Headache, body ache, malaise) & develops Flaccid Paralysis after 24–48 hours.
     Paralysis is asymmetrical, involves proximal parts of extremities, decreased muscle tone, reduced/absent reflexes.
     Paralysis persists as such or at reduced scale.
     Later gives rise to muscle wasting, skeletal deformities, limitation of joint movement, shortening of limb. No sensory loss.
     Cranial nerves involved in Bulbar & Bulbospinal Poliomyelitis – Facial asymmetry, swallowing difficulty, weakness or loss of voice.
     Respiratory Insufficiency can lead to death.

Treatment

No specific Treatment.
Good nursing care can minimise or prevent crippling.
Physiotherapy very important, can be initiated in affected limb immediately, helps weakened muscles to regain strength.
Child may require Calipers.

Prevention

Primary prevention – Sanitation
- Health education about cause, spread, immunization of infants.
- Immunization – IPV or OPV
- Human Immunoglobulins 0.25 ml/kg in very highly susceptible contact

Secondary Prevention – Early diagnosis and treatment
- Isolation, notification, symptomatic treatment, hot packs, analgesics, physiotherapy
- Aids eg. Slings, crutches.

Tertiary Prevention - Disability Limitation:
Affected muscles massaged, physiotherapy where all joints are put through full range of movements passively, then actively under warm bath.
Slings, crutches may be required.

Rehabilitation:
From 6 months - 2 to 3yrs
Arrangements made for schooling & training child in art, craft, occupation so that on growing he is able to lead independent life.

Differences between IPV & OPV

IPV (Inactivated Polio Vaccine) (Salk Type)	OPV (Oral Polio Vaccine) (Sabin Type)
1. Killed Formalised Virus	1. Live attenuated virus
2. Given IM or SC	2. Given orally
3. Only Humoral immunity	3. Humoral & Intestinal immunity
4. Prevents Paralysis but does not prevent reinfection by Wild Polio Viruses	4. Prevents Paralysis & also Intestinal Reinfection
5. Not useful in epidemics	5. Useful in epidemic
6. More difficult to manufacture	6. Easy to manufacture
7. Virus content is 10,000 times more than OPV. Hence costlier.	7. Cheaper
8. Cold chain not stringent	8. Cold chain required

Epidemiological Investigations

In Polio, occurrence of a single case is considered an epidemic therefore, Epidemiological Investigation should be carried out immediately.

1. Name of administrative area & locality
2. Date of first case reported from locality
3. Period of field investigation from   --------- to ---------- (dates)
4. No. of Paralytic Polio cases detected
   i.   Clinical diagnosis only
   ii. Laboratory confirmed
   iii. Type(s) of virus isolated
5. No. of Deaths from Paralytic Polio
6. No. of Paralytic cases of Polio by age

< 1yr	10–14years
1–4 years	15–19 years
5–9 years	20+ years.

7. No. of contacts of Paralytic Polio examined
   Household contacts
   Others (specify)
8. Brief description of investigations
9. History of previous vaccination practice in the locality including dates of last community vaccination programme & type of vaccine used.
10. Name of Principal Investigator & Laboratory

Samples of faeces from all cases/suspected cases of polio should be collected & sent to lab for virus isolation.

Where possible Paired Sera should be collected, first specimen at Acute Phase & second at Convalescence.

Strategies for Polio Eradication in India

i. Pulse Polio Immunization days every year until Poliomyelitis was eradicated.
ii. Sustained high levels of routine immunization coverage
iii. Monitored OPV coverage at District level & below
iv. Improved surveillance capable of detecting all cases of AFP due to Polio & Non-polio Aetiology
v. Ensured rapid case investigation, including collection of stool samples for virus isolation
vi. Arranged follow-up of all cases of AFP at 60 days to check for residual paralysis
vii. Conducted outbreak control for cases confirmed/suspected to be Poliomyelitis to stop transmission within 48 hours of notification

Line Listing of Cases

Line listing of reported cases started in 1989.

Helps to check for duplication (same case reported more than once), year of onset of illness (screen children who developed polio prior to year of reporting), identification of high-risk pockets (by analysis of residential status), documentation of high-risk age groups.

Line listing enabled to take appropriate follow up action in areas where cases were reported. It also helped for programme planning – Eg. Information on age at onset to understand urgency of completion of OPV immunization schedule.

All cases of AFP reported immediately to Chief Medical Officer/District Immunization Officer with following details:

- Name, age, sex
- Father's name, complete address
- Vaccination status

- Date of onset of Paralysis & date of reporting
- Clinical diagnosis
- Doctor's name, address, phone number

Mopping Up

This was done during the last stage of Polio Eradication. It involved door to door immunization in high-risk districts where wild Polio is known or suspected to be circulating.

Ring Immunization

It is the mopping up operation in cities where door-to-door OPV is given to < 5 years old children covering a radius of 5-km.

Pulse Polio Immunization in India

National Immunization days conducted since 1995.
Two Immunization days at 6-weeks apart in December and January (Low transmission season)

During PPIs Oral Polio Vaccine is given to children of 0–5years of age in the country on a single day, regardless of previous immunizations. As a result, Wild Polio virus strains got replaced by the harmless & protective OPV strain. Pulse denotes "sudden, simultaneous mass administration of OPV on a single day to all children of 0–5 years of age".

Since 1998 VVM – Vaccine Vial Monitors, colour monitors were put on the vaccine bottles. It has a deep blue circle & white square inside which changes colour & gradually becomes blue, if vaccine bottle is exposed to high temperature.
If the square in the centre is white or of lighter colour than the surrounding circle, it is effective & can be used (i & ii)

Day 1 - Fixed booth session
Days 2, 3 & 4 – Door-to-door session

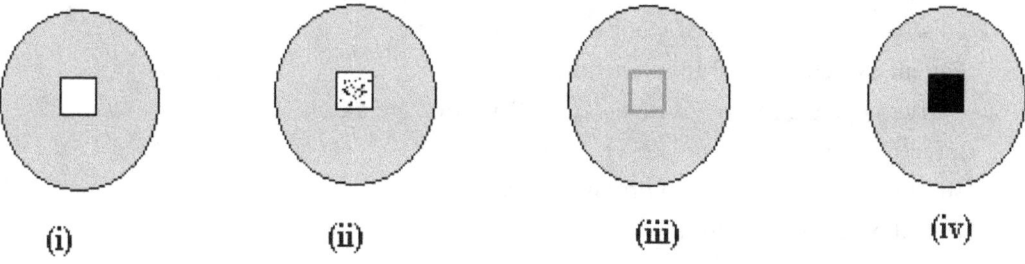

(i)　　　　(ii)　　　　(iii)　　　　(iv)

Polio eradication can be certified only when no cases of Clinical Poliomyelitis occurs for 3 years and when no Wild Polio Virus is found in the environment.

Cholera

An acute Diarrhoeal disease caused by V Cholerae (Classical or El Tor)

Epidemiology

Agent Factors

(i) Agent – V Cholerae 01 — Classical – Inaba, Ogawa, Hikojima
El Tor – Inaba, Ogawa, Hikojima

El Tor	Classical
1. Agglutinate Chicken & Sheep Erythrocytes	Do not agglutinate Chicken & Sheep Erythrocytes
2. Resistant to classical Phage IV	Not resistant to classical Phage IV
3. Resistant to Polymycin B 50-unit disc	Not resistant to Polymycin B 50 unit disc
4. VP Reaction & Hemolytic test do not give consistent results	

ii. Resistance – Resistant to cold; remains in ice 4–6 weeks
Sensitive to boiling, sunshine, drying, coal tar disinfectants eg. Cresol & bleaching powder
El Tor more resistant than classical Vibrios

iii. Toxin
Vibrios multiply in Small Intestines and produce Exotoxin
Toxin produces Diarrhea through effect on Adenyl Cyclase – Cyclic AMP system of Mucosal cells.

iv. Reservoir
Human Beings — Cases – El Tor mostly mild, asymptomatic
Carriers – Temporary, chronic

v. Infective Material
Stools & vomitus of cases & carriers
10^7–10^9 Vibrios per ml of stool
Patient excretes 10–20 liters of fluid
Carriers excrete fewer Vibrios – 10^2-10^5 Vibrios/gm stools

vi. Infective Dose
10^{11} Organisms required to produce disease

vii. Period of Communicability
Cholera case, 7-10 days
Convalescent carriers, 2-3weeks
Chronic carrier, 1 month - ≥ 10 years

Carriers in Cholera

An apparently healthy person who is excreting V Cholerae 01 (Classical or EI Tor) in stools.

These are of 4 types:
  i.   Incubatory carriers – During incubation period (1–5 days)
  ii. Convalescent Carriers – During convalescence (2–3 weeks), in patients who have not received adequate Antibiotic treatment, may become chronic carriers.
  iii. Contact/Healthy Carrier – Due to Subclinical infection from association with source of infection – case or environment
  iv. Chronic Carriers – 1-month $\geq$ 10 years, Gall Bladder infected.
       Investigations – Stools enrichment important in diagnosis since fewer Vibrios are excreted.

Host Factors

All ages
Both sexes
Gastric acidity – Effective barrier

Population Mobility – Pilgrimages, marriages, fairs, festivals increase risk of exposure. Country to country spread through air travel.
Economic Status - Low socio-economic status, due to poor hygiene, unsafe water, poor sanitation
Immunity:
Natural infection → Immunity
Vaccination, temporary, partial immunity for 3–6 months

Environmental Factors

Poor sanitation
Contaminated water
Contaminated food
Human habits – Indiscriminate defaecation, soil & water pollution,
Poor personal hygiene, lack of education

Mode of Transmission

Faecal–Oral Transmission ⟨ Indirectly – Contaminated water, food, drinks, flies
Directly – Contaminated fingers, linen & fomites

Incubation Period

1–5 days

Clinical Features

Majority – Mild, asymptomatic
Cases – Sudden profuse, effortless, watery Diarrhoea (Rice water stools), vomiting, rapid dehydration, muscular cramps, suppression of urine.

Typical case has 3 stages:

   i. Stage of Evacuation – Profuse, painless watery Diarrhoea followed by vomiting
  ii. Stage of Collapse – Due to dehydration, sunken eyes, dry lips & tongue, dry eyes, skin turgor decreased, pulse absent, BP unrecordable, shallow rapid respiration, subnormal temperature, restlessness, thirst, cramps in legs & abdomen, death possible due to dehydration & Acidosis
 iii. Stage of Recovery – BP begins to rise, temperature normal, urine secretion improves.

EI Tor differs from classical Cholera in following:

(a) Majority mild & asymptomatic infection
(b) Fewer secondary cases in affected families
(c) Occurrence of chronic carriers
(d) Survive longer in extra intestinal environment

Laboratory Diagnosis

1. Collection of Specimen
    (a) Stools – i. Rubber Catheter – Specimen collected onto transport media (Venkatraman–Ramakrishnan (VR) Medium, Alkaline Peptone water)
             ii. Rectal Swab – Dipped into transport medium before introduction into Rectum
    (b) Vomitus – Rarely used
    (c) Water – Suspect water 1–3L collected in sterile bottles or 9 vols sample water + 1 vol Peptone water sent to laboratory
    (d) Food Samples – Suspected 1–3g collected in transport media & sent to lab.
2. Transportation – In VR Media or Alkaline Peptone Water
3. Microscopy – With dark field illumination
    Vibrios - Shooting stars in a dark sky
    Motility ceases on mixing with Polyvalent Anticholera Diagnostic Serum.
4. Culture – 0.5-1 ml of material inoculated into Peptone Water Tellurite (PWT) for enrichment. 4–6 hours later Subcultured on Bile Salt Agar (BSA), overnight incubation
5. Characterisation
    Translucent, moist, raised, smooth, easily emulsifiable colonies which are 1-mm in diameter.
    The colonies tested i. Gram stain & motility. Gm –ve curved rods, scintillating movement in hanging drop preparations.

ii. Serological test – Slide Agglutination Test with Polyvalent Anticholera Diagnostic Serum. If agglutination positive, repeated test with Inaba & Ogawa Antisera

6. Biochemical Tests

Serologically positive colonies Subcultured in Mannose, Sucrose, Arabinose; production of acid in Sucrose & Mannose, not in Arabinose.

7. Further Characterisation:
   i. Direct Haemagglutination Test with Chicken or Sheep red blood cells
   ii. Polymyxin B Sensitivity Tests
   iii. Sensitivity to Cholera Phage IV
   iv. V – P Reaction
   v. Haemolysis Test

	El Tor	Classical
Chicken/Sheep RBC	Agglutinate	No agglutination
Phage IV	Resistant	Not resistant
Polymyxin B	Resistant	Not resistant
VP Reaction	Negative	Positive

Control of Cholera – WHO Guidelines

• Verification of Diagnosis – Case examination & laboratory diagnosis for Cholera as soon as suspicious case reported from community.
• Notification – Cholera is a notifiable disease locally, nationally, internationally. No. of cases & deaths to be reported daily & weekly to WHO by the National Government.
• Early Case Finding – Search for new cases (Mild, moderate, severe) & treatment initiated.
• Establishment of Treatment Centres – Mildly Dehydrated patients are treated at home with ORT. Severely dehydrated patients are sent to hospital or treatment centre for IV fluids. School or public building may be converted into temporary treatment centres.
• Rehydration Therapy – Rehydration may be Oral or Intravenous
• Antibiotics - Doxycycline   300mg stat
            Tetracycline   500mg QDS for 3 days
            Cotrimoxazole   160mg/800mg BD for 3 days
            Furazolidone   100 mg QDS for 3 days (in pregnant women)

• Epidemiological Investigations – Extent of outbreak, modes of transmission, effective & specific control measures applied.
• Sanitation Measures

   i.   Water Control   – Chlorination/boiling

   ii. Excreta disposal – Sanitary latrines

   iii. Food Sanitation – Sale of foods under hygienic conditions

                               Hot foods to be eaten

                               Safe food handling practices

                               Utensils cleaned & dried after use

   iv. Disinfection   – Concurrent & terminal disinfection

                               Cresol, bleaching powder used for patient's stools, vomitus, clothes, latrine

- Chemoprophylaxis
  Mass Chemoprophylaxis not advised
  Chemoprophylaxis only for household contacts or closed community
  Tetracycline BD for 3 days

- Vaccine – Phenol killed containing classical Ogawa, Inaba 6000 million each per ml.
     i.   Parenteral Vaccine – 1st Dose 0.5 ml
           2nd Dose 1.0 ml after 4 weeks
           Protective value 50% for 3–6 months
     ii. Oral Vaccine – This is of 2 types:
          i.   Killed whole cell V Cholerae 01+Recombinant B subunit
              2 doses 10–14 days apart
          ii. Live attenuated vaccine single dose
- Health Education
     i.   Oral Rehydration Therapy
     ii. Early reporting & prompt treatment
     iii. Food Hygiene
     iv. Foods cooked & hot
     v.   Hand washing
     vi. Safe water

Acute Diarrhoeal Diseases

Definition

Diarrhoea is defined as passage of loose/watery stools > 3 times per day.
Acute Diarrhea lasts 3–7 days.
Persistent Diarrhea continues more than 14 days.

Dysentery – Stools containing blood with or without mucus.

Epidemiology

Agent Factors

Agent

1. Viruses – Rotaviruses, Astroviruses, Adenoviruses, Calciviruses, Coronaviruses, Enteroviruses, Norwalk Group Viruses
2. Bacteria – Escherichia Coli, Campylobacter Jejuni, Shigella, Salmonella, Vibrio Cholera, Vibrio Para Haemolyticus, Bacillus Cereus
3. Others – E Histolytica, Giardia Intestinalis, Trichuriasis, Cryptosporidium, Intestinal Worms

Reservoir
Man – Eg. E Coli, Shigella, V Cholera, Giardia Lamblia, E Histolytica
Man & Animals – Campylobacter Jejuni, Salmonella, Y Enterocolitica

Host Factors

Age – Children
Nutritional Status – Malnutrition
Prematurity
Immuno-deficiency
Gastric Acidity
Poverty
Lack of personal hygiene
Incorrect feeding practices

Environmental Factors

Warm rainy season – Bacterial Diarrhoea
Winters – Rotavirus Diarrhoea
Indiscriminate Defaecation
Lack of Sanitation
Lack of safe water
Lack of food hygiene

Mode of Transmission

Faecal–oral route ⟨ Direct – Fingers, fomites
Indirect – Water, food

Clinical Features

Abdominal pain, Diarrhoea, vomiting, fever

Plague

Definition

Zoonotic infection primarily affecting rodents caused by Yersinia Pestis, transmitted by infected flea bites to humans. Known as "Black Death" due to high mortality in ancient times.

Problem in the World

Endemic countries - Africa, Asia, Americas

Return of Plague

Last reported cases in 1966, then reappearance in 1994 in Beed (Maharashtra) – Bubonic Plague & Pneumonic Plague in Surat (Gujarat). In 2004 - Bubonic Plague in Uttarkashi.

Epidemiology

Agent factors

Agent – Y Pestis, gram negative, non-motile, Coccobacillus with bipolar staining. Bacilli in abundance in Buboes, blood, spleen, liver, other viscera of infected persons & sputum of pneumonic cases.

Reservoir – Natural reservoir wild rodents (Tatera Indica) pass the infection to the normal reservoir (Rattus Rattus).

Source – Infected rodents & fleas in case of Pneumonic Plague.

Host Factors

All ages
Both sexes
Human Activities – Hunting, grazing, cultivation, harvesting, construction activities, outdoor recreation give opportunities for flea – man contact.
Movement of people – Plague associated with movement of people, cargo by sea, land. Rats & rat fleas transported this way.
Immunity – Man has no natural immunity and after recovery it is relative.

Environmental Factors

Season – September to May (North India). Disease decreased during hot weather when rodents commenced aestivation; closing themselves in their burrows & living on stored food reserves. No definite plague season in South India.

Temperature & Humidity
Temperature - 20–25⁰ C

Temperature - $20–25^0$ C
Relative Humidity $\geq 60\%$
Rainfall – Heavy rainfall floods rat burrows. Therefore, certain states (Bengal) free from Plague.

Areas
Rural areas mainly affected
Human Dwellings
Poor housing conditions

Vectors of Plague

* X Cheopis (Rat flea), X Astia, X Brasiliensis, Pulex Irritans.
Both sexes of fleas bite & transmit disease (Human flea)
Blocked Flea

A flea may ingest 0.5 cu mm blood which may contain 5,000 Bacilli. These multiply in the gut of the rat flea & may block Proventriculus so that no food can pass through. Such a flea is called "Blocked Flea".

Blocked flea eventually faces starvation and death because it is unable to obtain blood meal. It makes frantic efforts to bite and suck blood again and again. In the process it regurgitates the Plague Bacilli into the bite wound each time it bites.

Therefore, a Blocked Flea becomes an efficient transmitter of Plague. Partially Blocked Flea is more dangerous than a completely blocked one because it can live longer.

Infected fleas may live up to one year.
Certain species survive in burrows for 4 years.

Flea Indices

Flea Indices are useful measurements for density of fleas.

They are useful in evaluating the effectiveness of a spraying programme.

  i. Total Flea Index – Average number of fleas of all species per rat
  ii. Cheopies Index – Average number of X. Cheopies per rat.
                        It is a specific flea index.
                        If > 1 it is indicative of potential explosiveness if a Plague outbreak occurs.
 iii. Specific percentage of fleas – % of different species of fleas that are found on rats.
 iv. Burrow Index – Average number of free-living fleas per species per rodent burrow.

Flea Indices do not indicate imminent Plague Epidemic.

They warn that more stringent control measures are needed to protect the human population.

Mode of Transmission

i.   Commensal rats → Rat fleas → man eg. In Epidemic Bubonic Plague.
ii. Wild rodents → wild rodents' fleas/direct contact → man
     Disease is transmitted from rodent to rodent via wild rodent fleas or contaminated soil. Man contracts infection from infectious wild rodent fleas or by direct contact with infected rodents.
iii. Wild rodents, Peridomestic rodents, commensal rodents
     → Wild rodent fleas, Peridomestic rodent fleas, commensal rodent fleas → Man
     Plague Foci impinge on habitats of Peridomestic/commensal rodents.
     Interaction of rodents & their fleas convey infection to man.
iv. Man → Human flea (Pulex Irritans) → man
v.   Man → man
     When a primary case of Bubonic Plague develops Secondary Pneumonic Plague. Infections are contracted via the respiratory route.

Incubation Period

Bubonic & Septicaemic Plague 2–7 days
Pneumonic Plague 1–3 days

Clinical Features

3 main clinical forms

i. ***Bubonic Plague – Most Common***
    Infected rat fleas usually bite in the lower extremities & inoculate Bacilli. Patient develops fever, chills, headache, prostration, painful Lymphadenitis.
    Within a few days Buboes develop in Groin & less often – Axilla or neck depending on site of bite by rat flea → suppuration.
    Bubonic plague cannot spread person to person as Bacilli are locked in the Buboes - Dead end infection.

ii. ***Pneumonic Plague***
    Primary Pneumonic Plague is rare.
    Complication of Bubonic/Septicaemic Plague.
    Highly infectious & spreads from man to man by droplet infection. Plague Bacilli are present in the Sputum.

iii. Septicaemic Plague

Primary Septicaemic Plague is rare.

Bubonic Plague may develop into Septicaemic Plague.

Laboratory Investigations

i. Staining – Smears of clinical material (Eg. Bubo fluid, sputum) fixed with alcohol & stained with

Giemsa's or Wayson's stain to demonstrate Bipolar Bacilli.

ii. Culture – Blood, Bubo fluid or sputum cultured for isolation of Bacilli.

iii. Serology – Acute & convalescent specimens of blood Sera should be collected for Antibody studies.

iv. Other Methods

Inoculation of Guinea Pigs or mice or Immunofluorescent Microscopic Test.

Prevention & Control

1. Early Diagnosis

Clinical features of acute fever, painful lymph node enlargement developing into Bubos.

"Rat falls" (dead rats) provide useful warning of possible outbreak. Bacteriological exam to confirm diagnosis.

2. Notification

If human/rodent case is diagnosed, health authorities to be notified.

Notification required under International Health Regulations.

3. Isolation

Although Bubonic Plague is non-infectious, isolation is recommended. Pneumonic Plague should be isolated.

4. Treatment

Streptomycin (30mg/kg body weight) IM in 2 divided doses 7–10 days.

Tetracycline 30–40 mg/kg body weight.

Sulphonamides may be used.

5. Disinfection

Sputum in Pneumonic Plague should be received in sputum cups containing Antiseptics.

Patients' clothes should be boiled.

Mattresses & furniture should be Cyanogassed or put in hot sun.

Fleas die quickly on exposure to sun.

House should be sprayed with DDT.

Rat burrows insufflated with 10% DDT powder.

6. **Control of Rodents**

   Destruction of rodents

   Improvement of general sanitation, improvement of housing, quality of life.

7. **Vaccination**

   Mass inoculation with Plague Vaccine when an Epidemic is threatened and not as a control measure during an Epidemic.

   Vaccine given in 2 doses, Formalin killed vaccine of Y Pestis, 0.5 ml and 1.0 ml SC at interval of 7–14 days.

   In emergency, 3 ml single dose for adults SC, immunity starts 5–7 days after, inoculation lasts 6 months. Booster six monthly for at risk persons (Geologists, Biologists, Anthropologists).

8. **Chemoprophylaxis**

   In all plague contacts, Tetracyclic 500 mg 6 hourly for 5 days, or Sulphonamide 2-3g daily for 5–7 days.

9. **Surveillance**

   Surveillance of all aspects of rodent & human plague eg. Microbiology, Serology, Entomology, Mammalogy, Epidemiology and Ecology.

   Effective control measures must be carried out based on surveillance.

10. **Health Education**

    Education providing public with facts about Plague, mode of spread, rat control measures, sanitation.

11. **International Measures**

    WHO should be promptly informed of any outbreak.

    International Sanitary Regulations specify measures applicable to ships, aircrafts, land transport arriving from plague affected areas.

Human Salmonellosis

Definition

This is a Zoonotic disease; Salmonellosis, a group of food borne infections affecting man & animals.

World - Global problem, 60-80% of food borne diseases; aggravated by widespread use of animal feeds with Anti-microbial drugs favouring drug resistance.

Diarrhoeal diseases are widespread in developing countries.

Epidemiology

Agent Factors

Agent – Salmonellae Bacteria
Resistant to drying, salting, smoking, freezing
Sensitive to heat, will not survive > 70°C.

There are 3 main groups

i. Those which infect only man e.g. S. Typhi, S Paratyphi A & B.
ii. Those which infect animals eg. S. Cholera Suis in Swine, S. Dublin in Cattle, S. Abortus Equi in horses, S. Gallinarum in Poultry. S. Cholera Suis and S. Dublin are pathogenic for man also.
iii. Those with no particular host preference can infect both man & animals eg. S. Typhimurium and S. Enteritidis.

Reservoir – Intestinal Tract of man & animals

Foods – Foods of animal origin eg. Meat, poultry, eggs
Food can become contaminated eg. Chocolate, spices, coconut if processed in contaminated environment.
Multidrug resistant strains of Salmonella encountered (resistance to Fluroquinolones and 3rd generation Cephalosporins)
Animals are hosts & principal vectors of Zoonotic Salmonellosis eg. Cattle, swine, fowls, rodents. Bacilli are present in their tissues (meat), eggs, excreta.

Carriers – Man & animals

Environmental Factors

Dust, water, manure, sewage, sludge, vegetables, insects, birds, fish, rodents & other mammals harbour Salmonellae, can survive in soil for months.

Mode of Transmission

Fecal-Oral route ⟨ Direct – Contact with domestic animals eg. Dogs, rats, mice, insects, pigeons
Indirect – Through contaminated food or drink

Incubation Period

6–72 hours.

Clinical Features

i. Enteric Fever – S. Typhi, S Paratyphi A, B.
ii. Salmonella Enterocolitis (Gastroenteritis)

Fever, headache, nausea, vomiting, diarrhea 6–48 hours after ingestion of Salmonellae

Resolves in 2–3 days

Stool cultures positive for Salmonellae

Death rare & only in Neonates, infants or elderly

iii. Septicaemia with Focal Lesions

Non-Typhoid Salmonellae eg. S Cholera Suis may invade blood stream leading to generalised or localised infection presenting as PUO.

Focal infection may cause Osteomyelitis, Pyelonephritis, Arthritis, Meningitis, Cholecystitis, Endocarditis.

Investigations

First week - Blood cultures are positive

Second week - Weil Felix Test

Third week - Stool and urine cultures positive

Prevention & Control

Prevention of disease at farm level:

Disease control eg. Immunization of farm animals

Use of hygienic animal feeds

Ensuring sanitary environment for animals

Other approaches:

Hygienic slaughtering

Hygienic milking

Pasteurization of milk & eggs

Proper disposal of liquid & solid wastes

Cold storage

Health education & training

Dengue Syndrome

Caused by an Arthropod, it is a viral disease which may be:

1. Asymptomatic
2. Classical Dengue Fever
3. Dengue Hemorrhagic Fever
4. Dengue Shock Syndrome

Problem in the World

Globally 50 million Dengue infections annually, 500,000 with DHF require hospitalisation. 90% are children < 5years.

Mainly in Africa, Americas, Eastern Mediterranean, South East Asia, Western Pacific

Problem in India

Increased due to rapid urbanisation

Cases peak after monsoon

40,000 cases, 137 deaths in 2014, Case fatality rate 0.33%

States mainly affected - Maharashtra, Odisha, W Bengal, Karnataka, Tamil Nadu, Kerala, Gujarat

Epidemiology

Agent Factors

RNA virus

Agent – Den 1, 2, 3, 4 strains

Reservoir – Man – cases of DF

Transmission Cycle: Man – mosquito – man

Host factors

All ages

Both sexes

Immunity – Infection with one Dengue Serotype gives immunity against that serotype & partial protection against others.

International Air Travel – Contributes to worldwide dissemination of Dengue viruses

Environmental Factors

Rainy season

Temperature – Low temperature not favourable for mosquito breeding

Water scarcity

Inadequate Waste Management

Vector

Aedes Aegypti (main vector)
Aedes Albopictus
} Breeds in artificial collections of fresh water e.g. vases, plates below flower pots, water coolers; outside house – coconut shells, tyres. It is peridomestic, anthrophilous, day biting insect (tiger mosquito)

Mosquito becomes infected by feeding on patient from the day before onset to 5th day of illness (Viraemia Stage).

Extrinsic Incubation Period: 8–10 days, then mosquito becomes infective for life.

Transovarian Transmission.

Incubation Period

3–10 days

Clinical Features

Dengue Fever	DHF (Dengue Hemorrhagic Fever)	Dengue Shock Syndrome (DSS)
Break bone fever, high fever 39-40°C, chills, headache, Myalgia, Arthralgia, bone pain, Retroorbital pain, Photophobia. Also, extreme weakness, Anorexia, constipation, altered taste sensation, colicky pain, abdominal tenderness, sore throat Rash – Maculopapular or pin point on face, neck, chest on 3rd or 4th day. Fever - 5–7 days then complete recovery Case fatality rate low.	Severe form of Dengue Fever caused by >1 Dengue Virus; The first infection sensitises the patient, 2nd produces Immunological Catastrophe. High fever, headache, facial flushing. Anorexia, vomiting, Epigastric discomfort, generalised abdominal pain, tenderness right costal margin. Maculopapular rash less common. Pathophysiologic changes, Plasma leakage & abnormal Haemostasis. Clinical Diagnosis (a) Fever – Acute onset, high continuous lasting 2–7 days. (b) Hemorrhagic Manifestation – Positive Tourniquet Test (BP Cuff Method > 20 Petechiae per 2–5cm (1-inch) square Any of the following: - Petechiae, Purpura, Ecchymosis - Epistaxis, gum bleeding - Haematemesis &/or Malaena (c) Enlargement of Liver	Clinical Δ by: • All above criteria plus • Shock manifested by rapid weak pulse, narrowing pulse pressure hypotension, cold clammy skin, restlessness
Investigations DF Leucopenia WBC ≤5,000 cells/mm³ Thrombocytopenia Platelets <150,000 cells/mm³ Isolation of Dengue Virus 4-fold increased IgG, IgM Viral Antigen detection NS1	Grading of severity: Grade I – Fever, constitutional symptoms, Tourniquet Test Grade II – Spontaneous bleeding skin/other hemorrhages + Gr I manifestations. Grade III – Circulatory failure, pulse rapid, weak, narrowing of pulse pressure (≤20 mm Hg), Hypotension, cold clammy skin, restlessness. Grade IV - Profound shock with • Thrombocytopenia ≤ 100,000/mm³ • Haemoconcentartion Haemotocrit increase by 20% or more of basic value	

Primary Prevention

- Premises of houses to be cleared of small water containers (Breeding places of Aedes mosquito) eg. Broken glass bottles, tins, pots, discarded tyres, battery case, coconut shells, jars
- Water in animal water troughs, cisterns, barrels, drums etc should be emptied once a week (Weekly dry day method interrupts breeding of mosquitoes).
- Health education of community about Dengue Fever, its transmission & not to allow water puddles around houses.
- People advised to wear long sleeve shirts & apply DEET to exposed parts of the body.
- Dengue Vaccine - CYD-TDV Tetravalent live attenuated viral vaccine, 3 injections 0.5ml SC 6 monthly for 9-60 year-old people

Secondary Prevention

Rest
Antipyretics
Aspirin/NSAIDs contraindicated
Oral/IV fluids
Blood/Platelet Transfusion
Isolation of Cases - Under bed nets during first few days

Global Strategy for Dengue Prevention and Control 2012-2020

Goals

Reduce Dengue Mortality by 50% by 2020
Reduce Dengue Morbidity by 25% by 2020
Estimate true burden of disease by 2015

Strategy

Coordination and collaboration among multisectoral partners on Integrated Vector Management Approach
Sustained control measures at all levels

Malaria

Definition

Malaria is caused by the Plasmodium Group of Parasites transmitted to man by infected Female Anopheline Mosquito.

Problem in the World

Half the world's population is at risk of Malaria.
214 million cases; 438,000 deaths in 2015.
Sub-saharan Africa, Asia, Latin America, Middle East, parts of Europe are mainly affected.

Risk Groups: Young children, non-immune pregnant women, semi-immune pregnant women, semi-immune HIV infected pregnant women, HIV/AIDS persons, international travellers, immigrants and their children, poor underserved and marginalised populations, areas with poor health services.

Childhood deaths mainly from Cerebral Malaria and Anemia.

Problem in India

Major public health problem. Pl Falciparum main cause of deaths.

N Eastern states, Chattisgarh, Jharkhand, Madhya Pradesh, Odisha, West Bengal, Andhra Pradesh, Karnataka, Maharashtra, Gujarat, Rajasthan mainly affected.

Major Epidemiological Types

Tribal M	Rural M	Urban M	Project M	Border M	Forest M	Floods
Tribal areas	Rural Irrigated areas	Urban Poor sanitary conditions, low socio-economic groups	Construction Developmental Activities, Labourers non-immune, increased vector breeding, Chloroquine resistant Parasite	International or state borders Mixing population	Forests Temporary forest settlements, Malarial transmission difficult to control	Pools of water between floods and malaria 6-weeks
P Falciparum High morbidity, mortality High risk-Infants, young children, pregnant women, mobile population	P Vivax mainly P Falciparum during exacerbation					
Health infrastructure is limited	Health infrastructure moderately developed	Health infrastructure well developed	Health facilities limited	Poor administrative control		
Lack of drugs						

Agent Factors

Agent – P Vivax, P Falciparum, P Malariae, P Ovale

70% - P Vivax

25% - P Falciparum

4% - Mixed

1% - P Malaria (Tumkur, Hassan district in Karnataka)

P Ovale – Rare – Mostly in tropical Africa

Life History

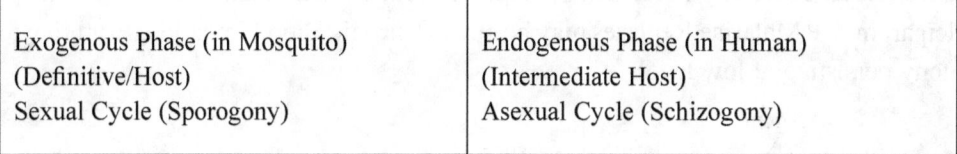

Exogenous Phase (in Mosquito) (Definitive/Host) Sexual Cycle (Sporogony)	Endogenous Phase (in Human) (Intermediate Host) Asexual Cycle (Schizogony)

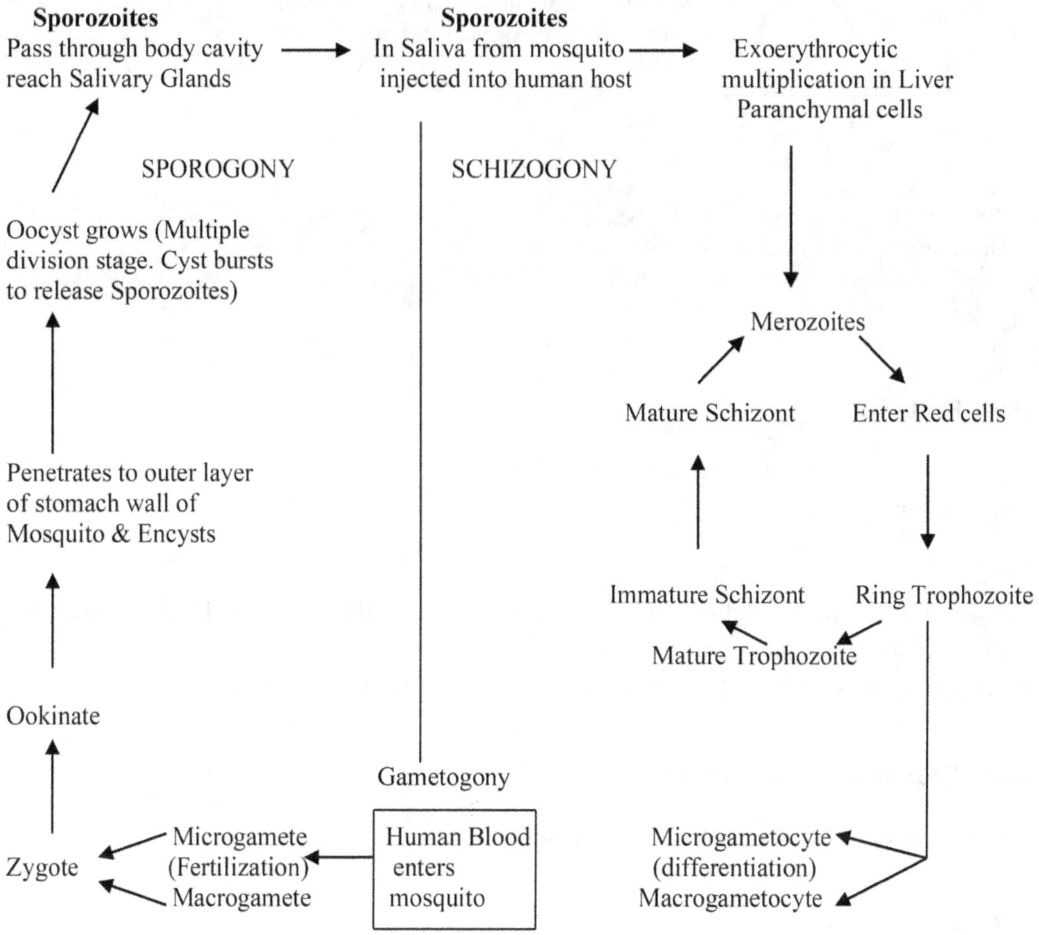

Sporozoites
Pass through body cavity ⟶ reach Salivary Glands

Sporozoites
In Saliva from mosquito ⟶ injected into human host

Exoerythrocytic
multiplication in Liver
Paranchymal cells

SPOROGONY

SCHIZOGONY

Oocyst grows (Multiple
division stage. Cyst bursts
to release Sporozoites)

Merozoites

Mature Schizont   Enter Red cells

Penetrates to outer layer
of stomach wall of
Mosquito & Encysts

Immature Schizont   Ring Trophozoite

Mature Trophozoite

Ookinate

Gametogony

Zygote

Microgamete
(Fertilization)
Macrogamete

Human Blood
enters
mosquito

Microgametocyte
(differentiation)
Macrogametocyte

Reservoir – Man – cases
Mosquito

Period of Communicability

Malaria is communicable as long as it is mature, viable Gametocytes exist in circulating blood in sufficient density to infect vector mosquitoes.

In Vivax infections – 5 days after appearance of Asexual Parasites.
In Falciparune Infections – 10 days after appearance of Asexual Parasites.

Relapses

In Vivax & Ovale, caused by Liver Schizonts which remained dormant.

In P Falciparum & P Malariae Replases may be due to Chronic Blood Infection, Erythrocyte Schizogony persisting at low level.

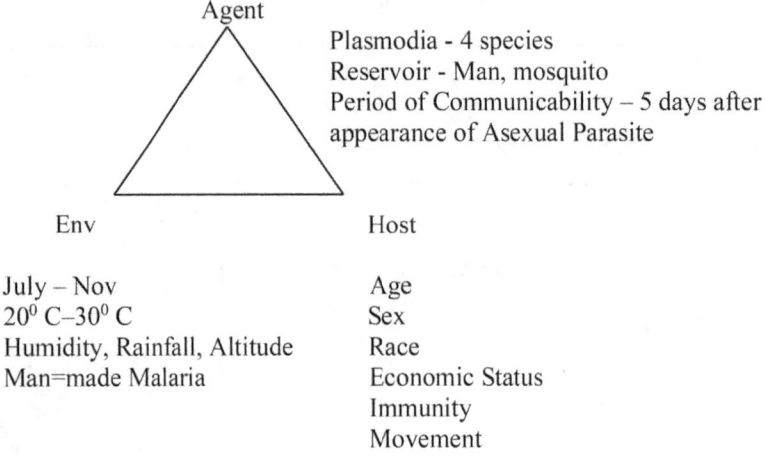

Agent

Plasmodia - 4 species
Reservoir - Man, mosquito
Period of Communicability – 5 days after appearance of Asexual Parasite

Env

July – Nov
20^0 C–30^0 C
Humidity, Rainfall, Altitude
Man=made Malaria

Host

Age
Sex
Race
Economic Status
Immunity
Movement

Host Factors

Age – All ages, Newborns' resistance to P Falciparum

Sex – M > F

Race:

People with AS Haemoglobin (Sickle Cell Trait), milder illness with Falciparum infection than those with normal (AA) Haemoblobin.

Persons whose red cells are Duffy negative, resistant to P Vivax Infection.

Socio Economic Development

Malaria has disappeared in most developed countries

Immunity

Immunity develops in the population where Malaria is Endemic.

Humoral & Cellular immunity present.

Infants born of immune mothers protected for 3–5 months by maternal IgG Antibody.

Active immunity is species specific, immunity against one strain does not protect against another.

Movement

People migrate from one country to another or from one part of a country to another.

Imported malaria is a public health problem in Europe, North America Labourers in various engineering, irrigation, agricultural projects, migration of nomads, tribes may import malarial parasites in their blood & reintroduce malaria to areas where it has been controlled or eliminated.

Housing

Ill ventilated, ill lighted houses

Occupation

Malaria is predominantly a rural disease related to agricultural practices.

Human Habits

Sleeping outdoors, no personal protection (bed nets), refusal for Spraying, replastering of walls after spraying.

Pregnancy

Increases risk of malaria. Malaria during pregnancy may lead to abortions, intrauterine death, premature labour.

Environmental Factors

Season: July to November
Temperature: 20^0C–30^0C
Humidity – 60%
Rainfall – Increases humidity therefore survival of mosquitoes, but heavy rainfall has adverse effect in flushing out breeding places.
Altitude – Anophelines not found > 2000–2500m.

Man Made Malaria

Burrow pits, garden pools, irrigation channels, engineering projects have led to mosquito breeding
& increase in malaria.
Malaria consequent on human undertakings is called Man-made Malaria.

Vector Bionomics

Rural Area – A. Culicifacies – Breeds in gentle flowing & stagnant water. Flight range 1-mile, causes Epidemic Malaria in project & irrigation areas
Urban Area – A. Stephansi, breeds in wells, cisterns, overhead tanks, causes Epidemic Malaria

Hilly Area – A. Fluviatitis, breeds in slow running water. Flight range ½ mile.

Sea Coast Area – A. Sundaicus, breeds in salt water

Tea Garden Area – A. Minimus, breeds in slow running water.

Water Logging Area – A. Phillipinensis, breeds where subsoil water level is high & in water stagnation between cracks of the soil.

Knowledge of Anopheline Biology essential for understanding Epidemiology of Malaria & its prevention.

Factors determining Vectorial importance of Mosquitoes:

(a) Density – Adequate density of mosquitoes required for transmission of disease. Each vector has a critical density below which effective transmission cannot be maintained.

(b) Life Span – Must be at least 10–12 days after an infective blood meal to become infective. Insecticides shorten the life span.

(c) Choice of Host – Anthrophilic – A. Fluviatilis, better vector of Malaria than A. Culicifacies.

(d) Resting Habits – Endophily – After blood meal mosquitoes rest indoors on walls. Residual spraying of Insecticides based on this knowledge.

Exophily – Some mosquitoes rest outdoors.

(e) Breeding Habits – A Stephansi breed in wells, cisterns, fountains, overhead tanks.

- A Fluvitilis breeds in moving water
- A Sundaicus breeds in brackish water

Knowledge of breeding habits is useful for Antilarval measures.

(f) Time of Biting – Anophelines have nocturnal feeding habits, between dusk & dawn.

(g) Vectorial Capacity – Combined effect of density, susceptibility to infection, life span and probability of feeding on man.

(h) Resistance to Insecticides – When there is DDT resistance, Malathion or Pyrethroids are used

Mode of Transmission

1. Vector Transmission – Infected Female Anopheline Mosquito with Sporozoites in Salivary Glands

2. Direct Transmission – Through IM or IV injections of blood or plasma eg. Blood transfusions, Malaria in drug addicts.

3. Congenital Malaria – Mother to child transmission leads to Congenital Infection of newborn.

Incubation Period

10 days between infective mosquito bite to fever.

Clinical Features

Paroxysms of fever correspond to development of parasites in RBCs.
Peaks of fever coincide with release of Merozoites into the blood stream.

Cold Stage – Lassitude, headache, nausea, vomiting, chills, rigors, Temperature 39–41° C
Hot Stage – Hot & dry skin
Sweating Stage – Fever comes down with sweating

Febrile Paroxysms occur with definite intermittent periodicity depending on species – Every 3rd day in Vivax & every 4th day in Malariae.

Splenomegaly & Secondary Anaemia
Complications of P. Falciparum Malaria – Cerebral Malaria, Blackwater Fever, Acute Renal Failure, Liver Damage

Diagnosis

BSMP – Blood Smear for Malarial Parasite
Thick film – For searching for Parasite   JSB stain
Thin film – Identifying species

Fluorescent Antibody Test – Used in Epidemiological Study to determine past infection
Rapid Dipstick Test to detect P. Falciparium

Measurement of Malaria

I Pre-Eradication Era

Magnitude of Malaria problem in the country is determined by:

(a) Spleen Rate - % of children 2–10 years showing enlargement of Spleen reflects endemicity of   malaria
(b) Average Enlarged Spleen
    Average size of enlarged spleen
(c) Parasite Rate - % of children 2–10 years showing Malarial Parasites in Blood Films
(d) Parasite Density Index - Indicates average degree of Parasitemia in a population
(e) Infant Parasite Rate -
    % of Infants (<1-year) showing Malaria Parasites in their Blood Films
    Most sensitive index of recent transmission of Malaria
    If Infant Parasite Rate is 0 for three consecutive years in a locality, it is regarded as absence of Malaria transmission even though Anopheline Vectors may remain.
(f) Proportional Case Rate - The number of cases diagnosed as Clinical Malaria for every 100 patients attending hospitals & dispensaries.

II Eradication Era

Microscopic Diagnosis main method of diagnosis

(a) Annual Parasite Incidence (API)

$$API = \frac{\text{Confirmed Cases during one year}}{\text{Population under surveillance}} \times 1000$$

(b) Annual Blood Examination Rate (ABER)

$$ABER = \frac{\text{No. of slides examined}}{\text{Population}} \times 100$$

WHO recommended 1% of population
In modified plan of operation minimum is 10% of population.
ABER is Index of Operational Efficiency.

(c) Annual Falciparum Incidence

$$AFI = \frac{\text{Confirmed cases of Falciparum during one year}}{\text{Population under surveillance}} \times 1000$$

(d) Slide Positivity Rate (SPR)
(e) Slide Falciparum Rate (SFR)

III Vector Indices

(a) Human Blood Index
     Proportion of freshly fed female Anopheline mosquitoes whose stomach contains human blood. Indicates degree of Anthrophilism.
(b) Sporozoite Rate
     The % of Female Anopheline with Sporozoites in their Salivary Glands.
(c) Mosquito Density
     Number of mosquitoes per man hour catch.
(d) Man – Biting Rate
     Average incidence of Anopheline bites per day per person determined by standardised Vector catches on human bait.
(e) Inoculation Rate
     Man Biting Rate x Infective Sporozoite Rate

Malaria Prevention & Control

Strategies

1. Surveillance
    (a) Case Detection (Active & passive)
    (b) Early Diagnosis and Treatment
    (c) Sentinel Surveillance

2. Integrated Vector Management
    (a) Indoor Residual Spray (IRS)
    (b) Insecticide treated Bednets (ITNs) & Long Lasting Insecticidal Nets (LLINs)
    (c) Antilarval measures including Source Reduction

3. Epidemic preparedness and Early Response

4. Supportive Interventions
    (a) Capacity Building
    (b) Behaviour Change Communication (BCC)
    (c) Intersectoral Collaboration
    (d) Monitoring & Evaluation
    (e) Operation Research & Applied Field Research

Treatment of Vivax Malaria

Chloroquine total 25mg/kg weight given as:

10mg/kg - Day 1

10mg/kg - Day 2

5mg/kg - Day 3

Primaquine 0.25mg/kg for 14days (Contraindicated in infants, pregnant, G6PD Deficiency)

Treatment of Falciparum Malaria (In states other than NE states)

Artemisinin based Combination Therapy (ACT-SP)

Artesunate (AS) - 50mg for 3 days

Sulfadoxine + Pyrimethanine (SP) - Day 1

(500 mg)   (25 mg)

Primaquine (PQ) 0.75mg/kg - Day 2

In North Eastern states

ACT-AL (Each Tab Artemether 20mg+Lumefantrine 20mg)

ACT-AL	5-14 kg 5m-3 yrs	15-24 kg 3-8 yrs	25-34 kg 9-14 yrs	>34 kg >14 yrs
Dose	20/120 BD for 3-days	40/240 BD for 3-days	60/360 BD for 3-days	80/480 BD for 3-days

Primaquine 0.75mg/kg on Day 2.

Treatment of Severe Malaria & Complicated Malaria

First 48 hours	Follow up
Quinine 20mg/kg on admission Followed by 10mg/kg 8-hourly infusion OR Artesunate 2.4mg/kgIV/IM 0, 12hrs & 24hrs then once/day OR Artemether 3.2mg IM on admission then 1.6mg/kg/day OR Arteether 150mg daily IM for 3days	Follow up 10mg/kg TDS with Doxy 100mg OD or Clindamycin pregnant & children < 8 yrs for 7 days Full course area specific ACT Other States ACT-SP for 3days PQ single dose Day 2 NE States ACT-AL 3days+ PQ Day 2

Dosage schedule for children

Pediatric Doses

Age (yrs)	Chloroquine	Primaquine
0 – 1	75 (1/2 tab)	Nil
1 – 4	150 (1 tab)	2.5
4 – 8	300 (2 tabs)	5.0
8 – 14	450 (3 tabs)	10
14 & above	600 (4 tabs)	15.0

Chemoprophylaxis

Chloroquine 300mg once a week starting 1-week before travel to Endemic Area to 4–6weeks after leaving Endemic Area.

Or

Sulphadoxine + Pyrimethamine combination 1 tab weekly.

Severe & Complicated Malaria – Artemisinine, Artesunate, Artemether, Artether IM/IV for 4–5 days

2. *Environmental Control*

Vector Control

(a) Antilarval Measures
   i. Larvicides – Oiling water collections, Paris Green, Temephos
   ii. Source Reduction – Techniques to reduce mosquito breeding sites – Drainage or filling, deepening or flushing, water level management, changing salt content of water, intermittent irrigation
   iii. Biological Methods – Guppy fish/Gambusia fish; Bacillus Thuringiensis in wells, irrigation channels

(b) Anti-Adult Measures
   i. Residual Spraying – Spraying indoor surfaces of houses with residual insecticides - DDT,

   Malathion, Fenitrothion
   ii. Space Spraying – Pyrethrum/Pyrethroid Spraying
   iii. Individual Protection

   Repellents, protective clothing, bed nets impregnated with insecticides, mosquito coils, screening of houses

(c) Integrated Vector Control Methods – Combined use of Bio-environmental, chemical & personal protection measures

3. *Protection of the Host*
   i. Keeping body well covered – Full sleeve shirts, socks
   ii. Sleeping under mosquito nets
   iii. Screening of windows & wire gauze doors
   iv. Applying mosquito repellents eg. DEET – Diethyltoluamide
   v. Spraying Pyrethrum & Synthetic Pyrethroids
   vi. Using electronic repellents
   vii. Antimalarial Vaccines

Sporozoites, Merozoites & Gametocytes are all antigenically distinct. Efforts are being made to develop vaccines against each of them.

Global Technical Strategy for Malaria (2016-2030)

2015 - World Health Assembly adopted it.

Target to reduce Global Malaria burden by 90% by 2030

Goals	Milestones		Targets
	2020	2025	2030
Reduce Malaria Mortality compared with 2015	40%	75%	90%
Reduce Malaria Incidence compared with 2015	40%	75%	90%
Eliminate Malaria from countries	10 countries	20	35
Prevent re-establishment of Malaria	Re-establishment prevented	Re-establishment prevented	Re-establishment prevented

Strategy

- Comprehensive Technical Guidance
- Increase investments for interventions
- Preventive measures
- Diagnostic Testing
- Treatment
- Disease Surveillance
- Innovations
- Research
- Strengthen Health Systems
- Address Multidrug Resistance
- Address Insecticide Resistance

Filaria

Lymphatic Filariasis caused by Wuchereria Bancrofti, Brugia Malayi, Brugia Timori and transmitted by mosquitoes.

Problem in World

It is a worldwide problem

Countries mainly affected are Africa, Asia, Western Pacific, parts of Americas.

Over 1-billion live in Endemic areas, 120 million are infected, 40 million overt disease - Lymphoedema, Hydrocele

Problem in India

It is a public health problem.

States mainly affected are Uttar Pradesh, Bihar, Jharkhand, Orissa, Andhra Pradesh, Tamil Nadu, Kerala, Gujarat

630 million at risk of infection, 12 lakh cases - Lymphoedema, Hydrocele

Epidemiology

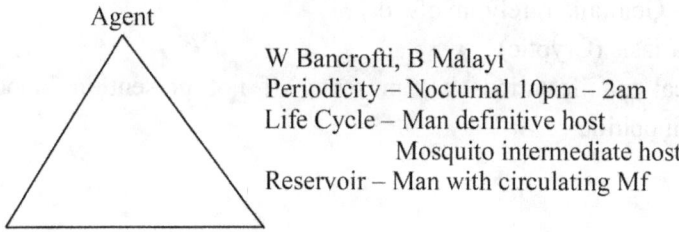

Agent

W Bancrofti, B Malayi
Periodicity – Nocturnal 10pm – 2am
Life Cycle – Man definitive host
　　　　　　Mosquito intermediate host
Reservoir – Man with circulating Mf

Environment

Temp 26–36⁰C

Humidity – 70%

Drainage – Bad

Lack of Town Planning

Mosquito Breeding

Cesspools, soakage pits,

Ill maintained drains

Septic tanks, open ditches,

burrow pits

Host

Age – All age

Sex – Males more

Immunity – Resistance to infection after many years

Migration – Movement of people leads to spread of disease

Social Factors – Urbanisation, industrialisation, migration,

illiteracy, poverty, poor sanitation

Vectors
C Quinquefasciatus for Bancroftian Filariasis
Mansonia for Brugian Filariasis

Mode of Transmission
By bite of infected mosquitoes

Type of Transmission
Cyclo-developmental

Incubation Period
8–16 months
Extrinsic Incubation period 10–14 days.

Clinical Manifestations
(a) Asymptomatic Amicrofilaraemia – Does not have Microfilaraemia nor Clinical Manifestation
(b) Asymptomatic Microfilaraemia – Asymptomatic, but Mf present in blood
(c) Stage of Acute Manifestations – Filarial Fever, Lymphangitis, Lymphadenitis, Lymphoedema of various parts of body, Epididymoorchitis in males

(d) Stage of Chronic Obstructive Lesions - Hydrocele, Elephantiasis, Chyluria, Brugian Filariasis – Genitalia rarely involved

(e) Occult Filariasis (Cryptic)

Classical clinical manifestations not present, Mf not present in blood. Eg. Tropical Pulmonary Eosinophilia

Filarial Survey

1. **Mass Blood Survey**
    i. Thick film
        Thick smear, blood collected between 8.30pm – 12 midnight.
    ii. Membrane Filter Concentration Methods (MFC)
        Most sensitive method, requires Venipuncture and filtering large volumes of blood
    iii. DEC Provocation Test
        Mf induced to appear in blood in daytime by administering Tab DEC 100mg & examining blood 1-hour later

2. **Clinical Survey**
    Clinical manifestations examined at the time of blood survey.

3. **Serological Tests**
    To detect antibodies to Mf using Immunofluorescent and Complement Fixing Techniques
    Detection of Parasite Antigens in patients' blood or urine

4. **Xenodiagnosis**
    Mosquitoes fed on patient & dissected 2 weeks later

5. **Entomological Survey**
    Mosquito collection from houses, dissection of female mosquitoes for detection of developmental forms of parasite, breeding places & bionomics of mosquitoes.
    Data assembled, analysed & results expressed as Clinical, Parasitological & Entomological parameters.

Assessment of Filaria Control Programme

Effect of Filarial Control Programmes assessed using Clinical, Parasitological & Entomological parameters

1. **Clinical Parameters**
    i. Incidence of Acute Manifestations
        Adenolymphangitis, Epididymoorchitis

ii. Prevalence of Chronic Manifestations
   Lymphoedema, Elephantiasis, Hydrocele, Chyluria

2. *Parasitological Parameters*
   i. Microfilaria Rate - % of persons showing Mf in peripheral blood.
   ii. Filarial Endemicity Rate - % of persons with Mf in blood/disease manifestations/both
   iii. Microfilarial Density – No. of Mf per unit vol (20cu mm) of blood.
   iv. Average Infestation Rate – Average No. of Mf per positive slide.

3. *Entomological Parameters*
   i. Vector Density per 10 man – Hour catch
   ii. % of mosquitoes positive for all stages of development
   iii. % of mosquitoes positive for infective (stage III) Larvae
   iv. Annual Biting Rate – For assessment of transmission
   v. Types of Larval breeding places.

1. Treatment for Uncomplicated Acute Dermato Lymphangio Adenitis (ADLA)
   (a) Analgesics eg Paracetamol 1g TDS/QDS
   (b) Antibiotics Amoxycillin 500 mg TDS/Oral Penicillin/Erythromycin for 8 days
   (c) Clean limb with Antiseptics
   (d) Check for wounds, cuts, abscesses, toes interdigital infection - Clean with Antiseptic, Antibiotic cream/Antifungal cream
   (e) Advice on prevention of Chronic Lymphoedema
   (f) Do not give Anti-filarial medication
   (g) Home Management - Drink plenty of water, rest, limb elevation, foot exercise, cooling the limb with cold water, washing the limb
   (h) Follow-up after 2 days. Refer to Physician if not improved.

2. Management of Severe ADLA
   (a) Refer to Physician - IV Benzyl Penicillin 5million units TDS/IM Procain Penicillin 5million units BD till fever subsides then Oral Phenoxymethylpenicillin (Pen V) 750mg-1g TDS for 8 days
   OR Erythromycin 1g TDS until fever subsides then Oral Erythromycin 1g TDS
   (b) Analgesics, Antipyretics eg Paracetamol
   (c) Do not give Anti-filarial medication
   (d) Surgery - Hydrocelectomy

Control Measures

   I. Chemotherapy
   II. Vector Control

Chemotherapy

- Dieethylcarbamazine 6mg/kg orally for 12 days in divided doses
- Mass Chemotherapy - Single dose with 2 drugs
- Albendazole 400mg + Ivermectin150-200mcg/kg once per year for 4-6 years
- DEC Medicated salt – Common salt medicated with 1-4g DEC per kg for 6-9 months
- Ivermectin 150-200 mcg/kg (Not used in India)

Vector Control

(a) Antilarval Measures - Sanitation and underground waste water disposal system
  Chemical control - Mosquito Larvicidal oil, Pyrosene oil E Organophosphorous (Temephos, Fenthion)
  Removal of Pistia plant, or using Herbicides eg. Shell Weed Killer
  Minor environmental engineering methods - Filling ditches, cesspools, drainage of stagnant water, maintenance of septic tanks
(b) Anti-adult Measures - Pyrethrum space sprays, Malathion
(c) Personal protection - Mosquito nets, screening, DEET, mosquito coils, mats
(d) Integrated Vector Control

Criteria for Control

WHO has fixed following criteria as indicators of adequate control:

- Mf rate should be < 5% in a community
- Children aged 1–10 years should be free from Microfilaria Infection

Zika Virus Disease

Mosquito borne Flavivirus disease

Problem in World

Countries affected mainly are Africa, Americas

India

Disease not reported in India
Mosquito - Aedes Aegypti

Agent

Zika Virus, Flavivirus

Mode of Transmission

Bite of infected Aedes mosquito

Clinical Features

Fever, skin rash, conjunctivitis, muscle and joint pain, malaise, headache 2-7 days
H/O travel to Endemic Areas

Diagnosis

PCR
Virus isolation from blood

Treatment

Mild - No treatment
Severe cases - Rest, plenty of fluids, Paracetamol for pain, fever
No vaccine available

Prevention

Aedes control:

(a) Source Reduction
(b) Insecticides
(c) Personal Protection

Kyasanur Forest Disease (KFD)

Zoonotic Febrile Disease with Hemorrhages caused by Arbovirus Flavivirus transmitted by Infective Ticks

Problem in India

Areas mainly affected are Shimoga district, North Karnataka, South Karnataka, Chikamagaloor Districts with 400-500 cases yearly

Epidemiology

Agent Factors

KFD Virus - Group B, Flavivirus
Reservoir – Rats, squirrels
Birds, bats
Monkeys – Amplifying hosts
Cattle – Important for maintaining Tick populations
Man – Dead end host (No part in transmission)

Host Factors:

Age – 20-40 years

Sex – Males > females

Occupation – Cultivators who visit forests accompanying cattle or cutting woods

Environmental Factors:

Season - Jan–June (Peak Nymphal activity of Ticks)

Forest activity

Vectors

Hard Ticks – Haemaphysalis – H. Spinigera &

H. Turtura

Mode of Transmission

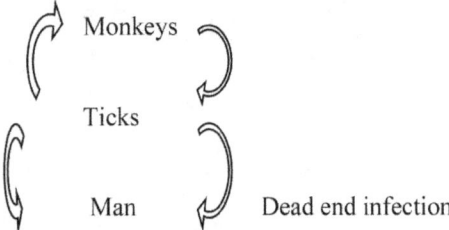

Monkeys

Ticks

Man   Dead end infection

Incubation Period

3–8 Days

Clinical Features

Fever, headache, severe Myalgia, Prostration, GI disturbance, Hemorrhages from nose, gums, stomach, intestine, Meningoencephalitis, mental disturbances, death

Case Fatality Rate - 5–10%

Investigations

Virus in blood

Serological Evidence

Control

1. Control of Ticks

Spraying operations

Power equipment or aircraft mounted equipment for dispensing Carbaryl, Fenthion, Propoxur at 2.24kg/hectare.

Spraying of **"hot spots"** areas where monkey deaths have been reported within 50m.

2. *Vaccination*

KFD Vaccine for population at risk

3. *Personal Protection*

Adequate clothing

Insect repellents Dimethyl Phthalate (DMP), DEET

Remove Ticks from body everyday

Health Education to discourage sitting or lying on ground

Surveillance

Karnataka Government has established surveillance system for monitoring cases & deaths due to KFD and monkey deaths

Japanese Encephalitis

It is a Zoonotic Disease caused by Group B Arbovirus (Flavivirus) and transmitted by Culex mosquitoes.

Problem in World

Countries mainly affected are Asia, Western Pacific, Bangladesh, India, Nepal, Pakistan, Thailand, Vietnam

Incidence <10 to >100/100,000 population yearly

68,000 cases globally per year, mostly children <15 years, 20,400 deaths

Problem in India

States mainly affected are Assam, Bihar, Haryana, UP, W Bengal, Karnataka, Tamil Nadu

About 8,000 cases and 1,100 deaths in 2015

Epidemiology

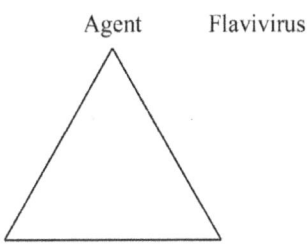

Agent   Flavivirus

Environment   Host   All susceptible

C Tritaeniorhynchus   Both sexes

C Vihsnui

Pig

Ardeid bird

Agent Factors

Agent – Flavivirus (Arbovirus Group B)
Reservoir – Pigs
Ardeid birds, Herons, Egrets, Ducks

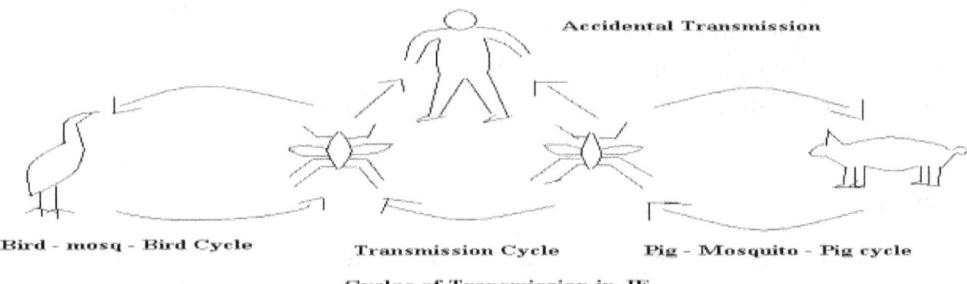

Cycles of Transmission in JE

LifeCycle

Period of Communicability

Viraemia in man is short lived therefore, no man-to-man transmission
Viraemia in birds 2–5 days.
Mosquitoes, once infected, remain infective lifelong.

Host Factors

All ages, more common < 15 years
Both sexes

Environmental Factors

It is mostly a Rural disease
Irrigated rice fields & ponds with vegetation breed the Culex mosquito
Pigs – Amplifier hosts
Cattle – Mosquito attractants
Only horses – Manifest the disease

Incubation Period

5–15 days
Extrinsic Incubation period
9–12 days

Vectors

C Tritaeniorhynchus ⎤
C Vishnui   ⎦ Generally breed in irrigated rice fields, ponds, shallow ditches, pools

Mosquitoes are Zoophilic

Female mosquitoes get infected after feeding on Viraemic host & after 9–12 days within the Extrinsic Incubation period can transmit virus to other hosts.

JE in man

After incubation period of 5–15 days, man may develop the disease.

For every overt case there are 300-1,000 subclinical cases (Tip of the iceberg)

Number of cases per village 1–2

i. Prodromal Stage

Acute onset – Fever, headache, malaise

ii. Acute Encephalitic Stage

High fever 38–40^0 C, Nuchal Rigidity, Focal CNS Signs, convulsions, Altered Sensorium, coma

iii. Late Stage & Sequelae

Temperature, ESR – Normal, neurological signs stationary or improve, Residual Neurological Deficit sometimes. 1/3 of cases die, 1/3 improve, 1/3 with residual deficit. Danger Signs - Fever with lethargy, unconsciousness, convulsions, paralysis, hypotension, feeble pulse, poor respiratory effort, Cyanosis

Investigations

Serology – Significant rise in Antibody Titre

Treatment

Fever- Sponging, paracetamol

Convulsions - Anticonvulsants

Secretions - Suction

Nil orally

Position patient - Prone/Semi-prone with head on one side

O$_2$

IV Fluids

Mannitol

Input - output Chart

Temperature, Pulse, Respiratory Rate (TPR), BP monitoring

Control

(i) Vectors

Mosquitoes controlled by

Antilarval measures – Filling up ditches, intermittent drainage, Gambusia fish in ponds.

Anti-adult measures - Insecticidal control for houses & animal Shelters

Spraying Malathion, Fenitrothion & for outside bushes & marshes by ultra-low volume (ULV) spraying of Malathion/Pyrethrum

Spraying of uninfected villages within 2–3 kms radius of infected village

Personal protection – Bed nets, DEET

ii. Vaccination

For high-risk groups & children < 15 years
Formalin Inactivated Mouse Brain JE Vaccine
3 doses, 1 ml (0.5ml < 3 years age) SC at intervals of 7–14 days between first and second doses
& 6 months between 2nd & 3rd doses, booster every 3 years.
Vaccination should be done during the Interepidemic Period
Vaccination of Pigs (Swine) is important in public health
It prevents Viraemia & hence eliminates their role as amplifiers of the virus

Rabies (Hydrophobia)

A Zoonotic disease, an acute fatal viral disease of CNS caused by Lyssavirus Type 1, transmitted by dogs and wild animals.

Global Picture

World – Rabies Free countries are Australia, New Zealand, Taiwan, Japan, Cyprus, Ireland, UK, Malta, Western Pacific, Finland, Norway, Sweden & Liberian Peninsula, Iceland, Andaman & Nicobar, Lakshadweep
(Water – A natural barrier to rabies)

Rabies is present in > 150 countries.
Rabies in dogs is the source of 99% of human infections.
Annually 55,000 deaths in Africa and Asia

Indian Picture

3 million dog bites
20,000 deaths

Epidemiology

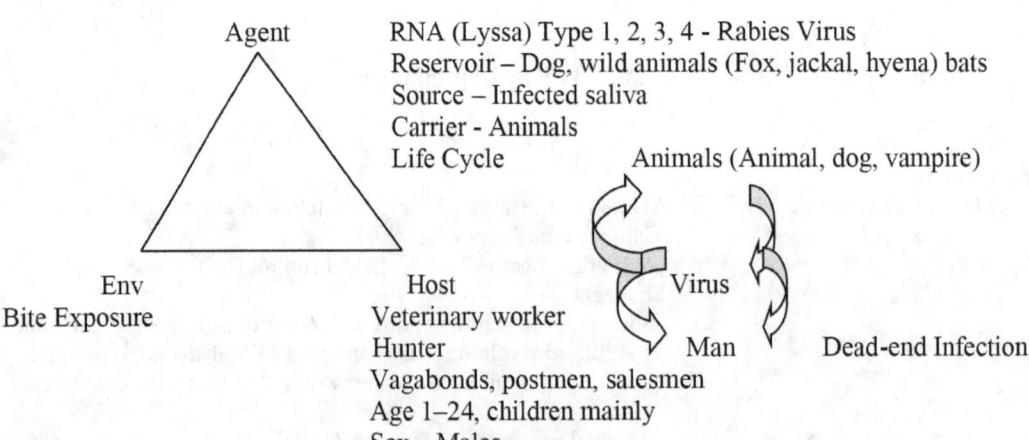

Agent   RNA (Lyssa) Type 1, 2, 3, 4 - Rabies Virus
         Reservoir – Dog, wild animals (Fox, jackal, hyena) bats
         Source – Infected saliva
         Carrier - Animals
         Life Cycle   Animals (Animal, dog, vampire)

Env   Host   Virus
Bite Exposure   Veterinary worker
                   Hunter   Man   Dead-end Infection
                   Vagabonds, postmen, salesmen
                   Age 1–24, children mainly
                   Sex – Males

Mode of Transmission

(a) Animal Bites – Dog bites, others – Cat, monkey, horse, sheep, goat
(b) Licks – Licks on abraded skin & mucosa
(c) Aerosols – Aerosol (Respiratory) transmission in caves with infected bats & in laboratory during Homogenisation of infected animal brains
(d) Person–to-Person – Rare (Child biting parents)

Incubation Period

2 weeks – 2 months
Depends on site of bite, number, severity, amount of virus injected, species of biting animal, protection provided by clothing & treatment undertaken.

Clinical Features

Prodromal – Fever, headache, malaise, sore throat
Sensory System – Intolerant to noise, bright light, cold, draught of air
Motor System – Hyperreflexia, muscle spasms
Sympathetic System – Pupillary Dilatation, Lacrimation, Salivation, Perspiration
Mental – Fear of death, anger, irritability, depression
Hydrophobia (Pathognomonic) – Mere sight/sound of water may provoke spasm of muscles of Deglutition
Aerophobia (Pathognomonic) - Fear of air – Fanning a current of air across the face causes violent spasms of Pharyngeal & Neck muscles.

Duration of illness - 2–3 days
Patient may die during convulsions or pass into Paralysis or Coma.
Intensive care may allow occasional patient to survive; To date 3 have survived.

Diagnosis

  i. Clinical – H/O Dog bite and symptoms & signs
 ii. Laboratory – Viral Isolation from Saliva
-    Negri bodies demonstration from brain

Treatment

Isolation in dark, silent room
Sedatives eg. Morphine
Muscle Relaxants eg. Curare like drugs
Supportive Therapy – IV Fluids
Intensive Therapy – Respiratory & Cardiac support

Vaccines

1. Nervous Tissue Vaccine – Now not recommended by WHO
2. Duck Embryo Vaccine (Has the risk of allergy)
3. Cell Culture Vaccine
   HDCV (Fibroblast cell)
   Non-Human (Dog kidney, chick embryo fibroblast)

Post Exposure Treatment

1. General
   Treated as a medical emergency
   Active and passive Immunization
2. Local
   (a) Wash wound
   Immediate flushing, washing with soap & water, catheters to irrigate punctured wounds
   (b) Chemical Treatment
   Virucidal agents – Alcohol, Tincture Iodine, Povidone Iodine
   Quaternary Ammonium Compounds (Eg. Savlon, Cetavlon) **NOT** recommended
   (c) No Immediate Suturing
   Bite wounds should not be sutured immediately to prevent spread of virus into deeper tissues.
   If suturing necessary, should be done only 24–48 hours later; To be done under Antirabies Serum locally
   (d) Local ARS/HRI
   Local application of Antirabies Serum around the wound or Human Rabies Immunoglobulin. ½ around wound, ½ IM
   (e) Antibiotic Treatment
   Antibiotic Medication
   (f) Antitetanus Treatment
   Tetanus Toxoid
   (g) Observation of Dog
   Observation of Dog/Animal for 10 days to estimate risk of infection

Wound Classification

Class I – Licks, scratches, unboiled milk consumption
(Slight risk)

Class II – Licks on fresh cuts, scratches with oozing of blood, all bites except on head, face, neck,
(Moderate risk), palms, fingers, minor wounds < 5

Class III – All bites, scratches with oozing of blood on head, face, neck, palms, fingers; lacerated wounds

(Severe risk) on any part of body; multiple wounds ≥ 5; bites from wild animals

Cell Culture Vaccine

A. IM schedule

6 doses IM 1ml each on days 0, 3, 7, 14, 28 & booster on day 90 in Deltoid (Not into Buttock)

Advantage – Efficacy, safety

Disadvantage – Cost

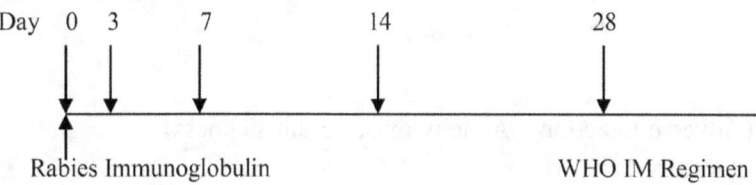

Rabies Immunoglobulin   WHO IM Regimen

B. Intradermal Schedule

(PVRV, PCECV, PDEV)

(Purified Vero Cell Vaccine, Purified Chick Embryo Cell Vaccine, Purified Duck Embryo Vaccine)

(a)   2–Site Intradermal Schedule

Multisite Intradermal vaccination used in India.

2 – 2 – 2 – 0 – 1 – 1   5 doses ID 0.1 ml.

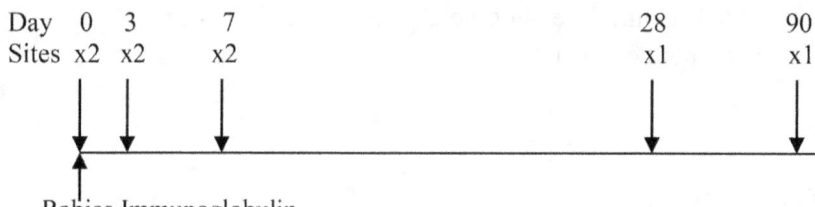

Rabies Immunoglobulin

(b)   8-Site Intradermal method (HDCV, PCECV)

Day 0 - 0.1 ml reconstituted vaccine given at 8 sites.

Deltoid, Lateral Thigh, Lower quadrant of Abdomen, Suprascapular Region

On Day 7 - 0.1 ml at 4 sites over Deltoid, Thighs

Day 28 - 0.1 ml at 1 site

Day 90 - 0.1 ml at 1 site

8 – 0 – 4 – 0 – 1 –1

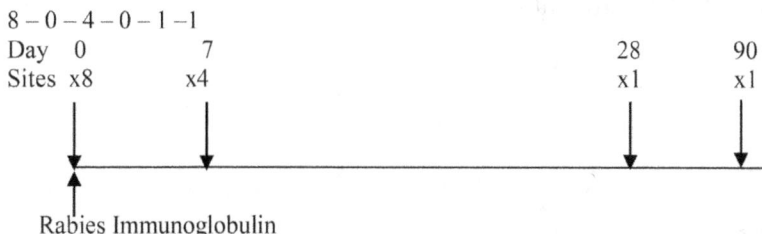

Rabies Immunoglobulin

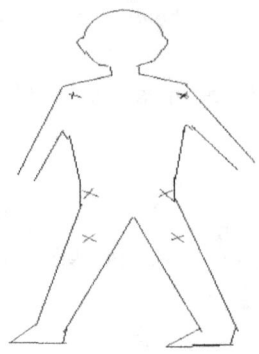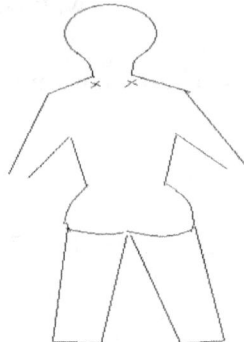

Anti-Rabies Serum

ARS (Horse) 40 IU/kg (Adverse Reaction – Anaphylaxis, Serum sickness)
HRI (Human) 20 IU/kg ½ locally & ½ IM

Pre-Exposure Prophylaxis

Indications – Occupations – Lab staff, Veterinarian, animal handlers, wild life officers
Cell Culture Vaccine – 1 ml IM or 0.1 ml ID on Day 0, 7, 28; Boosters at 2 yearly

Post Exposure Treatment of Persons who have been vaccinated previously:

Antibody Titre unknown – HDC Vaccine 1 ml IM day 0, 3, 7
Antibody Titre known – (>0.5 IU/ml), bite not severe, 2 doses – Day 0, 3
Passive Immunization should not be given

Rabies in Dogs

There are 2 types of manifestations:

(a) Furious Rabies – Furious type, behavioural change, running amuk, voice paralysis
(b) Dumb Rabies – Quiet, sleepiness stage, dies

Lab Diagnosis

Suspected dog's head sent to lab packed in ice, air tight container
If brain sent, should be in 50% Glycerol Saline

Dog Vaccine

5 ml single dose
2nd dose at 6th month
Revaccination once a year

Control of Rabies – Public Health Measures

Stray dogs – Elimination of stray dogs

Pet dogs – Registration, licensing, compulsory immunization, muzzling of pet dogs

- Destruction of dogs & cats bitten by rabid animals
- 6 months quarantine for imported dogs
- Health Education on Rabies and its prevention
- Oral vaccine placed in baits for oral vaccination of foxes, wild animals

Yellow Fever

A Zoonotic disease caused by Arbovirus transmitted to man by Culicine, Aedes mosquitoes
Mostly Tropical America & Africa are affected.

Epidemiology

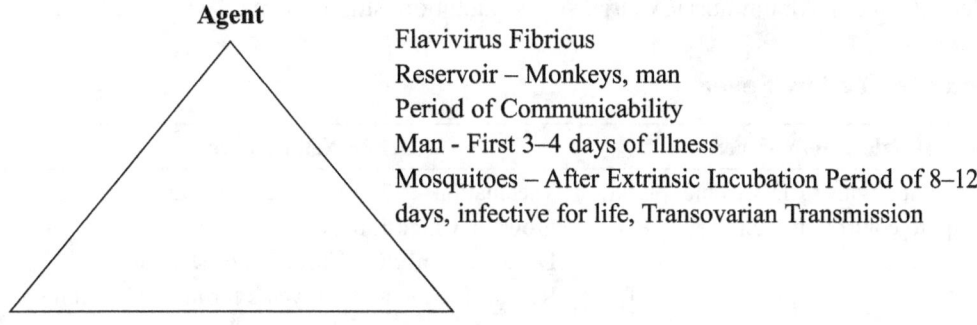

Agent

Flavivirus Fibricus
Reservoir – Monkeys, man
Period of Communicability
Man - First 3–4 days of illness
Mosquitoes – After Extrinsic Incubation Period of 8–12 days, infective for life, Transovarian Transmission

Env
Temp >24o C
Humidity > 60%
Global Travel, Urbanisation

Host
All Ages
Both sexes
Occupation – Wood cutters, hunters
Immunity - Life long

Modes of Transmission

   i. Jungle Cycle (Sylvan)

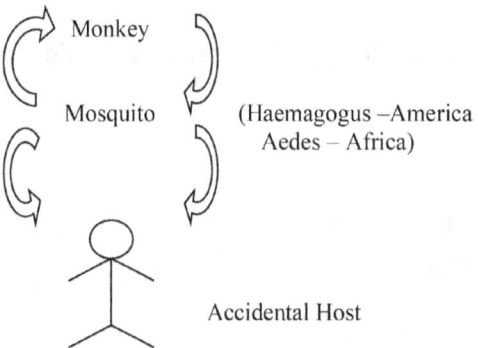

Monkey

Mosquito   (Haemagogus –America
                 Aedes – Africa)

Accidental Host

ii. Urban Cycle

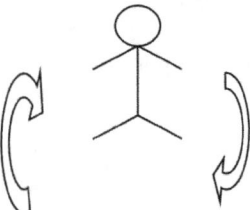

Mosquito (Aedes)

Incubation Period

3–6 days (International Health Regulations – 6 days)

Clinical Features

Viral Hemorrhagic Fever, severe cases - Jaundice, Hemorrhagic Manifestations (Hematemesis, Malena, Estaxis), Albuminuria/Anuria, shock, agitation, stupor, coma

Control of Yellow Fever

Jungle Yellow Fever	Urban Yellow Fever
Vaccination with 17 D Vaccine Mosquito control difficult	1. Vaccination – 17 D Vaccine, live attenuated vaccine grows in Chick Embryo Dose – 0.5 ml SC at insertion of Deltoid Re-vaccination after 10 years for international travel 2. Vector Control – Aedes mosquito - Antilarval measures – Source Reduction, artificial collections of fresh water - Anti-adult measures – Space sprays - Personal Protection – Repellents, mosquito nets, coils, Fumigation mats, screening 3. Surveillance – Clinical, Serological, Histopathological, Entomological

Surveillance

Aedes mosquitoes – Aedes Aegypti Index
The % of houses & their premises in an area showing breeding of Aedes Larvae should not be > 1% in towns & seaports

Yellow Fever-International Measures

India is Yellow Fever receptive area ie. Area where Yellow Fever does not exist but conditions permit its development if introduced because:

1. Susceptible Population (Unvaccinated)

2.   Vector – Aedes Aegypti Abundant
3.   Monkey (Macacus) is susceptible to Yellow Fever

Virus could be imported in 2 ways:

  i.   Infected travellers (Clinical & Subclinical cases)
  ii. Through infected mosquitoes

International Health Regulations

1.   *Travellers*
Vaccination for travellers exposed to risk of Yellow Fever or passing through Endemic zones.
International certificate of Vaccination

India and most countries require valid certificate of vaccination eg. Yellow Fever for travellers coming from infected areas. If no certificate, traveller is quarantined for 6 days from date of leaving infected area.

2.   *Mosquitoes*
Aerosol spraying with insecticides for:
Aircraft & ships from Endemic areas for destruction of Vectors
Airports & seaports kept free from breeding of Vectors in 400 m.
Aedes Aegypti Index kept < 1

Chikungunya Fever

Dengue like disease caused by GpA Arbovirus, transmitted by Aedes, Culex, Mansonia mosquitoes.
Mainly transmitted by Aedes.

Problem in the World

Subsahara Africa, India, Asia

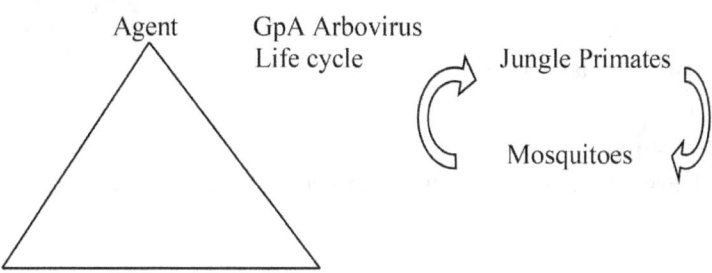

Agent   GpA Arbovirus
               Life cycle   Jungle Primates

                                   Mosquitoes

       Env   **Host**
Rainy season   All ages
Aedes, Culex, Mansonia mosquitoes.   Both sexes

Incubation Period:

4–7 Days

Clinical Features:

Fever, chills, Cephalalgia, Conjunctivitis, Lumbago, Anorexia, Adenopathy, rash, occasionally Purpura on trunk & limbs, Petechiae, coffee-coloured vomiting, Epistaxis.

Arthropathy – Chikungunya is a Tanzanian word meaning 'doubling up due to excruciating joint pain'. Pain, swelling, stiffness of Metacarpophalangeal, wrist, elbow, shoulder, knee, metatarsal joints from 3-5 days after onset of clinical symptoms & which can persist for months or years.

Investigations

Virus isolation from blood by Intracerebral Inoculation in Suckling Mice or VERO cells.

Serologic Diagnosis - Paired Sera rise in Antibody Titre in acute & convalescent Sera & ELISA can detect IgM.

RT – PCR or Nested PCR Technique for rapid diagnosis

Control

(a)   Vector Control
Aedes Aegypti control – Antilarval measures – Source reduction.
Community participation to eliminate breeding places eg. Coconut shells, tyres, tin cans.
Changing water once a week in vases, refrigerators, water coolers.

Insecticide Abate applied on sand granules

-    Antiadult measures
2 ULV spraying with Malathion or Sumithion, 10 days apart

-    Personal Protection
Wearing long sleeved clothes, DEET, mosquito coils, mats, screening.

(b)   Vaccine
No vaccine developed as yet.

Brucellosis (Undulant Fever, Malta Fever, Mediterranean Fever)

A Zoonotic Bacterial disease.

Problem in World

There is worldwide distribution wherever cattle, pigs, goats and sheep are reared.

Epidemiology

Agent Factors

Agent – Brucella Melitensis – Most virulent
　　　　B Abortus - Affects cattle
　　　　B Suis - Affects pigs
　　　　B Canis - Affects dogs
Reservoir – Cattle, sheep, goats, swine, buffaloes, horses, dogs
Source – Milk, urine, placenta, uterine & vaginal discharges

Host Factors

Adults
Males
Occupation – Farmers, shepherds, butchers, abattoir workers, veterinarians, laboratory workers
Immunity – Follows infection

Environmental Factors

Rainfall high
Lack of sunlight
Unhygienic practices in milk & meat productions, overcrowding of herds

Modes of Transmission

1. Contact Infection – Direct contact with infected tissues, blood, urine, vaginal discharge, aborted fetuses, placenta. Infection through abraded skin, mucosa or conjunctiva
2. Food Borne Infection – Indirectly by ingestion of raw milk or dairy products (cheese) from infected animals, fresh raw vegetables, contaminated water
3. Air Borne Infection – Infected dust from cowshed, slaughter houses, laboratories

Incubation Period

1 to 3 weeks.

Clinical Features

Fever - 40–41^{0}C, Rigors, sweating, headache, insomnia, Arthralgia or Arthritis involving larger joints (Eg. Hip, knee, ankle, shoulder)

Low back pain
Splenomegaly, Hepatomegaly
Leucopenia with relative Lymphocytosis

Investigations

Blood culture, bone marrow culture, exudates
Biopsy specimens
Serological tests

Control

In Animals	In Humans
(a) Test & slaughter Mass surveys with Skin Test or CFT. Cases slaughtered	(a) Early Δ & Rx Tetracycline 500 mg QDS for 3 weeks. Inj SM IM for cases with skeletal or other complications with Tetracycline.
(b) Vaccination Vaccination with strain 19 BA (B Abortus) for heifers yearly. Vaccination with B Melitensis for goats & sheep.	(b) Vaccination Human live vaccine of B Abortus Strain 19-BA
(c) Hygienic measures Sanitary environment for animals Sanitary disposal of urine, faeces Veterinary care of animals HE of occupationally involved persons	(c) Hygienic measures Farmers, shepherds, milkmen, abattoir workers should observe personal hygiene. Protective clothing, hand washing, exposed areas of skin washed. Soiled clothing removed. Care in handling placenta & disposal of foetus & discharges from aborted animal
	(d) Pasteurization of Milk Pasteurization/boiling of milk

Leptospirosis (Weil's disease)

A Zoonotic disease caused due to Leptospira (Spirochaete), transmitted through rats to humans resulting in clinical manifestation from inapparent infection to fulminant, fatal disease.

Problem in the World

>500,000 cases annually

Epidemiology

Agent Factors

Agent – Leptospira (Spirochaetes)
Source – Urine of infected rodents, animals
Reservoir – Rats, mice, voles, cattle, sheep, goats, water buffalo, pigs, horses, dogs

Host Factors

Age - Children get the infection from dogs
Occupation – Agricultural workers, livestock farmers, workers in rice fields, sugar cane fields, underground sewers, abattoir workers, meat & animal handlers, veterinarians. Leisure activities eg. swimming, fishing
Immunity –Follows infection

Environmental Factors

Environment contaminated by urine & faeces from carrier (reservoir) animal or infected animals, poor housing, limited water supply, inadequate waste disposal method, rural & urban slums, rainfall with floods.

Modes of Transmission

1. Direct Contact – Urine or tissue of infected animal, Leptospira can enter through Skin Abrasions or Intact Mucosa Membrane.
2. Indirect Contact – Through contact of broken skin with contaminated soil, water or vegetation or ingestion of food, water contaminated with Leptospirae
3. Droplet Infection – Through inhalation of air polluted with droplets of urine eg. When milking infected cows or goats

Incubation Period

1–2 weeks

Clinical Features

Fever, headache, Jaundice, Renal Dysfunction, Albuminuria, vomiting, abdominal pain, Purpura Haemorrhagic, Aseptic Meningitis.

Weil's Syndrome - Severe Leptospirosis causing Jaundice, Renal Dysfunction, Hemorrhagic Diathesis.

Diagnosis

Darkfield examination
Blood culture in 1st wk
Urine culture 2nd week onwards

Serological tests – Indirect Haemagglutination,
Immunofluorescent Antibody
ELISA – IgM ELISA in early diagnosis
Lepto Dipstick Test available

Control

1. Antibiotics – Penicillin, Tetracycline, Doxycycline
2. Preventing exposure to contaminated water
3. Protection of occupationally exposed population by providing protective clothing (Gum boots, gloves, aprons)
4. Prevention of environmental contamination by proper disposal of animal excreta
5. Rodent control in rural, urban, recreational areas, sugarcane field, rice field
6. Health awareness to occupationally exposed population about modes of transmission, avoidance of contaminated sources of water & protective clothing
7. Vaccination – Immunization of farmers & pets

Rickettsial Diseases

A Communicable Zoonotic disease caused by Rickettsial Organisms & transmitted to man by Arthropod Vectors (except Q fever)

Diseases	Rickettsial Agent	Insect Vectors	Mammalian Reservoirs
1. Typhus Group			
(a) Epidemic Typhus	R Prowazekii	Louse	Humans
*b. Murine Typhus	R Typhi	Flea	Rodents
*c. Scrub Typhus	R Tsutsugamushi	Mite	Rodents
2. Spotted Fever Group			
*a. Indian Tick Typhus	R Conorii	Tick	Rodents, dogs
(b) Rocky Mt. Spotted fever	R Rickettsia	Tick	Rodents, dogs
(c) Rickettsial Pox	R Akari	Mite	Mice
3. Others			
*a. Q fever	C Burnetii	Nil	Cattle, sheep, goats
(b) Trench fever	Rochalimaea Quintana	Louse	Humans

* Present in India.

Also serve as Arthropod Reservoir by maintaining Rickettsiae through Ovarian Transmission.

Clinical Features

Except Q fever (No skin lesion)
All others – Fever, headache, malaise, prostration, skin rash, Splenomegaly, Hepatomegaly

Diagnosis

Clinical features and

(a) Isolation of Rickettsia
(b) Serological Tests – IFA, CFT, Weil Felix Reaction
                ELISA, Fluorescent Antibody Staining

Treatment

Tetracycline
Doxycycline, Minocycline

Control

  i. Treatment with Tetracycline
 ii. Control of Vector – (BHC, Malathion)
iii. Rodent control
 iv. Vaccination

Murine Typhus

Agent – Rickettsia Typhi
Reservoir – Rats (Rattus Ratus, R Norvegicus)
Vector – Fleas (X Cheopis) once infected, remains so for life, Transovarian Transmission

Mode of Transmission

Rat ⟶ Rat flea ⟶ Rat ⟶ Rat flea ⟶ Rat
           ↓
          Man

Incubation period

1–2 weeks

Clinical features

As above

Control measures

As above
No vaccine

Scrub Typhus

Agent

Rickettsia Tsutsugamushi

Reservoir

Mite, rodents
Transovarian Transmission

Mode of Transmission

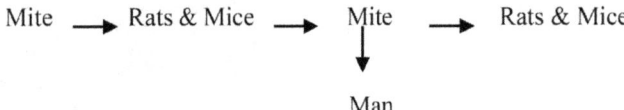

Incubation Period
1-2 weeks

Clinical Features

As above &
Eschar – Punched out ulcer with Black Scab, location of mite bite

Diagnosis

Weil Felix strongly positive with Proteus strain OXK

Control

As above
No vaccine

Indian Tick Typhus

Agent

Rickettsia Conorii

Reservoir

Tick (Transovarian Transmission)
Rodents, dogs

Mode of Transmission

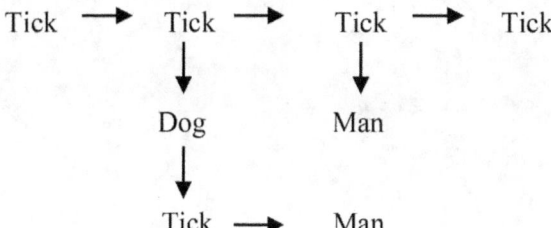

Incubation Period

1 week

Clinical Features

As above
+
Eschar

Control Measures

As above

Q Fever

Agent

Coxiella Burnetii

Reservoir

Cattle, sheep, goats, ticks

No vector
No rash

Mode of Transmission

(a) Respiratory route – Inhalation of infected dust from soil contaminated by urine/faeces of diseased animals
(b) Direct through Abrasions, Conjunctivae
(c) Ingestion of Contaminated foods – Meat, milk, milk products

Incubation Period

2–3 weeks

Clinical Features

As above
No rash
No local lesion

Control Measures

As above
+
Vaccines under development

Taeniasis (Tapeworm)

These are Parasitic Zoonoses.

Problem in the World

T Saginata - Africa, Eastern Mediterranean, Russia, Europe, India, Asia, Japan
T Solium - Latin America, Africa, Asia, Europe, Russia, India

Epidemiology

Agent Factors

Agent   i.   Taenia Saginata
          ii.   Taenia Solium

Host Factors

Hosts of Infection

Parasite	Definitive Host	Intermediate Host
1. T Saginata	Man	Cattle (C Bovis)
2. T Solium	Man	Pig (C Cellulosae)

Environmental Factors

Poor Sanitation
Unsafe Water
Lack of Food Hygiene

Mode of Transmission

(a)   Ingestion of Infective Cysticerci in undercooked beef or pork
(b)   Ingestion of food, water or vegetables contaminated with eggs
(c)   Reinfection through Retroperistalsis from bowel to stomach

Incubation period

2 – 3 months

Clinical Features

Majority no symptoms
Sometimes abdominal discomfort, Anorexia, Chronic Indigestion; Appendicitis, Cholangitis
Serious Complication – Cysticercosis
Eggs of T Solium in contaminated water or food or auto infection causes Human Cysticercosis
Intestine → Hepatic Portal System → Throughout body develop into Cysticerci

Neurocysticercosis – Cysticerci in CNS lead to space occupying lesion causing Epilepsy, increased Intracranial Tension, Hydrocephalus, Psychiatric Disease, death

Control

(a) Treatment of Patients
     Praziquantel – 10 mg/kg body weight, single dose
     Niclosamide – 2g (4 tabs), single dose
     For Cysticercosis
     Albendazole 400 mg BD for 2–4 weeks with fatty meal
     Praziquantel 50mg/kg/day in 3 divided doses for 2 weeks
(b) Meat Inspection
(c) Health Education on   i.   Transmission of disease
                            ii.   Handwashing
                           iii.   Proper cooking of beef/pork
                            iv.   Prevent pollution of soil, water, food with human faeces
(d) Proper sewage disposal
(e) Safe water

Hydatid Disease (Dog Tapeworm)

Parasitic Zoonoses caused by Metacestode Stage of Canine Tapeworm Echinococcus. Adult worms found in dogs and other carnivores.

Problem in the World

Global public health problem in sheep rearing countries – Australia, Tasmania, New Zealand, Middle East, Turkey, Greece, Russia, Cyprus, Latin America, Far East

Problem in India

Highest prevalence in Andhra Pradesh, Tamil Nadu

Epidemiology

Agent Factors

Agent – Echinococcus Granuloses
Life Cycle

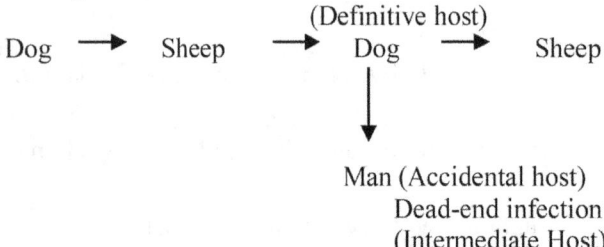

Dog – Sheep Cycle
Dog - Goat
Dog - Cattle
Dog – Camel

Host Factors

Children affected
Pets – Dogs, cats
Occupational Disease – Shepherds, shoe–makers

Environmental Factors

Poor sanitation
Unsafe water
Indiscriminate disposal of offal & carcasses

Mode of Transmission

(a) Ingestion of eggs of Echinococcus with food, unwashed vegetables or water contaminated with faeces from infected dogs
(b) Ingestion of eggs while handling/playing with infected dogs eg. Hand to mouth transfer of eggs or inhalation of dust contaminated with infected eggs

Incubation Period

Months to years

Clinical features

Cysts in Liver (R lobe) mainly
Other areas – Lungs, brain, peritoneum, kidney, long bones
Cysts Asymptomatic if small size
Large size cause pressure symptoms – Jaundice in Liver

Diagnosis

Clinical – H/O residence in Endemic area
Close association with dogs

Presence of slow growing Cystic Tumour

X- ray
U/S
CT Scan
Serological Tests – Indirect Immunofluorescent Test, ELISA, Casoni Test

Treatment

Surgical removal of Cysts – Risk of Anaphylactic shock if there is a spillage
Mebendazole

Prevention & Control

1. Preventing dogs from gaining access to raw offal at slaughter houses, farms & to dead animals i.e. Control of slaughter houses, meat inspection, destruction of infected viscera
2. Control of dogs
   Elimination of stray dogs, reduction of dog population, dog registration system, surveillance of dogs – Periodic stool examination, isolation & treatment of infected dogs
3. Health Education
   Health Education of the community especially dog owners, butchers, shepherds, animal breeders

Leishmaniasis (Kala Azar)

It is a Protozoal disease caused by Leishmania & transmitted to man by bite of Female Phlebotomine Sandfly

Problem in the World

Africa, Central America, South America, Asia, Mediterranean regions, India, Bangladesh, Nepal, Brazil, Ethiopia, Sudan.
Rural communities in India, Bangladesh, Nepal.
200,000-400,000 Visceral Leishmaniasis annually

Problem in India

Kala Azar (Visceral Leishmaniasis) in Bihar, Jharkhand, West Bengal, UP, Tamil Nadu
Cutaneous Leishmaniasis – North Western states, Amritsar to Kutch & Gujarat plains
Zoonotic Cutaneous Leishmaniasis – Rajasthan
Anthroponotic Cutaneous Leishmaniasis – Bikaner city

Epidemiology

Agent factors

Agent   L Donovani – Kala Azar
        L Tropica – Cutaneous Leishmaniasis
        L Braziliensis – Mucocutaneous Leishmaniasis

Reservoir – Indian Kala Azar - Man only reservoir (Non-Zoonotic Disease)
Animal reservoirs –Dogs, jackals, foxes, rodents, other mammals

Host Factors

All ages, peak between 5–9 years
M > F
Socio-economic status – Poor
Occupation – Farmers, forest workers, miners, fishermen
Population Movement – Migrants, labourers, tourists
Immunity – Infection gives lifelong immunity

Environmental Factors

Season – 2 peaks – November & March-April during & after rains
Altitude – Plains affected; does not occur > 2000 ft.
Rural areas

Vector

P Argentipes (Kala Azar)
P Papatasi, P Sergenti (Cutaneous Leishmaniasis)

Sandflies breed in cracks, crevices in soil, buildings, overcrowding, ill ventilation, tree holes, caves, accumulation of organic matter

Only females bite
Development Projects
Forest clearing, cultivation projects, colonization & resettlement programmes

Mode of Transmission

- Transmitted from person to person by bite of Female Phlebotomine Sandfly
- Contact by contamination of bite wound when insect is crushed during act of biting

Incubation Period

1–4 months
Extrinsic IP 6–9 Days

Clinical Features

(a) Kala Azar – Fever, Splenomegaly, Hepatomegaly, Anemia, darkening of skin of face, hands, feet, abdomen (Kala Azar = Black sickness). High mortality
PKDL – Post Kala Azar Dermal Leishmaniasis multiple nodular infiltrations of skin, Parasites numerous in Lesions

2. Cutaneous Leishmaniasis
Anthroponotic or Urban Cutaneous Leishmaniasis
Zoonotic or Rural Cutaneous Leishmaniasis
Diffuse Cutaneous Leishmaniasis
Painful ulcers on legs, arms, face (Exposed parts)

3. Mucocutaneous Leishmaniasis
Ulcers around margins of mouth, nose
Mutilate the face, victims may become social outcasts

Lab Diagnosis

1. Parasitological Diagnosis
Parasite LD bodies in aspirates of spleen, liver, bone marrow, lymph nodes, skin

2. Aldehyde Test

3. Serological Tests
ELISA Test
Direct Agglutination Test (DAT)
Rk 39 Dipstick Test
Indirect Fluorescent Antibody Test (IFA)

4. Leishmanin Test
Intradermal Test 0.1ml on forearm & read 48–72 hours later
Induration ≥ 5mm Positive: Distinguishes immune from non-immune person
Negative in active phase of Kala Azar

5. Haematological Tests
Leucopenia, Anemia, ESR increased
Reversed AG Ratio

Control

1. Control of Reservoir
Active & Passive case detection & treatment
Inj. Sodium Stibogluconate 20 mg/kg x 20 days, or
Pentamidine Isethionate 3mg/kg x 10 days.
If animal reservoirs present – Dog, Rodent Control Programmes

2. Sandfly Control
   (a) Insecticide DDT 1-2g/sq m in human dwellings, animal shelters & resting places; BHC, if resistant to DDT.

    (b) Sanitation – Elimination of breeding places
        Cracks in mud or stone walls, rodent burrows, removal of firewood, bricks or rubbish around houses, cattle sheds & poultry at distance from human dwellings
3.   Personal Prophylaxes
    (a) Avoid sleeping on floor
    (b) Use fine mesh nets around bed
    (c) Insect Repellants - DEET
    (d) Keeping environment clean
4.   Health Education

Trachoma (Preventable Blindness)

Chronic infectious disease of Conjunctiva, Cornea caused by Chlamydia Trachomatis

Problem in the World

Major preventable blindness.
1-9 million with visual impairment
1-2 million irreversibly blind
200 million at risk of infection

Epidemiology

Agent – C Trachomatis

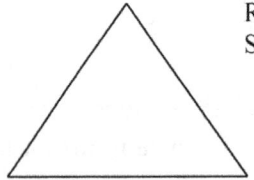

Reservoir – Children, adults
Source – Ocular Discharges, Fomites

Enviroment

Season – April-May; July-Sept – Fly season
Poverty, poor personal hygiene
Poor environmental hygiene, overcrowding

Custom – Kajal/Surma application

Host

Age – Children
Sex – Both in children; F > M in adults
Predisposing Factors – Sunlight, dust, smoke

Mode of Transmission

Direct contact with Ocular Discharges
Indirect Contact – Fomites eg. Infected fingers, towels, kajal/surma
Mechanical Transmission – Flies

Incubation Period

1–2 weeks

Clinical Features

Trachoma Infection – May undergo spontaneous resolution, or
Complications   – Inward deviation of eye lashes (Trichiasis)
                      – Inward deviation of lid margin (Entropion)
Corneal Ulcers
Corneal Scar
Blindness

Diagnosis

1. Follicles on the Upper Tarsal Conjunctiva
2. Limbal Follicles, Herbert's Pits
3. Conjunctival Scarring (Trichiasis, Entropion)
4. Vascular Pannus

Control

1. Assessment of problem
2. Trachoma is controlled with SAFE Strategy:
    S - Surgical treatment of Inturned Eyelids (Trichiasis, Entropion)
    A - Antibiotic application – Tetracycline ointment, Erythromycin ointment, Blanket Therapy/selective treatment
    F - Facial cleanliness, personal hygiene
    E - Environmental sanitation – Cleanliness of house, surroundings & control of Eye Gnats
3. Surveillance
4. Health Education
5. Evaluation

Tetanus

It is an Acute Bacterial disease caused by Clostridium Tetani Exotoxin

Problem in the World

Rare in developed countries
Maternal and Neonatal Tetanus are important preventable causes of maternal and neonatal mortality in developing countries by Maternal Immunization with TT, Aseptic Obstetric practices and Umbilical Cord care practices.

India

Maternal and Neonatal Tetanus has been eliminated in India

Strategies:
- Acceleration of TT Immunization coverage
- Strengthening routine Immunization of pregnant women
- Supplemental TT Immunization of women of child bearing age
- Promotion of institutional delivery
- Intensive Communication Program regarding 7 cleans
- Distribution of Disposable Delivery Kit (DDK) to skilled birth attendants

Epidemiology

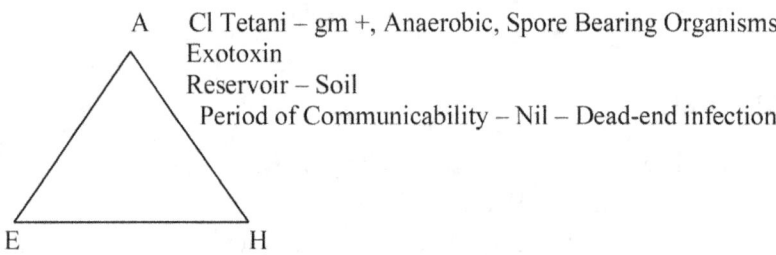

A   Cl Tetani – gm +, Anaerobic, Spore Bearing Organisms
     Exotoxin
     Reservoir – Soil
     Period of Communicability – Nil – Dead-end infection

E	H
Poverty	Age – 5-40 years, neonatal
Custom – Animal dung to wounds, Umbilical cord	Sex M>F; Puerperal Tetanus F
	Occupation - Agriculture
Delivery practices – Unsterile	Rural > Urban
Lack of Primary Health Care Services	Immunity - After Active Immunization

Mode of Transmission

Contamination of wounds with Tetanus Spores

Incubation Period

6–10 days

Clinical Features

Muscular Rigidity
Painful Paroxysmal Spasms
Masseters – Trismus or Lock Jaw
Facial muscles – Risus Sardonicus
Muscles of back, neck – Opisthotonus
Muscles of lower limbs & abdomen

Types

i.   Traumatic – Even from trivial wounds
ii. Puerperal – Postabortal, Pospartal by unsterile delivery practices

iii. Otogenic – Foreign bodies – Infected pencils, matches, beads
iv.   Idiopathic – Microscopic Trauma, Inhaled Spores
v.   Tetanus Neonatorum – 85% mortality, infection of umbilical stump due to cow dung application

Prevention of Tetanus After Injury

Wound cleaning
Wounds should be thoroughly cleaned.
Removal of foreign bodies, soil, dust, Necrotic tissue
(Anaerobic conditions favour germination of Tetanus Spores)

Immunization
Recommendations for prevention of Tetanus

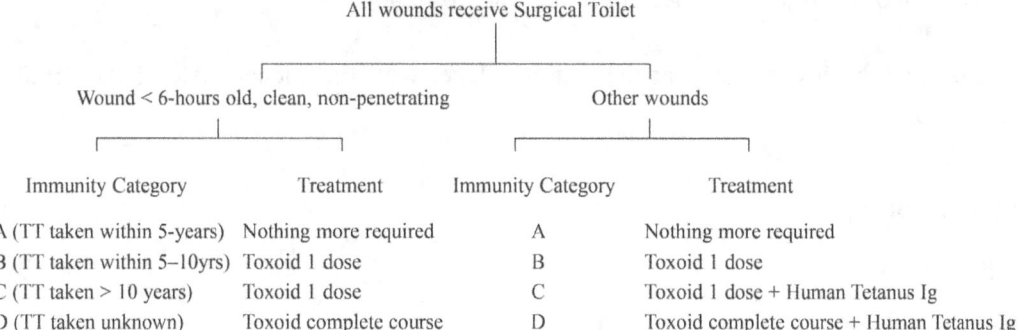

All wounds receive Surgical Toilet			
Wound < 6-hours old, clean, non-penetrating		**Other wounds**	
Immunity Category	Treatment	Immunity Category	Treatment
A (TT taken within 5-years)	Nothing more required	A	Nothing more required
B (TT taken within 5–10yrs)	Toxoid 1 dose	B	Toxoid 1 dose
C (TT taken > 10 years)	Toxoid 1 dose	C	Toxoid 1 dose + Human Tetanus Ig
D (TT taken unknown)	Toxoid complete course	D	Toxoid complete course + Human Tetanus Ig

Antibiotics

Penicillin or Erythromycin

Prevention

1. Active Immunization
    DPT/Pentavalent
    TT
2. Passive Immunization
    Human Tetanus Immunoglobulin   250-500 IU
    ATS (After Test Dose)   1500 IU
3. Active & Passive Immunization
4. Antibiotics – Benzathine Penicillin 1-2 mega units, or
    Erythromycin Estolate 500mg QDS x 7 days will kill vegetative forms of Cl Tetani
5. Neonatal Tetanus Prevention
    (a) TT in pregnancy
    (b) 7 cleans
    (c) Trained Birth Attendants

Leprosy (Hansen's Disease)

A Chronic infectious disease caused by M Leprae, affects mainly peripheral nerves. Also affects skin, muscles, eyes, bones, testes, internal organs

Problem in the World

Prevalence decreased from 2.1 cases/10,000 to 0.29/10,000
                    (1985)   (2015)
Eliminated from 119 out of 122 countries where it was a Public Health Problem.

Problem in India

It is widely prevalent but is unevenly distributed.
Prevalence of 57/10,000 has been decreased to <1/10,000.

Leprosy has been eliminated at the National level with Prevalence Rate of 0.69/10,000 population.

Epidemiology

Agent Factors

Agent - M Leprae
Source - Cases
Portal of Exit – Nose, skin
Infectivity – Highly infectious; low pathogenicity
Attack Rate - 4-12%

Host Factors

All ages
M > F
Migration - Rural to urban
Immunity - Cell Mediated and Humoral Immunity
Genetic - HLA linked genes influence type of response

Environmental Factors

Humidity
Overcrowding, Poor Housing, poor ventilation

Social Factors – Close contact, poverty, lack of education, lack of personal hygiene, prejudices, social stigma, social ostracism

Mode of Transmission

1. Droplet Infection
2. Contact Transmission - Direct skin-to-skin
   Indirect – Contact with soil, fomites (clothes, linen)
3. Others - Breast milk, Insect Vectors, Tattooing Needles

Incubation period

Long incubation period of 3 to 5 years

Classification

Indian Classification	Madrid Classification	Ridley-Jopling
Indeterminate type	Indeterminate	
Tuberculoid type	Tuberculoid	Tuberculoid (TT)
Borderline type	Borderline	Borderline Tuberculoid (BT)
Lepromatous type	Lepromatous	Borderline (BB)
Pure Neuritic type		Borderline Lepromatous (BL)
		Lepromatous (LL)

Indian Classification	Skin Lesion	Bacteriology
Indeterminate Type	1-2 Vague Hypopigmented Macules + Sensory Impairment	–
Tuberculoid Type	1-2 well defined Lesions, flat/raised; Hypopigmented/Erythematous, Anaesthetic	–
Borderline Type	> 5 Lesions, flat/raised, well/ill defined, Hypopigmented/Erythematous Sensory Impairment/loss	+/-
Lepromatous Type	Numerous flat/raised, ill defined	+
Pure Neuritic Type	Only Nerve involvement	–

Clinical Features

i. Hypopigmented patches
ii. Partial/total loss of sensation
iii. Thickened nerves
iv. Acid fact Bacilli in skin/nasal smears
   Signs of advanced disease - Nodules on skin of face & ears, Plantar ulcers, loss of fingers or toes, nasal depression, foot drop, claw toes

Diagnosis

  i.   Clinical examination
  ii. Bacteriological examination
 iii. Biopsy
 iv. Histamine Test

Bacteriological examination
Skin smears, nasal smears examined

Bacterial Index

Negative	No Bacilli in 100 fields
One plus (+)	One or < 1 Bacillus in each microscopic field
Two plus (++)	Bacilli found in all fields
Three plus (+++)	Many Bacilli found in all fields, add G if Globi present

Smears from 7 sites - R ear, L ear, nasal smear, 1st, 2nd, 3rd & 4th skin lesions

$$\text{Bacterial Index} = \frac{\text{Totaling the positives}}{\text{Number of sites}}$$

Paucibacillary BI= <2
Multibacillary BI= >2

Morphological Index

Solid Staining Bacilli:
Uniform staining of entire organism, Parallel sides, Rounded ends, Length 5 times the width
MI = % of Solid Staining Bacilli

Histamine Test

Detects the early-stage peripheral nerve damage.
Method 0.1ml of 1:1000 solution of Histamine Phosphate/Chlorohydrate Intradermally into Hypopigmented patches/Anaesthetic areas.
Wheal & flare in normal persons, but in Leprosy, Flare Response absent because nerve supply is destroyed.

Advantage - Can be used for Diagnosing Indeterminate Cases.

Lepromin Test (similar to Tuberculin Test in TB)

Method - Intradermal Injection 0.1ml Lepromin into Forearm
Reaction read at 48 hours and 21 days

Early Reaction	Late Reaction
Fernandez Reaction	Mitsuda Reaction
Inflammatory Response (redness, induration) within 24-48 hours	Appears after 1 week and maximum in 3-4 weeks
Test +ve if Red Area Diameter > 10mm	Test read at 21 days, positive >5mm nodule
Indicates - Sensitised to Leprosy Bacilli	Indicates Cell Mediated Immunity

Lepromin Test is not a diagnostic test

It is a useful tool in evaluating Immune Status (CMI) of cases

Helps in classification of the disease

Helps in estimating prognosis:

Lepromin –ve - Risk of progressive MB Leprosy

Lepromin +ve – Escape clinical disease or develop PB Leprosy

Sexually Transmitted Diseases & Reproductive Tract Infections

Syndromic Management of Sexually Transmitted Infections & Reproductive Tract Infections

Urethral Discharge/ Burning Micturition in Males	Genital Ulcers	Inguinal Bubo	Scrotal Swelling
Causative Organisms N Gonorrhoea C Trachomatis T Vaginalis	T Pallidum (Syphilis) H Ducreyi (Chancroid) H Simplex (Genital Herpes) K Granulomatis (Granuloma Inguinale) C Trachomatis	C Trachomatis (LGV) H Ducreyi (Chancroid)	N Gonorrhea Cl Trachomatis
History Urethral discharge Burning micturition Increased frequency Sexual exposure	Genital Ulcer/Vesicles Sexual exposure	Swelling Inguinal Region Preceding H/O Ulcer/discharge Fever, malaise Sexual exposure	Scrotal region swelling, pain Burning micturition/ pain Fever, malaise Sexual exposure
Examination: Redness, swelling Urethral Meatus Urethral discharge	Vesicles Genital Ulcer single/ multiple Inguinal Lymph Node	Lymph Node enlargement Skin over swelling Inflamed Multiple sinuses Presence of Genital Ulcer/Urethral Discharge	Scrotal swelling Skin overlying redness, oedema Tenderness Epididymis, Vas Associated Urethral discharge/Genital Ulcer/Inguinal Lymph Nodes

Lab Investigation: Gram stain – gm -ve Intracellular Diplococcic, Nongonococcal Urethritis >5 Neutrophils/ oil immersion field 1000x/ >10 Neutrophils/high power field	RPR for Syphilis Further Investigation Refer to higher centres	Diagnosis on clinical grounds	Gram Stain Non-Gonococcal Urethritis >5 Neutrophils/ oil immersion field 1000X/ >10 Neutrophils/High Power Field
Treatment: T Cefixime 400mg single dose +T Azithromycin 1g orally under supervision Advise to return after 7days If symptoms persist treat for T Vaginalis T Secnidazole 2g orally If symptoms persist refer to higher centres Partner treatment	Syphilis, Chancroid Inj Benzathine Penicillin 2.4million IU IM after TD/Doxy100mg BD 14 d+T. Azithro 1g orally single dose or T Cipro 500mg orally BD 3days (Chancroid) T Acyclovir 400mg orally TDS 7days (Herpes) Treat all partners	**Bubo should not be incised** Cap Doxy 100mg BD 21days (LGV) + T Azithro 1g orally single dose Or T Cipro 500mg orally BD for 3days (Chancroid) Partner treatment	Gonococcal + Chlamydial Infection T Cefixime 400mg BD 7 days + Cap Doxy 100mg BD 14 days Supportive Therapy (Bedrest, Scrotal elevation with T Bandage + Analgesics) Partner treatment

Vaginal Discharge in Women	Pelvic Inflammatory Disease in Women	Management of Oral & Anal STI
Causative Organisms **Vaginitis** T Vaginalis Candida Albicans G Vaginalis, Mycoplasma causing Bacterial Vaginosis (BV) **Cervicitis** N Gonorrhea C Trachomatis T Vaginalis H Simplex	N Gonorrhea C Trachomatis Mycoplasma Gardnerella Anaerobic Bacteria	N Gonorrhea C Trachomatis T Pallidum (Syphilis) H Ducreyi (Chancroid) K Granulomatis (G Inguinale) H Simplex (Genital Herpes)
Menstrual history to rule out pregnancy	Lower abdominal pain Fever	Unprotected oral sex with Pharyngitis

Discharge, amount, smell, colour, Genital Itching Burning micturition, increased frequency Ulcer, swelling, Vulval/ Inguinal Genital complaints in sexual partners Low backache	Vaginal discharge Menstrual irregularities -Heavy/irregular Dysmenorrhoea Dyspareunia Dysuria, Tenesmus Low backache Contraceptive use - IUCD	Unprotected anal sex with Anal discharge/Tenesmus Diarrhea, blood in stools Abdominal cramp, nausea, bloating
Examination: Speculum Examination -Vaginitis/Cervicitis	GE – Temperature, pulse, BP Speculum Examination Vaginal, Cervical discharge/ congestion/ulcers Abd Tenderness, Guarding Pelvic exam - Uterine/ Adnexal Tenderness	Oral ulcer, Pharyngeal Inflammation, General/Anorectal Ulcers -Single/multiple Vesicles Rectal Pus
Lab Investigations: Wet Mount Microscopy (TV) 10% KOH (CA) Gram Stain (Gonococci)	Wet Smear Examination Gram Stain - Gonococci CBC, ESR Urine microscopy	RPR/VDRL (Syphilis) Gram stain of Rectal Swab - gm-ve Intracellular Diplococcic (Gonorrhoea)
Treatment (TV+ BV+ Candida) **Vaginitis** T Secnidazole 2g orally single dose/T Tinidazole 500mg orally BD 5 days T Fluconazole 150mg orally single dose/local Clotrimazole **Cervicitis** Gono+ Chlamydia T Cefixime 400mg orally single dose+T Azithromycin 1g before lunch Partner treatment	N Gonorrhea, C Trachomatis, Anaerobes T Cefixime 400mg BD 7 days+ Cap Doxy 100mg BD 2 weeks+ T Metronidazole 400mg BD 2 weeks T Ibuprofen 400mg TDS 3-5 days T Ranitidine 150mg BD Remove IUCD if present Abstinence during treatment Partner treatment	T Azithromycin 1g+ T Cefixime 400mg+ Anti-diarrhoeal medicines Partner treatment

AIDS

Acquired Immuno Deficiency Syndrome (AIDS) – A fatal illness caused by the Human Immunodeficiency Virus (HIV) which breaks down the body's immune system therefore, the victim is vulnerable to life threatening opportunistic infections, Neurological Disorders or malignancy. AIDS refers to the last stage of the HIV infection.

Epidemiology

Modern pandemic since 1980s in developed and developing countries
People living with HIV 36.7 million; Adults 34.9 million; Children 1.8 million
Deaths 1.1 million; Adults 1.0 million; Children < 15years 110,000

India

People living with HIV - 2.1 million
Deaths   - 67,600

Epidemic shift from high-risk group (CSW, homosexual males, drug users) to bridge population (clients of sex workers, STD patients, migrant population, population in conflict areas, partners of drug users) to general population.

Prevalence	States
High Prevalence States	Karnataka, Tamil Nadu, Andhra Pradesh, Maharashtra, Manipur, Nagaland High Risk Group >5%; ANC 1%
Moderate Prevalence States	Gujarat, Goa, Pondicherry High Risk Group >5%; ANC < 1%
Low Prevalence States	Other States High Risk Groups < 5%; ANC <1%

Agent Factors

(a) Agent - HIV1, HIV 2
     Easily killed by heat; Inactivated by Ethanol 20%, Ether, Acetone, Beta Propiolactone
     Relatively resistant to ionizing radiation and UV light.
(b) Reservoir
     Cases, Carriers
(c) Source of Infection
     Blood, Semen

Host Factors

Age 20-49
Sex M>F

High Risk Groups
Male homosexuals, bisexuals, heterosexuals, IV drug users, transfusion recipients of blood and blood products, hemophiliacs, clients of STDs

(d) Occupation
     Truck drivers

Environmental Factors

Socio cultural practices eg. Belief that sex with virgin cures STDs; Homosexuality
Peer pressure
Poverty
Low educational status

Mode of Transmission in India

Transmission	%
Heterosexual	88.2
Parent to child	5
Injecting drug users	1.7
Homosexual	1.5
Blood & blood products	1
Unknown	2.7

Incubation Period

Few months – 10 years

Clinical Features

1. Initial Infection
2. Asymptomatic Carrier State
3. AIDS Related Complex (ARC)
4. AIDS

1. *Initial Infection*
   Mild illness (Fever, sore throat, rash) in some, most are Asymptomatic and look healthy though HIV positive and can transmit infection to others.
   HIV Antibodies appear 2-12 weeks in blood stream.
   "Window Period" is before Antibodies are produced, it is a highly infectious stage because high concentration of virus is in the blood, though he will test negative on standard antibody blood test.
   The Antibodies to HIV do not inactivate the virus.

2. *Asymptomatic Carrier State*
   Infected people have Antibodies but no signs of disease except persistent generalised Lymphadenopathy.

3. *AIDS Related Complex*
   Person with ARC have illnesses caused by damage to the immune system but without opportunistic infections and cancers;

May have persistent Diarrhea > 1month

Weight loss > 10%

Fever

Mild opportunistic infections eg Oral Thrush

Generalised Lymphadenopathy

Enlarged spleen

Diagnosis - 2 or more of above manifestations

+ decreased T Helper Lymphocytes

4. *AIDS*

End stage of HIV infection

Opportunistic Infections - TB, Candidiasis, Cryptococcus Meningitis, Pneumocystis Carinii Pneumonia,

T Gondi Encephalitis, Cytomegaloviral Retinitis, Herpes Zoster and Cancer - Kaposi's Sarcoma

It is a wasting disease therefore called "Slim disease" in Africa.

CD4 count < 200

Diagnosis

1. WHO case definition for AIDS surveillance (2 Major + 1 Minor for adult/children > 12 years)

Major Signs:

Weight loss $\geq$ 10% of body weight

Chronic Diarrhea > 1 month

Fever > 1 month

Minor Signs:

Persistent Cough > 1month

Generalised Pruritic Dermatitis

Herpes Zoster

Chronic Progressive Disseminated Herpes Simplex Infection

Oropharyngeal Candidiasis

Generalised Lymphadenopathy

The presence of either generalised Kaposi Sarcoma or Cryptococcal Meningitis is sufficient for the diagnosis of AIDS.

Children

2 Major + 2 Minor

Major Signs:

Weight loss or abnormally slow growth

Diarrhoea > 1 month

Fever > 1 month

Minor Signs:

Generalised Lymphadenopathy

Oropharyngeal Candidiasis

Recurrent common infections eg ear infections, pharyngitis

Persistent cough

Generalised rash

2.   Expanded WHO case definition for AIDS surveillance
     Adult or adolescent > 12years diagnosed as AIDS if:
     (a) Test for HIV Antibody is positive and
     (b) One or more of the following:
          Weight loss ≥10% with Diarrhoea, fever or both > 1 month
          Cryptococcal meningitis
          Pulmonary or Extrapulmonary TB
          Kaposi's Sarcoma
          Neurological Impairment (AIDS Dementia)
          Candidiasis of Oesophagus
          Life threatening or recurrent Pneumonia
          Invasive Cervical Cancer

Laboratory Diagnosis

  i.   ELISA Test for screening - TRI DOT Test
 ii.   Western Blot test for diagnosis
iii.   CD4 Count - For Prognosis (count < 200)

Control of AIDS

1.   Prevention
2.   Treatment
3.   Specific Prophylaxis
4.   Primary Health Care

1.   Prevention
     (a) Health Education
          A- Abstinence
          B - Be faithful

C - Condom

Avoid shared razors, tooth brushes

IV drug users to avoid sharing needles, syringes

Method – One-to-One interpersonal communication

Group method

Mass Media - TV, radio

(b) Prevention of blood borne HIV Transmission

High risk groups should not donate blood, body organs, sperm or other tissues

Blood to be screened for HIV-1, HIV-2

Heat treatment of Factor VIII, IX to prevent transmission to Hemophiliacs

Sterilisation of equipment in hospitals and clinics

Pre-sterilised disposable syringes and needles should be used

Should avoid injections unless absolutely necessary

2. *Treatment with Anti-retroviral drugs*

No cure for HIV/AIDS

No vaccine

Drugs suppress HIV infection

Therapy for asymptomatic persons with CD4 Lymphocyte Count < 200 Cells/mcL or Symptomatic HIV Disease

Post Exposure Prophylaxis (PEP)

ART - Antiretroviral Therapy started within hours following accidental exposure to virus

AZT (Zidovudine) for 4 weeks

Or combination drugs - AZT + Lamivudine/Nelfinavir/Stavudine

Preventing Perinatal Transmission – Zidovudine or Combination treatment

Breast Feeding: In poor socio-economic group to continue breastfeeding but if affordable better to give milk substitutes as rate of transmission is 10-20%

3. *Specific Prophylaxis*

Trimethoprim - Sulphamethoxazole to prevent Pneumocystis Carinii Pneumonia

Rifabutin against M Avium Intracellular, INH Prophylaxis against TB, Gancyclovir against CMV Retinitis,

Fluconazole against Cryptococcal Meningitis, Acyclovir for treatment of Herpes Simplex/Zoster

4. *Primary Health Care*

AIDS Control Programme incorporated into Primary Health Care

EMERGING AND REEMERGING INFECTIOUS DISEASES

Emerging Diseases	Re-emerging Diseases
Definition New diseases continue to occur Examples AIDS Hemorrhagic Fevers – Ebola Hanta Virus Pulmonary Syndrome Foodborne and Waterborne diseases - Cryptosporidium, new strains of E Coli, Cholera 0139 Influenza Virus - Avian H5N1, Swine Flu (H1N1) SARS	Infections thought to be conquered have returned: Mad Cow Disease - Bovine Spongiform Encephalopathy TB - MDRTB, XDRTB especially with increase in HIV/ AIDS Malaria - Resistance of Plasmodia to Chloroquine and resistance of Vectors to DDT Cholera Dysentery Pneumonia Staphylococcal Infections (skin infections, Endocarditis, Osteomyelitis, food poisoning) resistant to all antibiotics except Vancomycin Streptococci - Throat infection, middle ear infection, skin and wound infection, Gangrene increasingly resistant to antibiotics Pneumococci and H Influenza - Resistant to Penicillin, Cotrimoxazole N Gonorrhoea - Resistant to Penicillin, Tetracycline Shigella Dysentery - Results in severe Diarrhea Salmonella Typhi - (Enteric Fever) Resistant to Antibiotics E Coli resistant to Antibiotics

Factors responsible for emergence and re-emergence of infectious diseases

1. Unplanned and under-planned urbanisation
2. Overcrowding and rapid population growth
3. Poor sanitation
4. Inadequate public health infrastructure
5. Resistance to Antibiotics
6. Increased exposure of humans to disease Vectors and reservoirs of infection
7. Rapid international travel

Prevention and Control

i. Early diagnosis and treatment
ii. Efficient surveillance system
iii. International Health Regulation
iv. Personal Hygiene
v. Environmental Hygiene
vi. Immunization
vii. Health Education

viii. Strong National Disease Surveillance and Control Programmes
ix. Global networks of centres, organisations and individuals to monitor disease
x. Rapid information exchange through electronic links to guide policies, international collaboration, trade and travel

Hospital Acquired Infections

(Health Care Associated Infections)

Definition

Cross infection of one patient by another or by doctors, nurses and other hospital staff while in hospital is known as Hospital Acquired Infections.

Sources:

i. Patients – Viral, skin, respiratory, Urinary Tract Infections (UTI)
ii. Staff - Doctors, nurses, ward boys - Staphylococcal, Streptococcal, Salmonella infections
iii. Environment - Microorganisms in hospital dust, air, linen, bed clothes, furniture, sinks, basins, door handles

Routes of Spread:

i. Direct Contact
ii. Droplet Infection
iii. Airborne Particles
iv. Release of Hospital Dust into Air
v. Hospital Procedures - Catheterization, IV Procedures, Infected Catgut, Dressings, Sputum cups, bed pans, urinals

Recipients:

Patients - Especially in ICU, urology, geriatric, pediatric units

Preventive Measures:

1. Isolation
2. Hospital Staff with infections of Respiratory, Alimentary or Skin should be given leave till cured.
3. Hand washing
4. Dust Control
5. Disinfection - Urine, faeces, sputum, articles used by patient
6. Control of Droplet Infection
7. Nursing Techniques - Barrier nursing, Task nursing
8. Administrative Measures

Hospital Infection Control Committee

CHAPTER 17

NON-COMMUNICABLE DISEASES (NCDS)

Risk factors for Non-Communicable Diseases:

1. Tobacco - Active and passive smoking associated with Lung Ca, COPD, Cardiovascular Disease.

2. Alcohol - Cardiovascular Disease, Ca, Liver Cirrhosis, Domestic violence.

3. Physical Inactivity - Cardiovascular Disease, Hypertension, Diabetes, Breast Ca, Colon Ca, Depression.

4. Unhealthy Diet - Increased salt, Saturated fats, Trans fats.

5. Overweight/Obesity - Coronary Heart Disease, Stroke, Diabetes, Hypertension, certain cancers, Respiratory Diseases, Polycystic Ovary Disease. Childhood obesity leads to adult obesity.

6. Stress

7. Hypertension - Coronary Heart Disease, Stroke, Aneurysm Rupture, Dissecting Aneurysm of Aorta.

8. Raised Cholesterol - Cardiovascular Disease, Stroke.

9. Cancer Associated Infections - Human Papilloma Virus, Hepatitis B Virus, Hepatitis C Virus, Helicobacter Pylori.

Coronary Heart Disease

Impairment of Heart function due to inadequate blood flow to the Heart caused by obstructive changes in Coronary Circulation.

Magnitude of the Problem

Causes 25-30% of deaths globally
India - Prevalence 6.4% in urban; 2.5% in rural.

Risk Factors

Not Modifiable	Modifiable
Age	Cigarette Smoking
Sex	Alcohol
Race - Indian	High Blood Pressure
Family History	Elevated Serum Cholesterol
Genetic Factors	Diabetes
Personality - Type A	Obesity
	Sedentary Habits
	Stress

(a) Age - 51-60 years
(b) Sex - M > F
(c) Genetic Factors - Lipid levels -TC, LDL
(d) Family History - Increases risk of premature death
(e) Race - Indians are more prone to CHD than Western people
(f) Type A Personality - Competitive drive, restlessness, hostility, impatience, ambitious associated with CHD than Type B who are calmer, philosophical.
(g) Cigarette smoking –

   i. Carbon Monoxide induced Atherogenesis
   ii. Nicotine increases Adrenergic drive raising BP and demand for Myocardial Oxygen
   iii. Lipid Metabolism - Decrease in protective High Density Lipoprotein (HDL), increase in LDL, VLDL.
   iv. Is synergistic with other risk factors eg. Hypertension, Elevated Serum Cholesterol
   Risk of death from CHD decreases on cessation of smoking; declines substantially within 1 year and after 10-20 years it is same as non-smokers.
   Those who have suffered Myocardial Infarction, risk of fatal recurrence reduced by 50% after cessation.
(h) Hypertension - Accelerates Atherosclerosis. Systolic and Diastolic BP are both significant risk factors
(i) Serum Cholesterol > 220 mg/dl is an important risk factor; LDL, VLDL, TC levels influence Atherosclerosis;

   ii. HDL is protective; Cholesterol: HDL Ratio < 3.5 Clinical Goal
   iii. Plasma Apolipoprotein A-1 (The major HDL Protein), and Apolipoprotein B (the major LDL Protein) are better predictors of CHD than HDL, LDL.
(j) Diabetes
Risk of CHD higher in diabetics than in non-diabetics.

(k) Obesity
Obesity - Higher risk of CHD

(l) Physical Activity

Exercise - Decreases BP, improves glucose tolerance, decreases bad Lipoproteins (LDL, VLDL, TG), increases good Lipoprotein (HDL), Euphoria (Decreases stress). Sedentary lifestyle associated with CHD.

(m) Stress

Increases Adrenergic Drive, associated with increased CHD.

(n) Alcohol

High Alcohol intake (> 75g/day) risk for CHD, Hypertension, Cardiovascular Diseases

(o) Oral Contraceptives

OCPs increase risk of CHD, Hypertension

Prevention

Primordial Prevention

Prevention of unhealthy diet (High salt, fat), physical inactivity, smoking, alcohol, obesity, stress in the community.

Primary Prevention

1. Population Strategy

Prevention in the whole population - Specific Interventions

   i. Smoking – Goal – A smoke-free society
   ii. Hypertension – Control with tablets, diet, salt restriction, exercise, decrease weight
   iii. Diet - Decrease fat to 20-30% of total energy intake, saturated fats <10%, decrease Dietary Cholesterol < 100 mg/1000 kcal/day, increase complex Carbohydrates, decrease salt to $\leq$ 5g, Avoid alcohol
   iv. Physical Activity - Increase exercise from childhood

2. High Risk Strategy

   (a) Identifying Risk - BP, Serum Cholesterol, smoking, family history, Diabetes, obesity, women on OCPs
   (b) Specific Advice - Take positive action against above risk factors eg. Control BP with medication, diet, salt restriction, exercise, smoking cessation.

Secondary Prevention

Drugs - Beta-blockers, Nitrates, Aspirin

Angioplasty/Bypass Surgery/Pacemakers

Cessation of smoking, control Hypertension, control Diabetes Mellitus, diet, exercise

Hypertension

Prevalence

In the World - 40%;
In India - 17-21%

Types

Primary Hypertension - (Essential Hypertension)
Secondary Hypertension - (Kidney Disease - Chronic Glomerulonephritis, Chronic Pyelonephritis, Tumours of Adrenals, Congenital Narrowing of Aorta, Toxaemia of Pregnancy)

JNC 8-Classification of BP measurements

Category	Systolic BP (mm Hg)	Diastolic BP (mm Hg)
Normal	< 130	<85
Pre-Hypertension	130-139	85-90
Hypertension Stage 1 Stage 2 Stage 3	 140-159 160-179 >180	 90-99 100-109 >110

Complications

Classification of Hypertension by extent of Organ Damage

Stage 1	No organ damage
Stage 2	At least one of the following: Left Ventricular Hypertrophy, Generalised and Focal narrowing of Retinal Arteries, Microalbuminuria, Proteinuria &/slight elevation of Plasma Creatinine (1.2-2.0 mg/dl), U/S or Radiological evidence of Atherosclerotic Plaque (Aorta, Carotid, Iliac or Femoral)
Stage 3	Symptoms and signs due to Organ Damage: Heart - Angina Pectoris, MI, Heart Failure Brain - Stroke, TIA, Hypertensive Encephalopathy, Vascular Dementia Optic Fundi - Retinal Hemorrhages, exudates with or without Papilloedema Kidney - Pl. Creatinine > 2.0 mg/dl Renal Failure Vessel - Dissecting Aneurysm, Symptomatic Arterial Occlusive Disease

Rule of Halves

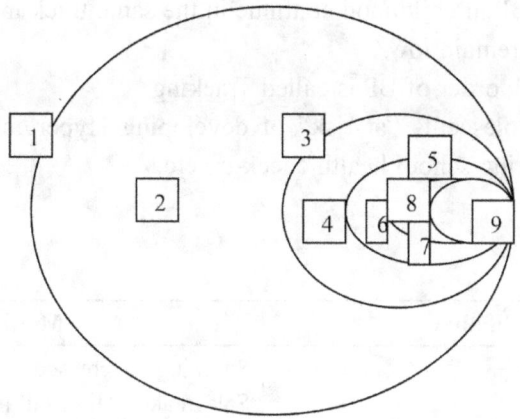

1. The whole community
2. Normotensive subjects
3. Hypertensive subjects
4. Undiagnosed Hypertension
5. Diagnosed Hypertension
6. Diagnosed but untreated
7. Diagnosed and treated
8. Inadequately treated
9. Adequately treated

*   Hypertension is an iceberg disease
*   Only half of Hypertensives in developed countries were aware of the condition.
*   Only half of those aware, were being treated.
*   Only half of those being treated, were adequately treated
*   In developing countries proportion treated would be much less.

Tracking of Blood Pressure

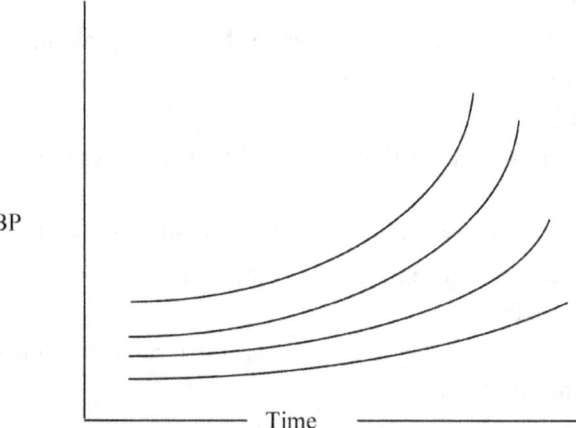

BP followed up over a period of years from childhood into adulthood.

Individuals with high BP in childhood continue in the same track into adulthood

Low BP levels tend to remain low.

This persistence of rank order of BP is called Tracking.

Thus, children and adolescents "at risk" of developing Hypertension as adults can be identified early eg. During school health check-up etc.

Risk Factors

Non-Modifiable	Modifiable
Age - BP rises with age	Smoking - Increased Adrenergic Drive
Sex - M>F	Salt Intake - High salt intake of 7-8g/day
Genetic Factors - Family history of parents, siblings	Indians take 12-16g salt/day
Ethnicity - Black Communities	Obesity - Positively correlated with High BP
	Physical Activity - Reduces body weight therefore indirect effect on BP
	Saturated Fats - Raises BP and Serum Cholesterol
	Dietary Fibre - Risk of BP and CHD is inversely related to Dietary Fibre
	Alcohol - High Alcohol Intake
	Stress - Leads to overactivity of Sympathetic Nervous System
	Socio Economic Status - Higher SES
	Heart Rate - Higher in Hypertensives
	Others - Oral Contraceptive pills associated with Hypertension

Prevention

1. *Primary Prevention*

   (a) *Population Strategy*

      i Nutrition

         Decrease salt <5g/day; moderate fat intake; avoid high alcohol intake; restriction of energy intake

      ii. Weight Reduction

         Prevention and correction of overweight, obesity; to maintain BMI < 23

      iii. Exercise

         Exercise decreases body weight, Blood Lipids, BP, improves Glucose tolerance, induces Euphoria, Reduces Stress

      iv. Smoking Cessation

         Decreases Hypertension, CHD, Cardiovascular problems

      v. Yoga and Meditation

         Reduces stress

vi. Health Education
   Preventive advice on risk factors and how to control them
vii. Self Care
   Patient is taught self-care ie. To take his own BP, maintain Log Book

(b) *High Risk Strategy*
   Detection of high-risk subjects ie. those with family history and tracking of BP from childhood and give above advice.

2. *Secondary Prevention*

Early Detection and Treatment
i. Early Detection
   Screening of persons ≥30 years for BP (National Programme for Prevention and Control of Cancer, Diabetes, Cardiovascular Disease and Stroke)
ii. Treatment
   Anti-Hypertensive drugs to be taken life-long.
   Patient compliance and regular follow up is important.

Rheumatic Heart Disease

Rheumatic Fever

A Febrile Disease affecting connective tissues particularly Heart and joints initiated by Throat Infection by Beta Haemolytic Streptococci.

Rheumatic Fever may lead to Rheumatic Heart Disease leading to damage to Heart, disabilities, repeated hospitalisation, premature death usually by 35 years.

Prevalence of Rheumatic Heart Disease in India

5-7/1000 in 5-15 years.
RHD cases one million.
Streptococcal Infection common in children of low socio-economic status.
Rheumatic Fever in 1-3% of Infections

Epidemiology

Agent Factors

Agent - Group A Beta Hemolytic Streptococci
Cases and Carriers (Convalescent, transient, chronic carriers)

Host Factors

Age - 5-15 years
Sex - Both
Immunity -Toxic - Immunologic Hypothesis

SES (Socio Economic Status) - Poverty, overcrowding, poor housing conditions, inadequate health services, low awareness of disease

High-risk Groups - School age children (5-15 years), slum dwellers, closed communities (eg. Barracks)

Environmental Factors

Overcrowding, poor housing, poor ventilation

Rheumatic Fever Clinical Features

Jones Major and Minor Classification - 2 Major or 1 Major and 2 Minor

Major Manifestations	Minor Manifestations
Carditis	Fever
Polyarthritis	Polyarthralgia
Chorea	Increased ESR
Erythema Marginatum	Leukocytosis
Subcutaneous Nodules	Prolonged PR Interval
	Increased ASO Titre
	Positive Throat Culture
	Rapid Antigen Test for Group A Streptococci
	Recent Scarlet Fever

Repeated attacks of Rheumatic Fever may lead to Rheumatic Heart Disease.

Prevention

1. **Primary Prevention**
   Prevent first attack of Rheumatic Fever:

(a) By identifying Streptococcal Throat Infection and treating with Penicillin 1.2 mega units for adults; 600,000 units for children or Penicillin V or Penicillin G orally.

(b) Non-Medical Measures
    Improve living conditions, improve SES, better housing condition, prevent overcrowding

2. **Secondary Prevention**
   Prevention of recurrences of Rheumatic Fever:

(a) Identifying those with Rheumatic Fever and giving Prophylaxis - Benzathine Penicillin (1.2 mega units in adults; 600,000 units in children) every 3 weeks for 5 years or up to 18 years

(b) Patients with Carditis (Mild Mitral Regurgitation or Healed Carditis) - Prophylaxis for 10 years or up to 25 years

(c) Patients with more severe Valvular Disease or Post Valve Surgery cases – Life-long Prophylaxis

Jai Vigyan Mission Mode Project on Community Control of RF/RHD

Components:

1. To study the Epidemiology of Streptococcal Sore Throat
2. Establish registers for RF & RHD
3. Vaccine development for Streptococcal Infection
4. Conducting advanced studies on pathological aspects of RF & RHD

Stroke

Rapidly developed clinical signs of focal or global disturbance of Cerebral Function lasting > 24 hours or leading to death with no apparent causes other than Vascular origin caused by Stenosis, Occlusion or Rupture of Arteries.

Transient Ischaemic Attack (TIA) - Focal, Reversible Neurological Deficit of sudden onset lasting < 24 hours

Magnitude of Problem

Worldwide problem.
Leads to morbidity, mortality, disability

Prevalence in India

1.5/1000 Population.

Risk Factors

Non-Modifiable	Modifiable
Age - Increase with age Sex – M > F Family History	Smoking Hypertension Diabetes Hypercholesterolemia Obesity Cardiac Abnormalities - LVH, Cardiac Dilatation

Stroke in young - <40 years, due to Rheumatic Heart Disease, Peripartum Ischaemic Stroke, Arteriopathies due to CNS Infections eg. Bacterial and TB Meningitis.

Clinical Features

Coma, Hemiplegia, Paraplegia, Monoplegia, speech disturbance, Paresis, Sensory Impairment

Prevention and Control

1. ***Primordial Prevention***
   Prevention of unhealthy diet (High salt, fat), physical inactivity, smoking, alcohol, obesity, stress in the community

2. ***Primary Prevention***
   Smoking Cessation
   Control of Hypertension
   Control of Diabetes
   Control of Hyperlipidemia

3. ***Secondary Prevention***
   Early diagnosis and treatment of TIAs

4. ***Tertiary Prevention***
   Disability limitation and Rehabilitation
   Physiotherapy

Cancer

A group of diseases characterised by:

   i.   Abnormal growth of cells
   ii. Ability to invade adjacent tissues and distant organs
   iii. Eventual death of patient

Magnitude of Problem

Second leading cause of death in developed countries.
Common Cancers - Breast, Cervical, Lung, Prostate, Colon and Stomach

World Incidence - 14 million/year
India Incidence - 10 lakh.

Men - Oral, Lung, Stomach, Colorectal, Oesophagus.
Women - Breast, Cervix Uteri, Ovary, Lip, Oral Cavity, Colorectum.

Causes

1. ***Environmental Factors***
   i. Tobacco
       Smoking, chewing can lead to Cancer of Lung, Larynx, Mouth, Pharynx, Oesophagus, Bladder, Pancreas, Kidney
       Cigarette smoking leads to 1 million premature deaths globally every year.

ii. Alcohol
Associated with Liver and Oesophageal cancer.
Beer may cause Rectal cancer.

iii. Customs, Habits, Lifestyles
Smoking associated with Lung cancer
Tobacco and Betel chewing with Oral cancer

iv. Occupational Exposure
To substances eg. Asbestos, Arsenic, Benzene, Cadmium, Chromium, Polycylic Hydrocarbons

v. Dietary Factors
Smoked fish associated with Stomach cancer
Fibre associated with Intestinal cancer
Beef associated with Bowel cancer
High fat diet associated with Breast cancer
Food Additives and Contaminants suspected to cause cancer

vi. Viruses
Hepatitis B and C associated with Hepatocellular Carcinoma
HIV and CMV associated with Kaposi's Sarcoma
Epstein Barr virus associated with Burkit's Lymphoma and Nasopharyngeal Carcinoma.
HPV associated with Cancer Cervix
Virus implicated in Hodgkin's Disease

vii. Parasites
Schistosomiasis associated with Bladder cancer in Middle East

viii. Others
Sunlight, radiation, air pollution, water pollution, medications (Oestrogens), pesticides associated with cancer

2. *Genetic Factors*
Retinoblastoma runs in families
Mongols associated with Leukemia

Cancer Control

1. *Primary Prevention*
    i. *Cancer Education*
        Danger Signals:

        (a) A lump or hard area in the Breast
        (b) Excessive loss of blood at monthly period or loss of blood outside usual dates
        (c) Blood loss from any natural orifice
        (d) Persistent change in Digestive and Bowel habits
        (e) Persistent Cough or Hoarseness
        (f) Swelling or Sore that does not get better

(g) Change in a Wart/Mole

(h) Unexplained loss of weight

ii. Control of Tobacco and Alcohol Consumption

This can reduce deaths due to Tobacco and Alcohol.

Norway has developed a plan to eradicate Tobacco Smoking

iii. Legislation

To control Tobacco, Alcohol, air pollution eg. "No Smoking in Public Places or Public Vehicles"

iv. Radiation

Efforts to reduce Radiation due to occupation or X-ray exposure during investigations.

v. Occupational Exposures

Industrial workers should be protected from exposure to Carcinogens

vi. Personal Hygiene

Important in Cancer Cervix

vii. Immunization

Hepatitis B Immunization prevents primary Liver Cancer.

viii. Foods, Drugs, Cosmetics

They should be tested for Carcinogens.

ix. Treatment of Pre-cancerous Lesions

Early diagnosis and treatment of Pre-cancerous Lesions eg. Cervical Tears, Chronic Cervicitis, Chronic Gastritis, Intestinal Polyposis, Warts, Adenomata, Leukoplakia

2. Secondary Prevention

Consists of:

i.   Cancer Registration

ii. Early Diagnosis

iii. Treatment

i. Cancer Registration

For Cancer Control Programme Cancer Registration forms the baseline for assessing magnitude of the problem and planning necessary services.

Cancer Registries - 2 Types

(a) Hospital Based Registries

Consists of Inpatients and Outpatients treated in an Institution.

Data according to WHO Handbook for Standardised Cancer Registers.

Advantage - Evaluation of diagnostic and treatment programmes possible in long term follow-up.

Disadvantage - Hospital patients are a selected population (Berkesonian Bias) therefore not useful for Epidemiology.

(b) Population Based Registries
   Aim - To cover the complete cancer situation in a given geographic area.
   Population size 2-7 million.

   Data can provide Incidence Rates of cancer, initiate Epidemiological enquiries into causes, surveillance of time trends, planning and evaluation of services.

   Population based cancer registries established at Bangalore, Mumbai, Chennai.

ii. *Early Diagnosis of Cases (Screening)*
   Cancer screening for early detection of Cancer at pre-invasive stage.
   Screening programmes available for Cancer Cervix, Breast Cancer, Oral Cancer.
   Cases detected should be sent to higher centres for further diagnostic investigations and treatment.

iii. *Treatment*
   Different types of cancers have different treatments.

   (a) Surgery
   (b) Radiotherapy
   (c) Chemotherapy
   (d) Combinations of above
   (e) Pain relief if no treatment is possible

Cancer Screening

Definition

Search for unrecognised Malignancy by means of Rapidly Applied Tests.

Methods of Cancer Screening

i. Mass Screening by Comprehensive Cancer Detection Examination
   Rapid clinical examination and examination of one or more body sites by a Physician
ii. Mass Screening at Single Sites
   Single site examined eg. Cervix, Breast or Lung
iii. Selective Screening
   High-risk groups selected for screening eg. Parous women > 35 years of low SES for Cancer Cervix, chronic smokers for Lung Cancer.

1. *Screening for Cancer Cervix*
   Pap Smear Test for Cancer Cervix Screening.
   Recommendation that Pap Smear should be done at the beginning of sexual activity, then every 3 years and periodic Pelvic Examination

2. **Screening for Breast Cancer**

Screening by:
   (a) Breast Self-Examination (BSE) by patient
   (b) Palpation by Physician
   (c) Thermography
   (d) Mammography

3. **Screening for Lung Cancer**
   (a) Chest X-ray
   (b) Sputum Cytology

Oral Cancer

Risk Factors

Tobacco - Smoking, chewing, reverse smoking (Chutta)
Alcohol
Pre-cancerous Lesions - Leukoplakia, Erythroplakia

Cultural Factors

Tobacco chewing, smoking - Beedi, Chutta, Chilum, Hookah, Snuff

Prevention

1. **Primary Prevention**
   Health Education
   Legislation - "Smoking is injurious to Health"

2. **Secondary Prevention**
   Precancerous Lesions detected and cured by cessation of Tobacco, Surgery, Radiotherapy

Cancer Cervix

Natural History

Normal Epithelium - Dysplasia - Ca in Situ - Invasive Ca
Agent - Human Papilloma Virus (HPV)

Risk Factors:

Age - 25-45 years
Marital Status - Multiple partners
Early Marriage - Early coitus, early childbearing, repeated childbirth

Oral Contraceptive Pills - Association with Ca Cx
Genital Warts
Socio-economic Class - Low SES

Prevention

1. *Primary Prevention*
    Personal Hygiene
    Family Planning

2. *Secondary Prevention*
    Screening, early detection
    Surgery or
    Radiotherapy

Breast Cancer

Risk Factors

Age 35-50 years
Family History

Age at Menarche, Menopause - Early Menarche and late Menopause
Hormonal Factors - Increased Estrogens, increased Progesterones, increased risk

Parity - Late first pregnancy, unmarried women high risk
Surgery - Prior Breast Biopsy

Diet - High fat diet, obesity
Socio-economic Status - High SES
Others – Radiation

Prevention

1. *Primary Prevention*
    Cancer Education
    Decreased fat diet

2. *Secondary Prevention*
    Screening, Early detection – BSE - Breast Self-Examination
    Surgery
    Radiotherapy
    Chemotherapy

Lung Cancer

Epidemiology

Age - One third cases < 65 years

Sex - M > F

Risk Factors

   i.   Smoking Tobacco - Active and passive smoking - Doll and Hill Prospective Study - Association of Smoking and Lung Cancer

  ii.   Air Pollution

 iii.   Radioactivity

 iv.   Occupational Exposure - Asbestos, Arsenic, Chromate, Polycyclic Aromatic Hydrocarbons

Prevention

Primordial prevention

Prevention of appearance of risk factors eg. Health education on smoking and ill effects in school health programmes

Primary Prevention

Public information and education

Legislation

Smoking Cessation activities

National and International Coordination

Secondary Prevention

Early Detection – X-ray and Sputum Cytology

Treatment - Surgery, Chemotherapy, Pain Relief

Stomach Cancer

Epidemiology

Agent Factors

Helicobacter Pylori

Smoked fish - Japanese

Prevention

Primary Prevention

Health Education

Secondary Prevention

Early Detection by Oesophagogastroduodenoscopy (OGDS) and Biopsy
Surgery
Chemotherapy

Obesity

Abnormal growth of Adipose Tissues due to:

(a) Enlargement of fat cell size (Hypertrophic Obesity) or
(b) Increase in fat cell number (Hyperplastic Obesity) or
(c) Both

Magnitude of Problem

World overweight - 1.9 billion; Obese 600 million adults; 41 million < 5 years
India - 1.3% males; 2.5% females $\geq$ 20 years obese

Epidemiology

Agent Factors

Diet - Dietary Habits - Eating in between meals, preference for chocolates, sweets, fatty foods

Host Factors

   i. Age - Any age - Childhood to old age
      Childhood obesity leads to adult obesity
  ii. Sex - F>M
      Women's BMI increases with every pregnancy
 iii. Education - Inversely associated with obesity in affluent societies
 iv. Genetic - Associated with obesity
  v. Exercise - Regular physical exercise prevents obesity eg. Brisk walking, gym exercises, swimming
 vi. SES - Inverse relationship between SES and obesity.
      Affluent countries, obesity more in lower socio-economic groups
 vii. Psychosocial - Depression, anxiety, frustration, loneliness.
      Obese people are self-conscious, lonely and secret eaters.
viii. Familial - Obesity runs in families
 ix. Endocrine - Cushing's Syndrome, Growth Hormone Deficiency, Thyroid Deficiency
  x. Drugs - Corticosteroids, oral contraceptives, insulin, Beta Adrenergic Blockers
 xi. Smoking - Smokers weigh < Ex-smokers or non-smokers
 xii. Alcohol - Increases obesity

Environmental Factors

i. Availability of Junk Food
ii. Advertisements, Marketing
iii. Lack of Recreational Facilities, Games
iv. TV, Computer
v. Culture, Fashion

Classification

1. **Body Mass Index (BMI) - Quetelet's Index = Wt/Ht^2**

Classification	Asia Pacific Classification	WHO Classification
Normal	18-23	18-25
Overweight	23-25	25-30
Obese	>25	>30

2. Broca's Index = Ht (cm) - 100
3. Ponderal Index = Ht (cm)/Cube root of body weight (kg)
4. Lorentz's Formula = Ht (cm) – 100 – Ht - 150/2 Women or 4 Men
5. Corpulence Index = Actual Weight/Desirable Weight (Should not exceed 1.2)
6. Waist Circumference - Asia Pacific Classification, males > 90 cm; females > 80 cm

Hazards of Obesity

Hypertension, Diabetes Mellitus, Coronary Heart Disease, Chronic Kidney Disease, Osteoarthritis (Hips, knees, spine), Infertility, Surgery risks (eg. Deep Vein Thrombosis and Pulmonary Embolism), Gall Bladder disease, Cancer (Breast, Colon), Hernia, Respiratory disease

Prevention and Control

Prevention of Obesity from childhood is important

1. *Diet*
   High energy foods eg. Sweets, chocolates, ice creams should be decreased.
   Sugar in coffees and teas should also be reduced.
   Fats and deep-fried foods to be taken within limits.
   Diet should consist of high fibre eg. Unpolished rice, whole wheat.
   For adults - 1000 kcal diet daily.
   Other nutritional requirements should be adequate.
   Lifestyle modification necessary.

2. *Exercise*
   Walking 1 hour per day or jogging, cycling, swimming, gym exercises.

3. **Both Diet and Exercise**
    Both are more effective together than separately.

4. **Drugs**
    Appetite Suppressant Drugs are available but have side effects.

5. **Surgery**
    Gastric Bypass Surgery, Gastroplasty, Laparoscopic Bariatric Surgery, Jaw Wiring, Liposuction

Diabetes

The Disease is characterised by Hyperglycemia due to defective production or action of insulin resulting in Defective Metabolism of Glucose, Fat and Amino Acid. Complications involve Ocular, Renal, Neurological, Cardiovascular, Recurrent Infections.

Magnitude of Problem

World prevalence - 422 million;
India prevalence - 65 million

Classification

1. Diabetes Mellitus
    i.   Type 1 Diabetes Mellitus
    ii. Type 2 Diabetes Mellitus
    iii. Malnutrition Related Diabetes Mellitus (MRDM)
    iv. Others (Secondary to Pancreatic, Hormonal, Drug Induced, Genetic, Other Abnormalities)
2. Impaired Glucose Tolerance (IGT)
3. Gestational Diabetes Mellitus

Epidemiology

Agent Factors

Insulin Deficiency - May be due to Inflammation, Genetic, Autoimmune

Host Factors

i.   Age – Type-1 DM in young and Type-2 DM in 40 years and older age group. With increased obesity Type-2 DM is seen in younger age group.
ii. Sex - Equal
iii. Genetic Factors - Twin studies have shown Genetic Link

iv. Genetic Markers - HLA B8, B15, DR3, DR4
v. Obesity - Especially Central Obesity Risk Factor for Type-2 DM
vi. Immune Mechanisms - Autoimmunity

Environmental Factors

i. Sedentary Lifestyle
ii. Diet - High Saturated Fats
iii. Dietary Fibre - Eg. Wholegrain Cereals, Millets, vegetables, fruits help to lower Blood Sugar levels
iv. Malnutrition - In infancy and childhood may result in damage to Beta cells
v. Infections - Rubella, Mumps, Coxackie Virus
vi. Chemical Agents - Alloxan, Streptozotocin, Cyanide producing foods, Cassava, certain Beans
vii. Alcohol - Excess intake damages Pancreas and Liver
viii. Stress - Surgery, Trauma
ix. Others - SES, Occupation, Urbanisation

Clinical Features

Polyuria, Polydipsia, Polyphagia, Recurrent Infections or Symptoms of Complications - Diabetic Retinopathy, Nephropathy, Neuropathy, Cardiovascular, Genitourinary, Gastrointestinal.

Diagnosis

Test	Normal	Prediabetic	Diabetes Mellitus
FBS	<110mg%	110-126mg%	>126mg%
PPBS	<140mg%	140-200mg%	>200mg%
HbA1c	<5.7%	5.7-6.5%	>6.5%

Syndrome X or Metabolic Syndrome - Hyperglycemia, Hyperinsulinemia, Obesity, Dyslipidemia, Hypertension leads to Coronary Heart Disease

Prevention

1. *Primordial Prevention*
   Prevention of risk factors
   Diet - High Carbohydrate, High fat
   Lack of physical activity
   Obesity
   Smoking
   Alcohol

2. **Primary Prevention**
   (a) Population Strategy
      i.   Normal body weight maintenance
      ii. Diet - Increase fibre, decrease sweet foods
      iii. Exercise
      iv. Avoid Alcohol

   (b) High Risk Strategy
      Identify High Risk persons - Overweight/Obese, Physical Inactivity, Family History, Hypertension, Gestational Diabetes, Birth of big babies > 4kg.

Strategy

   i.   Normal body weight maintenance
   ii. Diet - Increase fibre, decrease sweet foods
   iii. Exercise
   iv. Avoid Alcohol
   v.   Smoking Cessation
   vi. Control BP
   vii. Control Cholesterol and Triglyceride

3. **Secondary Prevention**
   (a) Screening
      i. Urine Examination
      ii. Blood Sugar

   (b) Diagnosis and Management
      FBS and 2 hours Post Glucose Test after 75g Glucose orally

      Diabetes Mellitus:
      FBS > 126 and PPBS > 200 mg/dl.

      Prediabetes:
      FBS 100-126 and PPBS 140-200 mg/dl
      Glycosylated Hb < 7% indicates control

      Self-Care - Diet, drugs, regular check-ups, self-administration of Insulin, maintenance of body weight, recognition of Hypoglycemic Symptoms and response, Blood Glucose monitoring with Glucometer, Identity Card with name, address, telephone number.

4. **Tertiary Prevention**
   Good control of Blood Glucose prevents complications - Blindness, Kidney Failure, Coronary Thrombosis, Stroke, Gangrene

Diabetic Clinics - Disability prevention and Rehabilitation eg. Laser for Microaneurysms in Eyes
Research
National Registries

Accidents and Injuries

Any unpremeditated event resulting in injury, disability or death.

Types of Accidents

1. **Road Traffic Accidents**
   Ranks first among fatal accidents.

   Causes in Developing Countries:

   i.   Mixed Traffic - Pedestrians, animals, slow moving vehicles (Bullock Carts) and fast moving vehicles (Trucks, Buses); No footpath for pedestrians.
   ii. Vehicles - Old, poorly maintained
   iii. Poor Public Transport System
   iv. 2-Wheelers in large numbers
   v.   Private vehicles in large numbers
   vi. Large number of overloaded buses
   vii. Low Driving Standards
   viii.Disregard for Traffic Rules
   ix. Roads - Potholes, defective layout of crossroads, plenty of humps
   x.   Poor Street Lighting
   xi. Unusual behaviour of people eg. Cross the road suddenly without looking left or right

2. **Domestic Accidents**

Definition
Accident in the home or immediate surroundings.

Causes

(a) Drowning
(b) Burns (Flame, hot liquid, electricity, fire crackers, chemicals)
(c) Poisoning (Drugs, insecticides, rat poisons, kerosene)
(d) Falls - Head injury, Colle's Fracture, fracture neck of Femur
(e) Injuries from sharp or pointed instruments
(f) Bites of animals

3. **Industrial Accidents**
   Workers in industries, agriculture, fisheries, home industries, small scale industries. Agricultural workers exposed to physical, chemical (Pesticides, Fertilizers), Biological (animal bites), Mechanical injuries.

4. **Railway Accidents**
   Train accidents take a large toll.

5. **Violence**
   Wars, Terrorist attacks, wife battering, child battering after consumption of alcohol. Self-violence - Suicide

Factors Causing Road Traffic Accidents

Human Factors	Environmental Factors
Age	Relating to Road
Sex	Defective, narrow roads
Education	Defective layout of cross roads & speed
Medical Conditions - Illness, Heart Attack,	breakers
Vision Impairment	Poor lighting
Fatigue	Lack of familiarity
Psychosocial Factors (Lack of experience, risk	Relating to Vehicle
taking, impulsiveness, defective judgement,	High speed
delay in decisions, aggressiveness, poor	Old, poorly maintained
perception, family dysfunction)	Large number of 2/3 wheelers
Lack of body protection (Helmet, Safety Belt)	Overloaded buses
	Low driving standards
	Bad weather
	Inadequate enforcement of laws
	Mixed traffic - Fast moving, pedestrians, animals

Increased Vulnerability
&/or
Risk Situation

Precipitating Factors
Tension
Alcohol, Drugs

Precipitating Factors
Special Traffic Conditions
Social Pressure
Use of Stolen Vehicles

ACCIDENT

Prevention

1. *Data Collection*
   Documentation of all accidents and their causes
   Data collection, analysis, interpretation, evaluation leading to effective prevention strategies.

2. *Safety Education*
   Should be taught to school children eg. Traffic rules, speed limits, how to cross the road. Training should be given to drivers on safe driving and maintenance of vehicles.

3. *Safety Measures*
   (a) Helmets
   (b) Seat belts
   (c) Children should be seated, prohibited from front seats, child restraints
   (d) Others - Door locks, design of vehicles, windscreen which is laminated, high penetration resistant
   (e) Leather clothing and boots - Prevents injuries to body, legs and feet

4. *Alcohol and Drugs*
   Persons on alcohol or drugs (Barbiturates, Amphetamines, Cannabis Cough Syrups, Antihistamines, Sleeping Medicines) should not drive.

5. *Primary Care*
   Emergency services during the "1ˢᵗ Golden Hour" - Ambulance service with First Aid can save lives.

6. *Elimination of Causative Factors*
   Eg. Roads, Vehicles, Human Factors should be eliminated.

7. *Enforcement of Laws*
   Enforcement of speed limits, proper driving test, medical fitness, compulsory helmets, seat belts, breath testing for alcohol.

8. *Early Diagnosis, Treatment, Rehabilitation of Accident Victims*
   IV Fluids, Blood Transfusion, Surgery, Rehabilitation (Medical, Surgical, Social, Occupational)

9. *Accident Research*
   Accidentology - Identifying causes including Human Behaviour and methods of Prevention of Accidents.

Visual Impairment & Blindness

Blindness – The inability to count fingers at a distance of 3-metres.

Types

1. Total blindness
2. Economic blindness
3. Social blindness

Magnitude of the Problem

World – 1-billion vision impairments which could have been prevented.

Causes

Cataract
Refractive Error
Glaucoma
Diabetic Retinopathy
Posterior Segment Pathology
Corneal Opacity
Vit A Deficiency
Trachoma
Unaddressed Presbyopia

Epidemiology

Age – Children - Vit A Deficiency, Refractive Error, Trachoma, Conjunctivitis
Old age - Cataract, Glaucoma, Diabetes
All ages - Accidents, Injuries

Sex - F>M (Trachoma, Conjunctivitis, Cataract)

Malnutrition - Vit A Deficiency especially with Measles, Diarrhea, PEM

Occupation - Factories, workshops, welding persons are more prone to injury.
Doctors exposed to X-rays, UV rays are prone to Cataract

Social class - Poorer classes

Social factors - Ignorance, poverty, poor personal hygiene, poor community hygiene, lack of health care services.

Control and Prevention of Blindness

Eye Health Care

Main objective is to reduce blindness to < 0.3%

1. Initial assessment of blindness in the country - Magnitude, distribution and causes

2. Intervention
    (a) Primary Eye Care - Infection control, foreign body removal, Vit A Prophylaxis by trained primary health care workers
    (b) Secondary Eye Care - Management of Cataract, Glaucoma, Trichiasis, Entropion, Ocular Trauma in PHCs and District Hospitals.
    (c) Tertiary Eye Care - Corneal Graft, Retinal Surgery at Medical College Hospitals and National or Regional Institutes.
3. Specific Programmes
    (a) Trachoma Control - Early diagnosis and treatment with Tetracyclines.
    (b) School Eye Health Services - School children screened for Refractive Error, Squint, Amblyopia, Trachoma.
    Health education on good posture, lighting, avoidance of glare.
    (c) Vit A Prophylaxis: 9 months – 5years children to prevent Nutritional Blindness
    (d) Occupational Eye Care - Health Education to prevent occupational hazards and use of protective devices eg. For welding.
4. Long Term Measures
    Improving quality of life, interventions to reduce eye health problems namely poor sanitation, lack of safe water, poor personal hygiene, poor intake of Vit A rich foods.
5. Evaluation
    This should be part of Intervention Programmes to measure the improvement after Ocular Programmes.
    National and International Agencies
    i.   National Association for the Blind (NAB)
    ii. Danish International Development Agency (DANIDA) - Funds provided for Cataract Operations.
    iii. WHO

CHAPTER 18

TRIBAL HEALTH IN INDIA

Tribals constitute 8.6% of India's population, 104 million

Triple burden of disease

1. Communicable and NCDs
2. Malnutrition
3. Mental Illness and Addictions
4. Animal Attacks and Violence

1. **Communicable Diseases**
   TB, Leprosy, Malaria, Vector-borne diseases.

2. **Non-Communicable Diseases**
   Hypertension, Diabetes, Blindness and Visual Impairment, Genetic Diseases - Sickle Cell Anemia, Thalassemia, G6PD Deficiency.

3. **Mental Health and Addictions**
   Tobacco, Alcohol

4. **Animal Attacks and Violence**
   Snake, dog, scorpion bite

Health Care Infrastructure and Tribal Development

Ministry of Tribal Affairs and Ministry of Health and Family Welfare are making efforts through educational, infrastructural and livelihood schemes.

Health Care Infrastructure:

Health Subcentre per 3,000 population
PHC per   20,000 population
CHC per   80,000 population

CHAPTER 19

VOLUNTARY HEALTH AGENCIES

An organization administered by an autonomous board which holds meetings, collects funds and expends money in conducting a programme to improve public health.

Functions

i. Supplementing the work of Government agencies through Manpower, Material (Equipment, Drugs) thus improving services.
ii. Pioneering Work eg. Family Planning Association of India (FPAI)
iii. Education
   Health education on prevention and control of diseases
iv. Demonstration
   Eg Bore Hole Latrines by Rockefeller Foundation to solve Hookworm Problem.
v. Advancing Health Legislation
   Mobilise public opinion and advance legislation on health matters.

1. ***Indian Red Cross Society***
   Established in 1920

Objectives:

i. Mitigation of suffering
ii. Improvement of health
iii. Prevention of diseases

Activities:

(a) Relief Work
   During disasters (Earthquakes, floods, drought, epidemics) rescues victims
(b) Milk and Medical Supplies
   Arrange milk powder, medicines, vitamins to hospitals, dispensaries, MCH Centres, schools and orphanages.
(c) Armed Forces
   Care of sick and wounded among the Armed Forces eg Red Cross Home in Bangalore for permanently disabled ex-servicemen

(d) Maternity and Child Welfare Services

Maternity and Child Welfare Centres throughout India are administered or affiliated to the Red Cross.

(e) Family Planning

Family Planning Clinics in several states are run by Red Cross.

(e) Blood Bank and First Aid

The Red Cross have started Blood Banks in some states.

First Aid is also taught by St John's Ambulance Association, India

2. *Hind Kusht Nivaran Sangh*

For Leprosy Services

Activities:

Financial assistance to Leprosy Homes, Clinics

Health Education through publications, posters

Training Medical Workers, Physiotherapists

Research and Field Investigations

Organising All India Leprosy Workers Conferences

Journal "Leprosy in India"

3. *Tuberculosis Association of India*

Activities:

Raising Funds for TB

Health Education

Training Doctors, Health Assistants, Social Workers

Organising Conferences

4. *Family Planning Association of India*

Branches throughout India

Activities:

Running Family Planning Clinics with Government Aid

Training Doctors, Health Assistants, Social Workers

IEC - On FP by correspondence or personal interview

5. *Indian Council for Child Welfare (ICCW)*

Activities to secure for children, opportunities and facilities necessary for them to develop physically, mentally, spiritually, morally and socially in a healthy and normal manner and in conditions of freedom and dignity.

6. *All India Women's Conference*

Activities:

Running MCH Clinics, Medical Centres, FP Clinics, Adult Education Centres, Milk Centres

7. *Kasturba Memorial Fund*

Activities:

To improve the lot of women in rural areas through Gram Sevikas.

8. *Central Social Welfare Board*

Activities:

Family and Child Welfare Services in rural areas for the welfare of women and children. Social education, literacy classes, maternity aid for women, distribution of milk, Balwadis and play centres for children.

9. *Bharat Sevak Samaj (BSS)*

Objective

To help people achieve health by their own actions and efforts.

Activities:

Improvement of sanitation

10. *All India Blind Relief Society*

Activities:

Organises Eye Relief Camps
Coordinates the work of various institutions for the blind.

11. *Professional Bodies*

Indian Medical Association, All India Dental Association, Trained Nurses Association of India

Activities:

Conducts Conferences
Arranges Scientific Sessions and Exhibitions
Set up standards of Professional Education
Organise relief camps during disasters

12. *International Agencies*

Rockefeller Foundation, Ford Foundation, CARE etc

CHAPTER 20

INTERNATIONAL HEALTH

International Health Organisations

World Health Organisation (WHO)

Specialised agency of the UN concerned with international public health with headquarters at Geneva.
It was started on 7 April 1948.

Objective

For all people of the world the attainment of a level of health that will permit them to lead a socially and economically productive life - HFA (Health For All) by 2000 AD.

Membership

194 Countries

Functions

1. *Prevention and Control of Specific Diseases*
    Communicable, non-communicable diseases, mental disorders, genetic disorders, drug addiction, dental diseases.

2. *Development of Comprehensive Health Services*
    Establish Primary Health Care and organize National Health Programmes in all countries.

3. *Family Health*
    MCH, human reproduction, nutrition and health education, improvement of life of the family.

4. *Environmental Health*
    Promotion of environmental health, safe water, sanitation, good air quality, food sanitation, health conditions of work, radiation protection.

5. **Health Statistics**
   Dissemination of morbidity, mortality statistics published in Weekly Epidemiological Record, World Health Statistics.

6. **Biomedical Research**
   WHO stimulates and coordinates research work.
   Six tropical diseases (Malaria, Filaria, Leprosy, Schistosomiasis, Trypanosomiasis, Leishmaniasis) for research and training programmes.

7. **Health Literature and Information**
   WHO publications and MEDLARS (Medical Literature Analysis and Retrieval System)

8. **Cooperation with Other Organisations**
   With UN and International Governmental Organisations.

Structure

1. The World Health Assembly - Health Parliament of Nations
2. The Executive Board - 31 Memberships
3. The Secretariat - Headed by Director General which provides technical and managerial support for National Health Programmes

Regions

Regions	Headquarters
South East Asia	New Delhi (India)
Africa	Brazzaville (Congo)
The Americas	Washington DC (USA)
Europe	Copenhagen (Denmark)
Eastern Mediterranean	Alexandria (Egypt)
Western Pacific	Manila (Philippines)

South East Asia Region (SEAR)

11 members - India, Sri Lanka, Nepal, Bhutan, Bangladesh, Myanmar, Thailand, Korea, Mongolia, Maldives, Indonesia.

UNICEF

United Nations International Children's Fund

It is one of the specialised agencies of the UN
It was established in 1946
It collaborates with WHO, UNDP, UNESCO, FAO

Headquarters - New York;
South Central Asian Region - New Delhi

Functions

i. *Child Health*
Immunization, infant and young child care, family planning, safe water, sanitation.

ii. *Child Nutrition*
Improving child nutrition, food supplementation, Applied Nutrition Programmes, Vit. A Supplementation Programme, Salt Iodization Programme, Iron and Folic Acid Supplements

iii. *Family and Child Welfare*
To improve care of children - Parent education, Day Care Centres, child welfare, youth agencies, women's clubs.

iv. *Education (Formal and Non-Formal)*
Collaborates with UNESCO and assists in teaching science - Laboratory equipment, workshop tools, library books, audiovisual aids to educational institutions.

Current Strategy (GOBIFFF)

G - Growth Charts to monitor child development
O - Oral Rehydration during Diarrhoea
B - Breastfeeding
I - Immunization
F - Fertility Control
F - Feeding
F - Female Literacy

UNDP

United Nations Development Programme

This was established in 1966
Member countries take help for National Development

Functions

- Fund poor countries
- Technical assistance

- Help:
  - o Agricultural development
  - o Industrial development
  - o Educational development
  - o Health development
  - o Social welfare

UNFPA

United Nations Fund for Population Activities

(a) Helps in development of Family Welfare Infrastructure, and
(b) Availability of Family Welfare Services

Functions:

- Development of Contraceptive manufacture
- Development of Population Education Programmes
- Introducing innovative approaches to FP, MCH

FAO

Food and Agricultural Organisation

Founded in 1945 with headquarters in Rome

Functions:

- Helps nations to raise living standards to improve nutrition
- Development of farming, forestry, fisheries
- Recent campaign - Freedom From Hunger (1960)
- To combat Malnutrition and to disseminate information and education
- WHO and FAO collaboration for nutritional surveys, training courses, seminars, research programmes

Non-Governmental Agencies

Rockefeller Foundation

John D Rockefeller started a Philanthropic Organisation in 1913.

Objective

To provide well-being to mankind throughout the world.

Functions

Improvement of public health, medical education, life sciences, control of Hookworm through construction of latrines in rural areas, establishment of All India Institute of Hygiene and Public Health in Kolkata, training of competent teachers and research workers, development of medical college libraries, population studies, assistance to Research Projects and Institutions, improvement of agriculture, family planning, Rural Training Centres and medical education.

Ford Foundation

Helps Rural Health Services and Family Planning

i. Established Orientation Training Centres in Singur, Poonamallee, Najafgarh.
ii. Research cum Action Project for Environmental Sanitation.
iii. Gandhigram Pilot Project in Rural Health Services.
iv. Establishment of NIHAE - National Institute of Health Administration and Education at Delhi
v. Calcutta Water Supply
vi. Family Planning Programme

CARE

Cooperative for Assistance and Relief Everywhere

Founded in North America
Non-profit, non-sectarian international relief and development organisation.

Provides emergency aid and long-term development assistance
Provides food for children - ICDS (Integrated Child Development Services) Programme, Integrated Nutrition and Health Project, Better Health and Nutrition Project, Anemia Control Project, Improved Health Care for Adolescent Girls' Project, Improving Women's Health Project, Child Survival Project, Improving Women's Reproductive Health and Family Spacing Project.

ILO

International Labour Organisation

Established in 1919

Objective

To improve the working and living conditions of workers throughout the world.

Functions

Development of policies, justice and codes of Labour
Promotion of Social Justice
Improve Occupational Health through health and welfare of workers

WORLD BANK

A specialised agency of the UN.
Gives loans for projects which will lead to Economic Growth - Projects connected with electric power, roads, railways, agriculture, water supply, education, health, family planning. In India, programmes funded by World Bank – NRHM (National Rural Health Mission), RCH (Reproductive and Child Health), IPP (India's Population Project), DOTS (Directly Observed Treatment, Short-course) Programme.

Health Work of Bilateral Agencies

USAID

United States Agency for International Development

Helps in projects to improve health of Indians:

(a) Control of Communicable Diseases
(b) Malaria Eradication
(c) Medical Education
(d) Nursing Education
(e) Health Education
(f) Nutrition
(g) Family Planning
(h) Water Supply
(i) Sanitation, Agriculture

COLOMBO PLAN

Objective:

To improve the living standards of South and South East Asian countries.

Members

20 Developing countries and 6 Non-Regional members (Australia, New Zealand, UK, USA, Canada, Japan).

Activities

Mainly Industrial and Agricultural Development and Health Promotion.

SIDA

Swedish International Development Agency

Helps in RNTCP (Revised National TB Control Programme) - DOTS Programme, assistance for procuring equipment eg. X-ray units, Microscopes, Anti TB Drugs.

DANIDA

Danish International Development Agency

Activity

Development of services under the National Programme for Control of Blindness

INTERNATIONAL RED CROSS

Founded by Henry Dunant, a Swiss businessman.

When travelling through North Italy, during the Battle of Solferino, he saw the plight of wounded, dying soldiers and organised volunteers from nearby villages to help relieve their suffering.

In his book, "Un Souvenir de Solferine" and interviews with eminent persons he urged voluntary national societies to be founded which in time of war would render aid to the wounded without distinction of nationality.

Functions

Humanitarian service for Victims of War
Relief during Natural Disasters
Service to Armed Forces, service to War Veterans
First Aid, nursing, health education, maternity and child welfare services

CHAPTER 21

HEALTH PLANNING AND MANAGEMENT

Health planning is required to improve health services.

Purpose of Planning

i.   To match limited resources with many problems
ii. Eliminate wasteful expenditure
iii. Develop best course of action to accomplish a defined objective

Planning Cycle

Steps in Planning

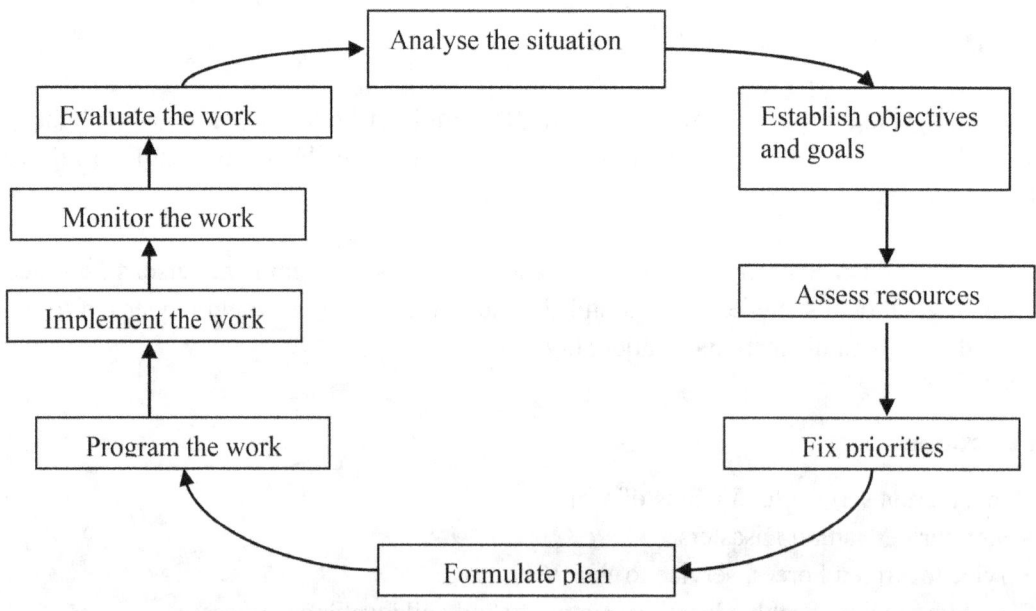

1. ***Analyse Health Situation***
   Health situation assessed by collecting data and interpreting information:
   (a) Population, age, sex structure
   (b) Morbidity, Mortality

(c) Epidemiology of Diseases
(d) Medical Care facilities available - Public and private
(e) Technical Manpower
(f) Training Facilities available
(g) Attitudes and beliefs of population towards disease, cure, prevention

Analysis of above brings out Health Problems, Health Needs and Health Demands of the population.

2. **Establishment of Goals and Objectives**
    Goals and objectives are required to guide efforts.
    General and specific objectives, short term and long-term objectives.

3. **Assessment of Resources**
    Resources are manpower, money, materials, skills, knowledge and techniques needed for implementation of health programmes.
    Balance is struck between resources required and what is available.

4. **Fixing Priorities**
    Priorities are established in order of importance because resources always fall short of total requirement.
    Next, alternate plans for achieving them are formulated and assessed and plans with greater effectiveness are chosen.

5. **Write up of Formulated Plan**
    Detailed plan is prepared.
    For each proposed health programme, resources (inputs) required are related to results (outputs) expected.
    Each stage of the plan is defined, costed, and time needed to implement is specified.
    Plan must have working guidance to all responsible for the execution.
    A built-in system of evaluation should be incorporated.

6. **Programming**
    Sequence of action in health activity should be specified.

7. **Implementing**
    Delegation of authority and fixation of responsibility of all team members for achieving objectives during the scheduled period.

8. **Monitoring**
    Day-to-day follow up of activities during implementation to ensure they are proceeding as planned and on schedule.

9. **Evaluation**
    Evaluation to see whether objectives have been achieved; Mid-term and end-term evaluation to be done.

Management

The effective use of resources (Manpower, materials, money) for fulfilling a predetermined objective is called Management.

Activities

  i. Planning
 ii. Organising
iii. Communicating
 iv. Monitoring

Management Methods

I Methods Based on Behavioural Sciences (Qualitative Methods)

  i. *Organisational Design*
  Flexible and effective organisation since concepts and technology are changing.

 ii. *Personnel Management*
  Skillful use of human resources.
  Proper methods of selection, training, motivation, division of responsibility, distribution of roles, incentives, opportunities for professional advancement.

iii. *Communication*
  Good communication leads to strong health management.
  Vertical and horizontal communication channels to be established.

 iv. *Information Systems*
  Information is required for day-to-day management.
  Information system comprises of collection, classification, transmission, display and provides data for monitoring and evaluation.
  Health Information System (HIS), improved with computers.

  v. *Management by Objectives*
  Objectives set forth at the start of a programme and each unit prepares its own plan of action.

II Quantitative Methods

  i. *Cost Benefit Analysis*
  Commonly used in health field.
  Cost invested and benefits obtained from the programme are compared.
  Benefits are expressed in monetary terms

ii. **Cost Effective Analysis**
Suitable in health field; cost invested and effect obtained are compared.
Effect eg. Number of lives saved, number of days free from disease.

iii. **Cost Accounting**
Cost invested is accounted in each step and in each purpose.

iv. **Input-Output Analysis**
Units of input and units of output are compared.

v. **Model**
It is an aid to understand how factors in a situation affect one another.

vi. **Systems Analysis**
Health system is analysed for objectives, finding alternate solutions, cost effectiveness.

vii. **Network Analysis**
Graphic plan of all events and activities to be completed in order to reach an objective

(a) **PERT**
Programme Evaluation and Review Technique

A Management Technique where logical sequence is followed with diagrammatic representations.
It is possible to calculate the time by which each activity must be completed and identify activities that are critical.
All concerned will know what is expected of them and minimise any delays or crises in implementation of plan.
PERT aids in planning, scheduling, monitoring and evaluation of the project.

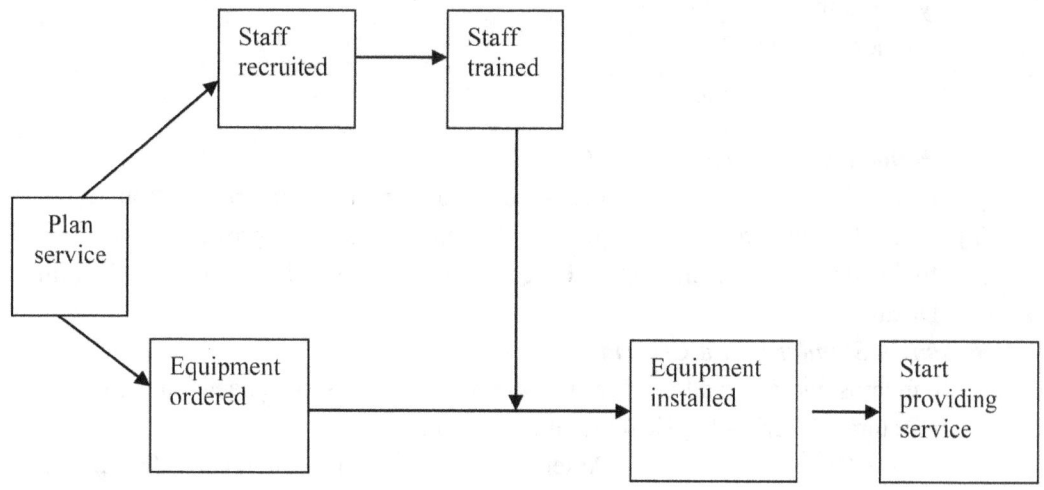

(b) Critical Path Method (CPM)

The longest path. If any activity along critical path is delayed, the entire project will be delayed.

viii. Planning Programming Budgeting System (PPBS)

Plan, program, budget involved.

Helps decision makers to allocate resources so that resources used in cost effective ways to achieve objectives.

Zero Budget Approach - All budgets start at zero, no one gets any budget that he cannot justify on year-to year basis.

ix. Work Sampling

Periodic, random check in health management on Doctors, nurses, pharmacists, laboratory technicians.

x. Decision Making

Decisions made regarding development of resources, optimum work load for medical and paramedical workers, strategies for providing health care.

EVALUATION

General Steps in Evaluation of Health Services

1. Determine what is to be evaluated
2. Establish Standards and Criteria
3. Plan Methodology
4. Gather Information
5. Analyse Results
6. Take Action
7. Re-evaluate

1. Determine what is to be evaluated

   (a) Evaluation of Structure - Facilities, equipment, manpower, organisation

   (b) Evaluation of Process - Recognition, diagnosis, treatment, prevention

   (c) Evaluation of Outcome-5Ds - Disease, Discomfort, Dissatisfaction, Disability, Death

2. Establish Standards and Criteria

   • Standards and criteria to determine whether objectives have been attained

   • Structural Criteria - Physical facilities, equipment

   • Process Criteria - Eg ANC- 4 Antenatal check-up; Lab technician - 100 Smears

   • Outcome Criteria - Health status - Cured, disability, death

   • Health care behavior - Satisfaction, dissatisfaction

   • Educational Process - Smoking cessation, acceptance of small family norms

3. *Plan Methodology*

Format prepared based on objectives and criteria for evaluation.

4. *Gather information*

Data collection including political, cultural, economic, environment, administrative factors.

5. *Analyse Results*

Analysis, interpretation, feedback to all stakeholders.

6. *Take Action*

Reviewing objectives, modify services and develop new programmes.

7. *Re-evaluate*

Evaluation is ongoing aimed at more efficient, effective health services

CHAPTER 22

DISASTER MANAGEMENT

Any occurrence that causes damage, ecological disruption, loss of human life and deterioration of health and health services on a scale sufficient to warrant an extraordinary response from outside the affected community

Classification

I Natural Disasters

Meteorological Disasters: Storms (Cyclones, Hailstorms, Hurricanes, Tornadoes, Typhoons, Snowstorms), cold spells, heat waves, Droughts

Typological Disasters: Avalanches, Landslides, Floods

Telluric & Teutonic Disasters: Earthquakes, Tsunamis, Volcanic Eruptions

Biological Disasters: Insect Swarms (eg Locusts), Epidemics of Communicable Diseases

II Manmade Disasters

Civil Disturbances: Riots, Demonstrations

Warfare:

Conventional Warfare: Bombardment, Blockage, Siege

Non-conventional Warfare: Nuclear, Biological, Chemical

Refugees: Forced movement of large number of people across frontiers

Accidents: Transportation Calamities (Land, air, sea), collapse of buildings, dams, mine disasters

Technological Failures: Mishap at Nuclear Power Stations (Chernobyl), leak at a chemical plant

(Bhopal gas tragedy), breakdown of public sanitation system.

Effects of Disasters

Deaths

Morbidity - Gastrointestinal Diseases, Typhoid, Cholera, Tetanus, Plague, Hepatitis, Leptospirosis

Injuries - Mild, moderate, severe, fractures, Pneumothorax

Emotional stress

Damage to Health Facilities

Damage to Water Systems
Poor Sanitation
Food Shortage
Major Population Movements

Disaster Management

There are 3 main aspects:
1. Disaster Response
2. Disaster Mitigation
3. Disaster Preparedness

Disaster Cycle

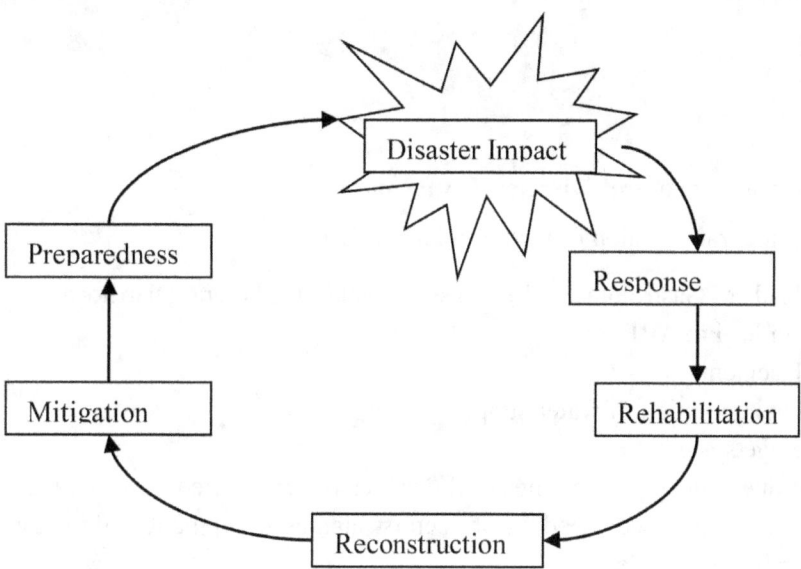

1.   Disaster Impact and Response
First few hours - Greatest need for Emergency Care (Golden Hours)

Management of mass casualties divided into:

  i.   Search, Rescue, First Aid
 ii.   Field Care
iii.   Triage and Stabilisation
       Category I - Immediate treatment required - Red
       Category II - Delayed treatment required - Yellow
       Category III - Minimal treatment required - Green
       Category IV - Severely injured; Moribund Cases - Black
 iv.   Hospital Treatment
  v.   Redistribution to other Hospitals if necessary

Relief Phase

Assistance from outside reaches disaster areas

(a) Drug supplies for treatment of casualties
(b) Supplies for preventing spread of Communicable Diseases
(c) Food
(d) Clothing, blankets
(e) Shelter
(f) Sanitary engineering equipment
(g) Construction material

Disaster Managers

There are 4 principal components in managing supplies:

i. Acquisition of supplies
ii. Transportation
iii. Storage, and
iv. Distribution

Epidemiological Surveillance and Disease Control

Disasters can increase the transmission of Communicable Diseases:

1. Poor sanitation leads to Gastrointestinal Diseases - Typhoid, Cholera, Diarrhoea
2. Overcrowding can lead to ARI
3. Population displacement
4. Disruption and contamination of water supply
5. Damage to sewerage system
6. Disruption of routine control programmes as funds, personnel diverted for relief work
7. Ecological Changes - Increased breeding of vectors, increased population of vectors leading To vector borne diseases
8. Displacement of domestic and wild animals – Zoonoses - Domestic animals (Leptospirosis, Rickettsioses); wild animals (Equine Encephalitis, Rabies)
9. Provision of emergency food, water, shelter itself may be a source of infectious diseases

Principles of Prevention and Control

(a) Implement public health measures
(b) Organise reliable disease reporting system to identify outbreaks and promptly initiate control measures
(c) Investigate all reports of disease outbreaks rapidly

Vaccination

WHO does not recommend Typhoid, Cholera, Tetanus vaccines during disasters.
Safe drinking water & proper disposal of excreta.

Mass vaccination against Tetanus is unnecessary.

Best protection: Maintain high level immunity by routine vaccinations and adequate wound cleaning and treatment

Maintenance of on-going National Control/Eradication Programmes

Nutrition

At risk groups - Infants, children, pregnant women, lactating mothers, sick persons

Nutritional problems eg PEM, Vit A Deficiency may occur

Immediate Steps

(a) Assessing food supplies
(b) Gauging nutritional needs
(c) Calculating daily food rations and need for large population groups
(d) Monitoring nutritional status

Rehabilitation

Important issues:

Water Supply

Basic Sanitation

Food Safety

Vector Control

2. *Disaster Mitigation (Decreasing Severity)*

Emergency prevention and mitigation involves:

Measures to prevent hazards causing emergency or

Lessen likely effects of emergency

Eg Flood mitigation works, appropriate land use planning, improved building codes, protection of vulnerable populations, protection of structures

3. *Disaster Preparedness*

Goal - To strengthen the overall capacity and capability of a country to efficiently manage all types of emergencies.

Policy Development - Formal statement of course of action.

Disaster Training - Of manpower eg Health care personnel, police department, fire brigade, ambulance services on Disaster Management.

Disaster Drill - Simulation Exercise on disaster and action to be taken during emergencies.

CHAPTER 23

HOSPITAL WASTE MANAGEMENT

Hospital waste (Biomedical waste) - Any waste generated during Diagnosis, Treatment, Immunization of human beings/animals or from Research Activities.

Sources of Health Care Waste

Government hospitals, Private hospitals, Nursing homes, Physician's clinics, Dentist's clinics, PHCs, Vaccination centres
Blood Banks
Mortuaries
Animal Houses
Laboratories
Medical Research & Training Centres
Biotechnology Institutions

Public Health Importance

Waste generated from hospitals:
85% - General waste
15% - Infectious waste

If the 15% Infectious Waste is not segregated from the 85% General Waste, then 100% will become infectious waste!

Infectious Waste (15%) + General Waste (85%)→100% Infectious waste

Therefore, Infectious Waste should be properly segregated and disposed.

Health Hazards of Health Care Waste

1. Hazards from infectious waste & sharps
    Pathogens eg., HIV, Hepatitis B, C
2. Hazards from Chemical & Pharmaceutical waste
    Chemicals & pharmaceuticals can be toxic, genotoxic, corrosives, flammable, reactive, explosive

3. Hazards from Genotoxic waste
   Cytotoxic drugs, chemicals may be inhaled, ingested or enter through skin
4. Hazards from Radioactive waste
   Radioactive waste can lead to headache, dizziness, vomiting, cancer, chromosomal anomalies
5. Public sensitivity
   General public is sensitive to see health care waste e.g., Anatomical waste

At Risk Persons

Medical doctors, nurses, paramedicals, housekeeping personnel
Patients
Visitors
Workers in support services allied to health care establishments eg. Laundry, waste handling & transportation
Workers in waste disposal facilities eg. Landfills, incinerators

Biomedical waste - Categories, Segregation, Collection, Treatment, Processing & Disposal

Category	Type of Waste	Type of Bag/ Container	Treatment & Disposal
YELLOW	a) Human Anatomical Waste (b) Animal Anatomical Waste (c) Soiled Waste	Yellow coloured, non-chlorinated plastic bags	Incineration/Plasma Pyrolysis/ Deep Burial
	Items contaminated with blood/ body fluids eg Dressings, plaster cast, cotton swabs, bags containing discarded blood & blood components	Yellow coloured, non-chlorinated plastic bags	Incineration/Plasma Pyrolysis/ Deep Burial In absence of above: Autoclaving/Microwaving/ Hydroclaving followed by shredding/mutilation/ combination of sterilisation & shredding Treated waste to be sent for energy recovery

Category	Type of Waste	Type of Bag/ Container	Treatment & Disposal
	(d) Expired/ Discarded medicines Pharmaceuticals, Cytotoxics and glass, Ampoules, vials All other discarded medicines shall be either sent back to manufacturer or disposed by incineration	Yellow coloured, non-chlorinated plastic bags	Expired Cytotoxics returned to manufacturer or supplier for incineration at >1200°C or common Biomedical Waste Treatment Facility or Hazardous Waste Treatment Facility and Incineration >1200°C or Encapsulation or Plasma Pyrolysis>1200°C Incineration/Plasma Pyrolysis/ Encapsulation
	(e) Chemical Waste: Chemicals and Disinfectants		
	(f) Chemical Liquid Waste: chemical liquid waste, disinfectants, X-ray film liquid, formalin, infected secretions, aspirated body fluids, liquid from floor washings	Separate collection system leading to effluent treatment system	After resource recovery, chemical liquid waste pre-treated and discharged with other waste water
	(g) Discarded linen, mattress, beddings, contaminated with blood/body fluids	Non-chlorinated yellow plastic bags/suitable packing material	Non-chlorinated Chemical Disinfection followed by incineration/Plasma Pyrolysis for energy recovery In absence of above: Shredding/mutilation/ combination of sterilisation & shredding. Treated waste to be sent for energy recovery or incineration or Plasma Pyrolysis
	(h) Microbiology, Biotechnology, other clinical laboratory waste		

Category	Type of Waste	Type of Bag/ Container	Treatment & Disposal
		Autoclave safe plastic bags/ containers	Pre-treat to sterilise with non-chlorinated chemicals as per NACO/WHO Guidelines thereafter incineration
RED	Contaminated waste (Recyclable) Tubes, bottles, IV tubes, catheters, urine bags, syringes without needles, vacutainers with their needles cut, gloves	Red colour non-chlorinated plastic bags/containers	Autoclaving/Microwaving/ Hydroclaving followed by Shredding/mutilation or combination of sterilisation and shredding Treated waste to be sent to registered/authorised recyclers or energy recovery or plastics to diesel/fuel or road making Plastic waste should not be sent to landfill sites
WHITE (translucent)	Waste sharps including metals: Needles, syringes with fixed needles, needles from needle tip cutter/ burner, scalpels, blades, contaminated sharp objects including metal sharps	Puncture-proof, leak-proof, tamper-proof containers	Autoclaving/Dry heat sterilisation followed by Mutilation/Encapsulation in metal container/cement concrete, combination of shredding cum autoclaving, sent for final disposal to iron foundries/ sanitary landfills/designated concrete waste sharp pits
BLUE	a) Glassware: Broken/discarded and contaminated glass including medicine vials, Ampoules, except those contaminated with Cytotoxic wastes (b) Metallic body implants	Cardboard boxes with blue coloured marking Cardboard boxes with blue coloured marking	Disinfection (By soaking the washed glass waste after cleaning with detergent and Sodium Hypochlorite treatment) or through Autoclaving/ Microwaving/Hydroclaving and then sent for Recycling

Categories of Biomedical Waste

Legislation
It was passed in 1998, modified in 2016 – Biomedical Waste (Management & Handling) Rules by Government of India.

CHAPTER 24

PRIMARY HEALTH CARE

Essential Health Care made universally accessible to individuals and acceptable to them through their full participation and at a cost the community and country can afford.

Elements

- Education concerning prevailing health problems and methods of preventing and controlling them
- Promotion of food supply and proper nutrition
- Adequate supply of safe water and basic sanitation
- Maternal and Child Health Care and Family Planning
- Immunization against major infectious diseases
- Prevention and control of locally Endemic Diseases
- Appropriate treatment of common diseases and injuries
- Provision of essential drugs

Principles

1. *Equitable Distribution:*
   Health Care should be available to rural as well as urban; to poor as well as rich.

2. *Community Participation:*
   Community involvement is important for planning, implementation, maintenance of health services and for local resources (Manpower, money, materials) eg. ASHA under NRHM, dais, Anganwadi workers in villages; in China barefoot doctors.

3. *Intersectoral Coordination:*
   Among various sectors eg. Agriculture, animal husbandry, food industry, housing, public works, communication, education.

4. *Appropriate Technology:*
   Technology which is scientifically sound, adaptable to local needs, acceptable to those who apply it and for whom it is used and can be maintained by people themselves with the resources the community and country can afford eg. ORS for Diarrhea.

HEALTH FOR ALL

In 1977, World Health Assembly launched a movement called Health For All (HFA) by 2000.

Definition

Attainment of a level of health that will enable every individual to lead a socially and economically productive life.

In 1978, Alma Ata International Conference stated that the key to attaining HFA 2000 is through Primary Health Care, specially to underserved rural and urban poor people.

1983 National Health Policy

Goals to be achieved by 2000

(a) IMR <60/1000 live births
(b) CBR 21/1000 population
(c) Life expectancy raise to 64 years
(d) CDR - 9/1000 population
(e) To achieve NRR of 1

UN's Millennium Development Goals Indicators:

Indicators for Children:

Proportion of underweight children under 5 years
Infant Mortality Rate
Under 5 Mortality Rate
Proportion of 1-year-old children immunized for Measles
Proportion of population below minimum level of Dietary Energy Consumption

Indicators for Mothers:

Maternal Mortality Rate
Proportion of births attended by skilled health personnel

For HIV, Malaria, TB:

HIV prevalence among young people (15-24 years; 15-49 years)
Condom use in high-risk populations
Ratio of children orphaned/non-orphaned in schools (AIDS Orphans)

Malaria Death Rate per 100,000 children of 0-4 years
Malaria Death Rate per 100,000 in all age groups
Malaria Prevalence Rate per 100,000 population

Proportion of under 5 population with fever being treated with Antimalarial drugs
Proportion of under 5 population in Malaria risk areas using Insecticide treated bed-nets

TB Death Rate per 100,000
TB Prevalence Rate per 100,000

Proportion of Smear Positive PTB cases detected and under DOTS treatment
Proportion of Smear Positive PTB cases detected cured under DOTS

For Environment

Proportion of population using Biomass Fuel
Proportion of population with sustainable access to an improved water source - Rural and urban
Proportion of urban population with access to improved sanitation

For Essential Drugs

Proportion of population with access to affordable essential drugs

Sustainable Development Goals (SDGs)

In September 2015, the UN General Assembly adopted a new Development Agenda: Transforming Our World - The 2030 agenda for Sustainable Development comprising 17 goals.

Goal 1 - No Poverty
Goal 2 - Zero Hunger
Goal 3 - Good Health & Well-being
Goal 4 - Quality Education
Goal 5 - Gender Equality
Goal 6 - Clean Water & Sanitation
Goal 7 - Affordable & Clean Energy
Goal 8 - Decent Work & Economic Growth
Goal 9 - Industry, Innovation, Infrastructure
Goal 10 - Reduced Inequalities
Goal 11 - Sustainable Cities & Communities
Goal 12 - Responsible Consumption & Production
Goal 13 - Climate Action
Goal 14 - Life Below Water
Goal 15 - Life on Land
Goal 16 - Peace, Justice & Strong Institutions
Goal 17 - Global Partnership

SDG 3 - Health has 13 Targets and 26 Indicators

Goals & Targets	Indicators
3.1 - By 2030 reduce Global MMR <70/100,000 LB	3.1.1 - MMR 3.1.2 - Proportion of births attended by skilled health personnel
3.2 - By 2030 end preventable deaths of newborns & children < 5 years Neonatal Mortality < 12/1000 LB Under 5 Mortality < 25/1000LB	3.2.1 - Neonatal Mortality Rate 3.2.2 - Under 5 Mortality Rate
3.3 - By 2030 end Epidemics of AIDS, TB, Malaria, & neglected Tropical Diseases & combat Hepatitis, Water Borne Diseases & other Communicable Diseases	3.3.1 - No. of new HIV/1000 uninfected population 3.3.2 - TB incidence/1000 persons/year 3.3.3 - Malaria incidence/1000 persons/year 3.3.4 - Hepatitis incidence/100,000 population/year Hepatitis B vaccination coverage 3 doses 3.3.5 - No. of people requiring interventions against neglected Tropical Diseases
3.4 - By 2030 reduce by one third Premature Mortality from NCDs through prevention, treatment & promote mental health and well-being	3.4.1 - Mortality of Cardiovascular Disease. Ca, Diabetes or Chronic Respiratory Diseases 3.4.2 - Suicide Mortality Rate
3.5 - Strengthen the prevention & treatment of substance abuse including Narcotic Drug Abuse & harmful rise of Alcohol	3.5.1 - Coverage & treatment interventions for substance use disorders Harmful use of Alcohol
3.6 - By 2020 halve the no. of Global Deaths & injuries from RTA (Road Traffic Accidents)	3.6.1 - No. of road traffic fatal injury deaths within 30 days/100,000 population
3.7 - By 2030 ensure universal access to sexual & reproductive health care services including FP information & education and introduction of Reproductive Health into national strategies & programmes	3.7.1 - % women of reproductive age (15-49 years) who have their need for FP satisfied with modern methods 3.7.2 - Adolescent Birth Rate (10-14; 15-19 years) per 1000 women in that age group
3.8 - Achieve Universal Health Coverage including Financial Risk Protection, access to quality essential health care services, access to safe effective quality affordable essential medicines & vaccines	3.8.1 - Coverage of Tracer Interventions eg. Child full immunization, ART, TB treatment, Hypertension treatment, Skilled birth attendant at birth 3.8.2 - Proportion of population protected against catastrophic out of pocket health expenditure

3.9 - By 2030 substantially reduce no. of deaths & illness from hazardous chemicals & air, water and soil pollution & contamination	3.9.1 - Mortality Rate due to household & ambient air pollution/lakh population Mortality Rate due to hazardous chemicals, water and soil pollution and contamination
3.10 - Strengthen implementation of WHO Framework Convention on Tobacco control in all countries	3.10.1 - Age standardised prevalence of current Tobacco use among persons 15 years and older
3.11 - Support Research & Development of vaccines & medicines for Communicable & Non-Communicable Diseases	3.11.1 - Proportion of population with access to affordable medicines & vaccines 3.11.2 - Total net official development & assistance to medical research & basic health sectors
3.12 - Substantially increase Health Financing & Recruitment Development Training and Retention of health workforce in developing & least developed countries and small island developing states	3.12.1 - Health worker density & distribution per 10,000 Population
3.13 - Strengthen capacity of all countries for early warning, risk reduction & management of national & global health risks	3.13.1 - % of attributes of 13 core capacities that have been attained at a specific point in time

Health Status and Health Problems

For planning Health Care Services, community diagnosis regarding Health Status and Health Problems is required.

Data Required

Morbidity, Mortality statistics
Population Demography
Environmental conditions
Socio-economic factors
Cultural factors
Medical & Health Services available
Other services available

Analysis of above data will help to identify health needs of the community.

Health Problems in India:

- Population problem
- Communicable diseases
- Non-communicable diseases

- Nutritional problems
- Environmental Sanitation problems
- Health Care problems

Resources

Manpower
Money
Material
Time

Health Care Services

Services

(a) Curative
(b) Preventive
(c) Promotive

Primary Health Care to achieve Health For All by 2000.

Village Level (1000 Population)   AWWs, Dais, ASHAs
Sub-centre Level (5,000 Population)   Health Worker Males, Health Worker Females
Primary Health Centre (PHC)
30,000 Population

Indian Public Health Standards (IPHS)

Objectives

- To provide comprehensive health care to community through PHCs
- To achieve & maintain acceptable standard of care quality
- To make services more responsive & sensitive to needs of the community
- Services – Preventive, Promotive, Curative, Rehabilitative

    1. Medical Care – OPD – 4 hours morning,
       2 hours afternoon/evening
       40 Patients/day
       24-hours Emergency Services
       Referral Services
       Inpatient Services - 6 Beds
    2. MCH - ANC, INC, PNC (Mother & infant)
    3. Family Planning
    4. MTP
    5. Health Education for prevention & management of RTI/STI
    6. Nutrition Services
    7. School Health Services

8. Adolescent Health Care
9. Disease Surveillance & control of Epidemics
10. Collection & reporting vital events
11. Promotion of Sanitation - Use of toilet, garbage disposal
12. Testing water quality, disinfection of water
13. National Health Programs
    RNTCP, NPCB, NVBDCP, NACP etc
14. Referral
15. Record vital events
16. Training - Health workers, health assistants, ANMs, ASHAs, Pharmacists, AYUSH Doctors
17. Laboratory Services - Basic
18. Monitoring & Supervision
19. Selected Surgical Procedures - Tubectomy, Vasectomy, MTP, Cataract Surgery, Hydrocelectomy
20. Mainstreaming of AYUSH

Staffing Pattern

Staff	Existing	Recommended
Medical Officer	1	3 (1 female)
Ayush Practitioner	-	1 (AYUSH/ISM)
Accounts Manager	-	1
Pharmacist	1	2
Nurse Midwife	1	5
Health Worker Female	1	1
Health Educator	1	1
Health Assistant (M+F)	2	2
Clerks	2	2
Lab Technician	1	2
Driver	1	Optional
Class - IV	4	4
TOTAL	**15**	**24**

Under ROME (Re-Orient Medical Education) Program, 3 PHCs attached to 148 medical colleges each.

Job Responsibilities

Medical Officer

- Leader of Health Team
- OPD patients, In-patients
- Referral to CHC/FRU

- National Health Programmes - RCH, UIP, FP, IDSP, IMNCI, RNTCP, NLEP, NBCP, NPCDCS
- Organise & conduct Tubectomy & Vasectomy camps
- Visit sub-centres, supervise, guide
- School Health Programme - August yearly
- Training AWWs, Dais, ASHAs
- Monthly meetings at PHC
- Attends monthly meetings conducted by DHO

Second Medical Officer - Same duties

Health Assistant

Common	Male	Female
Supervision of Health Workers Guidance Meetings Camps Campaigns	Malaria Leprosy TB UIP FP Nutrition Blindness Control Epidemic measures Vital events	RCH UIP Training

Health Worker

Common	Male	Female
Multi-Purpose Worker (MPW) (5,000 Population) Hilly/Tribal - 3,000 Population	Records, Registers Maps Malaria Leprosy TB UIP FP Nutrition Blindness Control Epidemic measures Sanitation	Records, Registers Maps, Survey **Care at Home:** MCH ANC PNC FP MTP Advice Infants & Children Supervise Dais Training of Dais First Aid Referral Notifiable Diseases Vital Statistics **Care at Clinic:** Arrange MCH & FP clinics at sub-centres

Common	Male	Female
		Investigations - Hb, Urine Conduct deliveries Refer complicated cases for institutional delivery Health Education on MCH & FP **Care In Community**: Identify & Train women leaders Identify Depot Holders for Condom Distribution & Train Participate in Mahila Mandal Meetings Educate on Family Welfare

Community Health Centre (CHC)

Population - 80,000-120,000
Beds - 30
Specialists - Surgery, Medicine, OBG, Paediatrics
X-Ray facilities
Laboratory facilities

Indian Public Health Standards (IPHS)

Services to be provided by CHC:

Care of routine & emergency services in Surgery

I&D, Hernia, Hydrocele, Appendicitis, Hemorrhoids, Fistula operations
Emergencies - Hemorrhage, Intestinal Obstruction

Care of routine & emergency services in Medicine

Emergencies in National Programmes
DHF, DSS, Cerebral Malaria

OBG
Delivery Services 24-hours.
Care of routine & emergency Obstetric Care - LSCS

FP

Services including Laparoscopic Sterilisation

Safe Abortion Services

Infants & Children

Newborn Care
Routine & emergency care of sick children

Other Management

Nasal Packing, foreign body removal, Tracheostomy

All National Health Programs

RNTCP, NACP, NVBDCP, NLEP, NPCB, IDSP

Blood Bank Facility

Laboratory Services

Referral Services

Manpower at CHC:

Medical Personnel	Strength
Block Health Officer	-
Surgeon	1
Physician	1
OBG Specialist	1
Pediatrician	1
Anaesthetist	1
Public Health Manager	1
Eye Surgeon	1
Dental Surgeon	1
General Medical Officers	6 (At least 2 females)
AYUSH Specialist	1
AYUSH Medical Officer	1
Total	**16**

Paramedical Personnel	Strength
Staff Nurse	19
Public Health Nurse	1
ANM	1
Pharmacist	3
AYUSH Pharmacist	1
Lab Technician	3
Radiographer	2
Ophthalmic Assistant	1
Dresser	2
Ward boys	5
Sweepers	5
Chowkidar	5
Dhobi	1
Mali	1
Ayah	5
Peon	2
OPD Attendant	1
Registration Clerk	2
Statistical Assistant	2
Accountant	1
OT Technician	1
Total	**64**

CHAPTER 25

ESSENTIAL MEDICINES & COUNTERFEIT MEDICINES

Essential Medicines

Those that satisfy the priority health care needs of a population.
These should be available in all PHCs in adequate amounts, doses and quality at all times.

Counterfeit Medicines

Medicines produced with the intention to cheat. eg Mislabeling of expiry date; decreased or no active ingredient or wrong ingredient; unregistered or unlicensed medicines.

Branded and generic drugs too can be counterfeited.
They may contain Corn Starch, Potato Starch or Chalk.

10% of medicines are substandard; Contribute to Antimicrobial Resistance.
Suspicious medicines have to be reported to National Medicines Regulatory Authority.

List of Essential Medicines

Anesthetic Agents - General & local anesthetics, preoperative medications, sedatives

Analgesics, Antipyretics, NSAIDs, Antigout - Disease modifying agents

Antiallergics & Anti-anaphylactics

Antidotes & Substances used for poisoning

Anticonvulsants & Antiepileptics

Anti-infectives - Antihelmintics, Antifilarials, Antischistosomal, Antibacterial, Antileprosy, Anti TB, Antimalarial, Antifungal, Antiviral, Antiherpes, Antiretroviral, Antihepatitis B, C, Antiprotozoal, Antileishmaniasis
Antimigraine medicines

Anti-neoplastic, Immuno-suppressives
Hormones & Antihormones

Anti-Parkinsonism

Medicines Affecting Blood – Anti-anemic medicines, Anticoagulation
Blood products & Plasma substitutes

CVS Medicines

Medicines for Dementia

Dermatological medicines - Antifungal, anti-infective, anti-inflammatory, anti-pruritic,
Scabicides,

Pediculicides

Dialysis solutions

Disinfectants, Antiseptics

Diuretics

ENT Medicines

Ophthalmology medicines

GI medicines
Hormones, Endocrinology Medicines, Contraceptives

Immunologicals
Muscle Relaxants & Cholinesterase Inhibitors

Medicines for Neonatal Care
Oxytocics & Anti-oxytocics

Psychotherapeutic medicines

Respiratory Tract medicines

Solutions correcting water - Electrolyte disturbances and acid-base disturbances

Vitamins & Minerals

Miscellaneous medicines

CHAPTER 26

HEALTH PLANNING IN INDIA & NATIONAL PROGRAMMES

Bhore Committee

Formulated in 1946 – A Health Planning & Development Committee
Founded by - Sir Joseph Bhore, Chairman
The committee surveyed health conditions and health organisations

"If the nation's health is to be built, a Health Programme should be developed on a foundation of preventive health work & such activities should proceed side by side with those concerned with treatment of patients"

Recommendations:

i.   Integration of preventive and curative services at all administrative levels
ii. Development of PHCs in two stages
(a) Short Term - PHC for 40,000 population
(b) Long Term – Plan for 3 million population
PHCs with 75 beds for 10,000-20,000 population,
Secondary Units with 650 beds,
District Hospitals with 2500 beds

iii. Formation of Village Health Committee
iv. Provision for Social Doctor, Intersectoral Approach to Health Services Development
v.   Major changes in Medical Education, 3 months Preventive & Social Medicine Training to prepare Social Physicians

Mudaliar Committee

A Health Survey & Planning Committee
Formulated in 1962 by Dr AL Mudaliar

It reviewed the progress made in the Health Sector

Recommendations:

- PHCs should be strengthened
- Strengthening Sub-divisional & District Hospitals
- Regional Organisations in each state
- Limit population served by PHC to 40,000
- Improve quality of Health Care
- Integration of Medical & Health Services
- Constitution of All India Health Service on the IAS pattern

Chadah Committee

This was formulated in 1963 by Dr MS Chadah

The aim was to study arrangements for maintenance phase of National Malaria Eradication Programme (NMEP)

Recommendations:

- Vigilance Operations of NMEP the responsibility of PHCs
- Basic Health Workers for Vigilance Operations through monthly home visits - 1 BHW for 10,000 population
- To look after Vital Statistics and Family Planning
- FP Health Assistants to supervise 3-4 BHWs
- At District Level - Responsibility of General Health Services

Mukherjee Committee

It was formulated in 1965 by Sri Mukherjee – The Secretary of Health

Recommendations:

- Delink Malaria activities from Family Planning
- Family Planning Programme should have separate staff
- Family Planning Assistants – To take care of family planning duties only
- Details of Basic Health Service at the Block level & strengthening of Supervisory Levels

Jungalwalla Committee

It was formulated in 1967
A Committee on Integration of Health Services
It was founded by Dr N Jungalwalla

Integrated Health Services:

i. Service with a unified approach for all problems instead of segmented approach for different problems

ii. Medical care of sick & Public Health Programmes under a single administrator & operating in an unified manner.

Recommendations:

- Unified Cadre
- Common Seniority
- Recognition of extra qualifications
- Equal pay for equal work
- Special pay for specialised work
- Abolition of private practice by Government Doctors
- Good service conditions

Kartar Singh Committee

A Committee on MPW under Health & Family Planning
Formulated by Sri Kartar Singh, the Additional Secretary of Health

Recommendations:

- ANMs to be replaced by Female Health Workers
- Basic Health Workers, Malaria Surveillance Workers, Vaccinators, Health Education Assistants, Family Planning Health Assistants to be replaced by Male Health Workers.
- 1PHC for 50,000 population
- 16 Sub-centres with 3,000-3,500 population each
- Sub-centre - 1 MHW & 1 FHW
- 1 Male Health Supervisor for 3-4 MHWs
- 1 Female Health Supervisor for 3-4 FHWs
- Medical Officer - Overall in-charge of Supervisors & Health Workers

Shrivastav Committeee

It was formulated in 1975 – A Group on Medical Education & Support Manpower

Recommendations:

- Creation of para-professionals & semi-professional health workers from within the community to provide promotive, preventive, curative health services
- Establishment of 2 cadres of Health Workers - MPWs & HAs

- Referral service complex establishment - Linkages between PHC, higher level referral and service centres - Taluka, District, Regional, Medical College Hospitals
- Medical & Health Education Commission for planning and implementing reforms needed in Health and Medical Education on the lines of University Grants Commission

Rural Health Scheme

This was formulated in 1977 - Community Health Volunteer Scheme - Village Health Guides It was launched based on the recommendations of Shrivastav Committee.

Recommendations:

- Training of Community Health Volunteers
- Reorientation Training of MPWs
- Linking Medical Colleges to Rural Health

Health For All 2000 AD

In 1981 - Report of the Working Group
Headed by Secretary, Ministry of Health & Family Welfare
For Health Planning during VI 5-year plan
Framed Indices and Targets to be achieved by 2000 AD

1981 Report of Working Group on HFA by 2000
Broad approach to Health Planning
Targets fixed

Health System in India

28 States + 7 Union territories

At Central Level	At State Level	At District Level
1. Ministry of Health & Family Welfare 2. DGHS 3. Central Council of H & FW	1. State Ministry of Health 2. State Health Directorate	District is the principal unit of Administration There are 593 districts 6 types of Administrative Aeas:

1. Union Ministry of H & FW
Functions
Union List:
International Health
Regulations
Administration of Central
Institutes
	1. State Ministry of Health
	  Minister of H & FW
	  Deputy Minister of H &
	  FW
	2. State Health Directorate
	Director of H & FW - Chief
	Technical Advisor
		1. Subdivisions
		2. Tehsils (Talukas)
		3. Community Development
		  Blocks
		4. Municipalities &
		  Corporations
		5. Villages
		6. Panchayats

At Central Level	At State Level	At District Level
Medical Education, Dental Education, Nursing, Pharmacy Promotion of Research Drug Standards Census and other Statistics Data Coordination with states Concurrent List: PFA Control of Drugs and Poisons Labour Welfare Population Control & FP Vital Statistics 2. DGHS Functions General: Surveys, planning, programming, appraisal of all health matters Specific: International Health Regulations and Quarantine Drug Standards Medical Store Depots PG Training Medical Education Medical Research CGHS National Health Programmes Central Health Education Bureau National Medical Library Health Intelligence 3. Central Council of H & FW Policy of Health Legislation Grant in Aid Cooperation with State		CMOs &Deputy CMOs for all Health, Family Welfare and MCH Programmes Panchayati Raj System: 1. Panchayat - Village level 2. Panchayat Samiti - Block level 3. Zilla Panchayat - District level At Village Level: Trained Birth Attendant Anganwadi Worker ASHA At Sub-centre: 1 Health Worker Female 1 Health Worker Male At PHC: MO + Team At CHC: Specialists + Team Health Care Facilities: i. Primary Care: PHC for 30,000 population Sub-centre for 5,000 population Village for 1,000 population ii. Secondary Care: CHCs and Hospitals where Surgeon, Physician, OBG, Pediatrics specialists are available iii.Tertiary Care: Teaching Hospitals, Super-speciality Hospitals (Cancer, Neurology, Cardiology), Regional Hospitals (Railway Hospital) Present Satus: Medical Colleges 146 CHCs 2,962 PHCs 23,266 SCs 137,027

NITI AAYOG

On 01 January 2015 the National Institution for Transforming India (NITI) was launched. It is a Think Tank, providing Central and State governments with Technical Advice and Monitor and Evaluate the implementation of programmes.

Health Goals to be achieved by 2020

- Decrease MMR to 120/100,000 Live Births
- Decrease IMR to 30/1000 Live Births
- Decrease U5MR to 38/1000 Live Births
- Decrease TFR to 2.1
- Decrease TB Incidence to 130/100,000 Population
- Decrease Malaria Incidence API to <1/1000 in 90% districts
- Eliminate Kala Azar and Lymphatic Filariasis
  Reduce Premature Mortality from Cardiovascular Diseases, Cancer, Diabetes, Chronic Respiratory Diseases by 25%
- Reduce out-of-pocket spending to 50% of the total health expenditure

National Health Policy

The National Health Policy was formulated in 1983.

The Policy is a system which provides logical framework and rationality of decision making for achievement of intended objectives. It sets priorities and guides resource allocation. Policy adequacy may be measured by its impact on population health.

Present Scenario

(a) Major concerns are Population Explosion, Urbanisation and Urban Health Problems.

(b) Communicable Diseases - Malaria resurgence, insecticide resistant Malarial vectors, drug resistant Plasmodia, other vector borne diseases (Dengue fever, Japanese Encephalitis), TB - (MDR TB, XDR TB), HIV/AIDS, water borne infections - Gastroenteritis, Cholera, Typhoid, Hepatitis A and E.

(c) Lifestyle Diseases - Diabetes, Hypertension, Cardiovascular Diseases, Cancer.

(d) Geriatric Health Care need.

(e) Health Care for trauma patients required.

(f) MCH - Women's health problems, child health problems, macro and micronutrient deficiencies, decreasing sex ratio.

(g) Mental Health Disorders

(h) Escalating Cost of Health Care

(i) Inadequate Health Statistics

(j) Poor Information, Education and Communication

(k) 35% Illiterate Population

Achievements of India from 1951-2000

Indicator	1951	2001
Demographic Changes		
Life Expectancy (years)	36.7	63
CBR (per 1000 Population)	40.8	25.5
CDR (per 1000 Population)	25	8.4
IMR (per 1000 Live Births)	146	70
Couple Protection Rate (%)	-	46
Total Fertility Rate	6.0	3.8
Epidemiological Shifts		
Malaria (Cases in millions)	75	2.0
Smallpox (No. of cases)	> 44,887	Eradicated
Guinea Worm	-	Eradicated
Polio	-	265
Infrastructure		
Sub-centres	725	137,311
Dispensaries/Hospitals	9,209	43,322
Beds (Private & Public)	117,198	870,161
Doctors (Allopathic)	61,800	1:1,800
Nurses	18,054	1:5,600

National Health Policy 2002

A new policy framework for accelerated achievement of Public Health Goals was formulated in 2002.

Objectives:

- To achieve an acceptable standard of good health among the general population.
- To increase access to decentralised public health system by establishing new infrastructure in deficient areas and upgrading the infrastructure in existing institutions.
- To ensure a more equitable access to health services across social and geographical expanse of the country.
- To increase the aggregate Public Health Investment through a substantially increased contribution by the Central Government.
- To strengthen the capacity of Public Health Administration at the State Level to render effective service delivery.
- To enhance contribution of the private sector in providing health services for population groups which can afford to pay for services.
- To rationalise the use of drugs within the Allopathic System.
- To increase access to Traditional medicines

Goals to be achieved within 2000-2015

Year   Goals to be achieved

2003   Enactment of legislation for regulating minimum standard in Clinical Establishments/ Medical Institutions

2005   Eradicate Poliomyelitis and Yaws

Eliminate Leprosy

Establish an Integrated System of Surveillance, National Health Accounts & Health Statistics

Increase State Sector Health spending from 5.5% to 7% of the budget

1% of total Health Budget for Medical Research

Decentralisation of implementation of Public Health Programmes

2007   Achieve zero level growth of HIV/AIDS

2010   Eliminate Kala Azar

Reduce Mortality by 50% due to TB, Malaria and other Vector and water borne diseases

Reduce IMR to 30/1000 Live Births and MMR to 100/lakh Live Births

Reduce Blindness Prevalence to 0.5%

Increase utilisation of Public Health Facilities from <20 - >75%

Increase health expenditure by Government from 0.9% to 2% of GDP

Increase of State sector health spending to 8%

2015   Eliminate Lymphatic Filariasis

Policy Prescriptions

1. *Financial Resources*
    Central Government from 0.9 to 2%
    State Government from 5.5 to 7% to 8% by 2010

2. *Equity*
    Increased allocation for primary, secondary and tertiary health sectors.

3. *Delivery of National Health Programmes*
    Policy ensures financial resources, technical support, monitoring and evaluation of National Health Programmes.

4. *AYUSH*
    Ayurveda, Yoga, Unani, Siddha and Homeopathy included to expand the pool of Medical Practitioners.

5. *Role of Local Self Government*
    Great emphasis is laid upon implementation of Public Health Programmes through Local Self-Government Institutions.

6. **Education of Health Care Professionals**
   Envisages setting up a Medical Grants Commission for funding new Government Medical/Dental colleges and for upgradation of existing colleges.
   The policy also recommends Continuing Medical Education (CME)

7. **Need for Specialists in Public Health and Family Medicine**
   Increased Postgraduate seats in Public Health and Family Medicine

8. **Nursing Personnel**
   Training Institutes for training nurses and training courses for super-speciality nurses required for Tertiary Care Institutions.

9. **Generic Drugs and Vaccines**
   Essential drugs of Generic nature will be promoted.

10. **Urban Health**
    Setting up of Urban Primary Health Care Structure with a 2-tier system, PHC as first tier and Government General Hospital as secondary tier.
    Also envisages Trauma Care networks to decrease Accident Mortality.

11. **Mental Health**
    Decentralised Mental Health Services where Medical Officer PHC would be able to prescribe medicine.

12. **IEC**
    Information, Education and Communication with focus on interpersonal communication, folk and traditional media.
    Development of modules for information dissemination.
    School Health Programmes for preventive health education, providing regular health checkup, promotion of health seeking behavior and family life education.

13. **Health Research**
    2% of total health spending for Medical Research.
    Research on new Therapeutic Drugs, Vaccines for Tropical Diseases eg. TB, Malaria, HIV/AIDS

14. **Role of Private Sector**
    Participation of Private Sector including Private Insurance in primary, secondary and tertiary health care.
    Social Health Insurance Scheme funded by the Government.
    Quality accreditation of Clinical Establishments/Medical Institutions.

15. **Role of Civil Society**
    To include NGOs and Civil Society in implementation of Disease Control Programmes.

16. **National Disease Surveillance Network**
Integrated Disease Control Network by 2005.

17. **Health Statistics**
Baseline estimates for incidence of common diseases – TB, Malaria, Blindness, Hepatitis and Japanese Encephalitis.
Baseline estimates for Non-Communicable Diseases - CVD, Ca, Diabetes, Accidental injuries.

18. **Women's Health**
Highest priority of Central Government funding for programmes related to women's health.

19. **Medical Ethics**
Common patient should not be subjected to profit driven medical regimens.

20. **Quality Control**
Enforcement of quality standards for Food and Drugs and Laboratory facilities.

21. **Standards in Paramedical Disciplines**
Establishment of Statutory Professional Councils for Paramedical Disciplines to register practitioners, maintain standards of training and monitor performance.

22. **Environmental & Occupational Health**
Environmental Health policies to be included with programmes of the health sector.
Periodic screening of health conditions of workers associated with their occupations.

23. **Medical Tourism**
National Health Policy 2002 strongly encourages providing medical facilities to users from overseas.

24. **Impact of Globalisation on the Health Sector**
The policy envisages securing for the country, affordable access to the latest medical and other therapeutic discoveries.

National Health Policy 2017

The Primary aim of NHP is to inform, clarify, strengthen, prioritise the Government's role in moulding health system eg. Investment in health, prevention of disease, promotion of good health through cross sectoral actions, organisation of health care services.

Specific Quantitative Goals & Objectives

A. Health Status and Programme Impact
B. Health Systems Performance
C. Health System Strengthening

A. Health Status and Programme Impact

1. *Life Expectancy and Healthy Life*
    (a) Increase Life Expectancy from 67 to 70 years
    (b) Regular tracking of DALY (Disability-Adjusted Life Year)
    (c) Decrease TFR to 2.1

2. *Mortality by Age and/Cause*
    (a) U5MR to 23 & MMR to 100
    (b) IMR to 28
    (c) Neonatal Mortality Rate to 16

3. *Reduction of Disease Prevalence/Incidence*
    (a) HIV/AIDS achieve 90:90:90 target
    (b) Achieve and Maintain elimination status of:
        Leprosy
        Kala Azar
        Lymphatic Filariasis
    (c) TB - Cure Rate >85% in new sputum positive patients and decrease incidence of new cases to elimination level
    (d) Blindness - Decrease prevalence of Blindness to 0.25/1000
    (e) Decrease premature Mortality from Cardiovascular Disease, Ca, DM, Chronic Respiratory diseases by 25%

B. Health Systems Performance

1. *Coverage of Health Services*
    (a) Increase utilisation of Public Health facilities by 50% by 2025
    (b) ANC coverage >90% & skilled birth attendance >90%
    (c) Over 90% of newborn fully immunized by 1-year of age
    (d) Meet need of Family Planning > 90%
    (e) 80% of known Hypertensives and Diabetics maintain controlled disease

2. *Cross Sectoral Goals Related to Health*
    (a) Reduction in use of Tobacco by 15% by 2020 and 30% by 2025
    (b) Reduction of 40% in Stunting of under five children
    (c) Access to safe water and sanitation (SWACHH BHARAT MISSION)
    (d) Reduction of Occupational Injury by half
    (e) National/State level Tracking of selected Health Behaviour

C. Health System Strengthening

1. *Health Finance*
    (a) Increase health expenditure by government from 1.15% to 2.5% of GDP
    (b) Increase state sector spending to > 8% of their budget
    (c) Decrease the proportion of households facing catastrophic health expenditure by 25%

2. *Health Infrastructure & Human Resource*

    (a) Ensure availability of Paramedics and Doctors as per IPHS in high priority districts

    (b) Increase Community Health Volunteers to population ratio as per IPHS

    (c) Establish primary and secondary care facilities as per norms in high priority districts by 2025

3. *Health Management Information*

    (a) Ensure district level electronic database of information on health system components

    (b) Strengthen health surveillance system and establish registers for diseases of public health importance

    (c) Establish federated integrated Health Information Architecture, Health Information Exchanges and National Health Information Network by 2025

National Health Mission

Ministry of Health & Family Welfare initiated National Programmes to provide access to quality health care in rural areas and urban slums.

National Rural Health Mission, 2005

Rural Population - 70% and has direct impact on health indicators. However, best health services and infrastructure is located in urban areas.

Before NRHM	Rural	Urban
IMR	62	39
Government beds	31.9%	68.1%
Beds/1000 population	0.2	1.1
Graduate Doctors Distribution	28%	74%

Following challenges were identified for Public Health in rural areas:

- Integration of sanitation, hygiene, nutrition and drinking water
- Population stabilisation
- Striking Regional Inequalities
- Undue importance to curative services favouring non-poor
- For every Re 1 spent on the poorest, 20% of population spends Rs 3 on richest quintile
- Only 10% Indians had Health Insurance
- On 12 April 2005 the Union Government launched NRHM because of inequalities in distribution of health services.

Goals

The Mission is expected to achieve the goals set under National Health Policy and Millennium Development Goals.

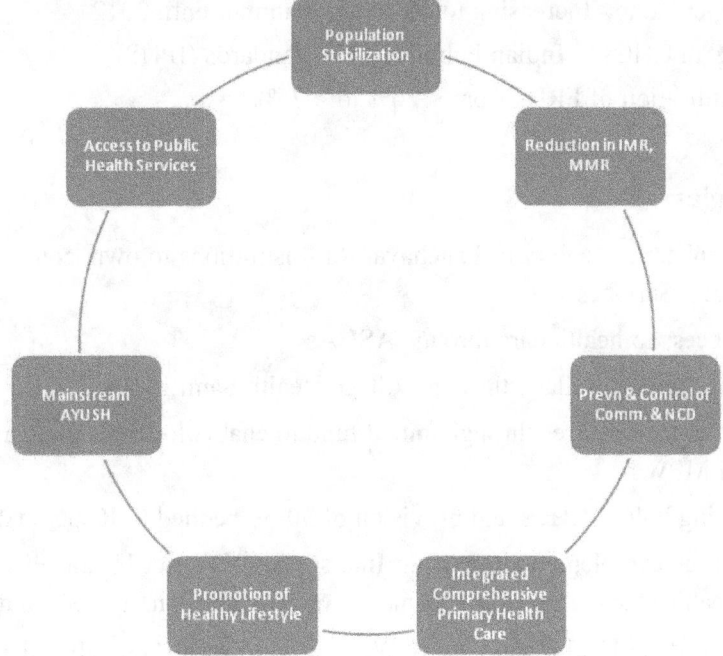

Objectives

- ASHA - Trained Accredited Social Health Activist at the village level
- Health Action Plan - Preparation of health action plans by Panchayats as mechanism for involving community in health care
- IPHS - Strengthening SC/PHC/CHC by developing Indian Public Health Standards
- FRU - Increase utilisation of FRUs from <20% to >75%
- District - Institutionalising and strengthening District level management of Health
- AYUSH - Strengthening sound local health traditions and local resource-based health practices

Expected Outcomes

- IMR reduced to 30/1000 live births by 2012
- MMR reduced to 100/100,000 live births by 2012
- TFR reduced to 2.1
- Malaria Mortality Reduction Rate 50% by 2010, additional 10% by 2012
- Filaria Reduction Rate 70% by 2010, 80% by 2012
- Kala Azar Mortality Reduction Rate 100% by 2010, sustaining elimination until 2012
- Dengue Mortality Reduction Rate 50% by 2010 and sustaining that level till 2012

- JE Mortality Reduction Rate 50% by 2010 and sustaining that level till 2012
- Leprosy Prevalence Rate reduced from 1.8/10,000 in 2005 to <1 per 10,000
- TB DOTS maintain 85% cure rate
- Cataract operations - Increasing to 46 lakh per annum until 2012
- Upgrading all CHCs to Indian Public Health Standards (IPHS)
- Increase utilisation of FRUs from < 20% to > 75%

Core Strategies

- Train and enhance capacity of Panchayat Raj Institutions to own, control and manage Public Health Services
- Promote access to health care through ASHAs
- Health Plan for each village through Village Health Samiti
- Strengthening sub-centres through untied fund to enable local planning and action and training of MPWs
- Strengthening PHCs, CHCs and provision of 30-50 bedded CHC per lakh population
- Preparation and implementation of an Intersectoral District Health Plan prepared by District Health Mission including drinking water, sanitation, hygiene and nutrition
- Integrated Vertical Health and Family Welfare Programmes at National, State, District levels
- Technical support to National, State, District Health Missions for Public Health Management
- Strengthening capacities for data collection, assessment and review for evidence-based planning, monitoring and supervision
- Ensure transparent policies for deployment and career development of human resources for health
- Developing capacities for preventive and promoting health care at all levels such as healthy lifestyles, reduction in consumption of Tobacco and Alcohol
- Promoting non-profit sector especially in underserved areas
- IEC regarding availability and access to quality health care for poor in rural areas to encourage health seeking behaviour

Supplementary Strategies

- Promotion of Public Private Partnerships (PPP) for achieving Public Health Goals
- Mainstreaming AYUSH - Revitalising local health traditions
- Reorienting Medical Education to support rural health issues
- Health Insurance to provide health security to the poor by ensuring accessible, affordable, accountable and good quality hospital care

National Urban Health Mission - NUHM, 2013

Objective

To improve health status of Urban Slum Population by facilitating access to quality health care.

Focus on:

1. Urban poor population in slums
2. All other vulnerable populations - Homeless, rag pickers, street children, rickshaw pullers, construction and brick kiln workers, sex workers, temporary settlements.
3. Public health thrust on sanitation, clean drinking water, vector control
4. Strengthening public health capacity of Urban Local Bodies (ULBs)

Facilities:

Urban PHCs (U-PHCs): 5,000-10,000 up to 75,000 population, OPD services - 12 noon to 8 pm
Urban CHCs (U-CHCs): For every 4-5 U-PHCs, 250,000 population, 30-50 bedded facility
Metrocities: U-CHCs - 5 lakh population,100 beds

Manpower:

ANMs, ASHAs

Services by ASHA:

*   Promoter of good health practices
*   Create awareness on RCH services, age at marriage, ANC, PNC, safe delivery, FP, immunization, nutrition
*   Escort pregnant women and children requiring treatment to U-PHC/secondary/tertiary health care facility
*   Facilitate access to health services at Anganwadi, U-PHC, U-Local Body
*   Formation of Mahila Arogya Samitis - Focus on preventive and promotive care, risk pooling fund, health insurance
*   Reinforcement of community action for Immunization, prevention of water borne diseases and common diseases eg. TB, Malaria, Chikungunya, Japanese Encephalitis
*   Carrying out preventive and promotive health activities with Anganwadi worker, Mahila Arogya Samitis
*   Management Information System - Information and records on vital statistics, immunization, ANC
*   Provision for a minimum package of curative care, depot holders for ORS, IFA, Chloroquine, OCP, Condoms

National Population Policy

Population Explosion
Rapid increase in population when BR>DR

11 May 2000 - 1 billion population (16% of world's population on 2.4% of global land area)
Population has increased from 238 million (1901) to 1.3 billion (2011).
Population control is one of the biggest challenges facing the country.

Facts

- Every 6th person in the world is an Indian.
- India adds 10 lakh persons to its population every fortnight.
- India adds one Australia every year.
- By 2045, India will overtake China as the world's most populous nation.
- 49% of increase in population is from 4 states - Bihar, Madhya Pradesh, Rajasthan and Uttar Pradesh (BIMARU states)

Causes of Population Explosion

1. Widening gap between Birth Rate (BR) and Death Rate (DR)
2. Low age at marriage
3. High illiteracy especially female illiteracy
4. Low socio-economic status
5. Unfavourable religious attitude towards FP
6. Preference for male child
7. Lack of information
8. Lack of choice of contraceptives
9. Poor services of FP

Effects of Population Explosion

1. Homelessness
2. Illiteracy
3. Malnourished children and adults
4. Overcrowding
5. Lack of Safe Water
6. Lack of Sanitation
7. Breakdown of transport, electricity, telephone
8. Unemployment
9. Rise in crime and violence
10. Environmental degradation - Air, water, soil pollution

National Population Policy 2000

Objectives

Immediate

- To meet the unmet need of contraception
- Strengthening health infrastructure
- Strengthening health manpower
- Promote integrated service delivery for RCH care

Mid term

To bring TFR to replacement level of 2 by 2010

Long term

Stable population by 2045

National Socio Demographic Goals for 2010

1. Address unmet needs for RCH services, supplies and infrastructure
2. School education up to 14 years free and compulsory and reduce drop-outs
3. Reduce IMR <30/1000 Live Births
4. Universal immunization against vaccine preventable diseases
5. Reduce MMR <100/lakh Live Births
6. Marriage age for girls not <18, preferably 20 years
7. Achieve 80% institutional delivery and 100% by trained personnel
8. Achieve100% registration of births, deaths, marriages and pregnancy
9. Containment of AIDS and greater integration between management of AIDS & STDs
10. Prevention and control of communicable diseases
11. Achieve universal access to information, counseling services for fertility regulation and contraceptives with a wide basket of choices (Cafeteria method)
12. Integration of Indian System of Medicine in provision for RCH services
13. Promote small family norm
14. Bring about convergence in implementation of Social Sector Programmes so that Family Welfare becomes People Centred Programme

Strategies

1. ***Decentralised Planning and Programme Implementation***
Village Panchayat Raj Institutions in charge of health and family welfare and education.

2. ***Convergence of Service Delivery at Village Levels***
Promoting RCH through Mobile Clinics and Counseling Services.

NGOs in partnership with Government for providing services.
At least 2 Trained Birth Attendants (TBA) per village proposed.

3. ***Empowering Women***
Women empowered through information, education and communication on Health and Nutrition.

4. ***Child Health and Survival***
IMR is a sensitive indicator of human development.
Priority to intensify Neonatal Care.
National Technical Committee should be set up comprising consultants in Obstetrics, Pediatrics, Family Health, Medical Research and Statistics.

Aim

- To set up Perinatal Audit Norms, developing quality improvement activities with monitoring schedules and CMEs for medical and nursing personnel.
- Baby Friendly Hospital Initiative (BFHI) should be extended to all hospitals, clinics and sub-centres.
- Child Survival Interventions - Universal immunization, control of Diarrheal Diseases, ARI, Vit A Supplementation, food supplements in Anganwadis have helped to decrease mortality and morbidity.
- With IPPI Polio has been eradicated in 2014.

5. ***Meeting Unmet Needs for Family Welfare Services***
At village, sub-centre, PHC levels to improve facilities for services, referrals and for social marketing schemes.

6. ***Greater Emphasis for Underserved Population***
Urban slums, Tribal communities, Hill area population, Migrant population need special basic health and RCH services.
Mobile clinics can cover these areas.
Adolescents - Programmes should encourage delayed marriage and child bearing and education on risks of unprotected sex.
Participation of men in Planned Parenthood, re-popularising Vasectomies especially No-Scalpel Vasectomy and IEC for men to promote small family norms.

7. ***Involvement of ISM***
Practitioners of Indian Systems of Medicine to promote RCH.

8. ***Collaboration with Private Agencies and NGOs***
Private practitioners and NGOs for RCH to achieve Public Health Goals.

9. ***Research***
Contraceptive Technology, Research and Behavioural Science.

10. **Management Information System**
    MIS to ascertain impacts and outcome through district surveys.

11. **Providing Health Care and Support for Older Population**
    Promoting old age health care and support will help reduce desire to have large families.

12. **Information Education and Communication**
    Need to undertake massive National Campaign on population issues by involving artists, film stars, doctors, vaidyas, hakims, nurses, midwives, women and youth organisations.

National Health Programmes in India

➢ **Disease Eradication Programmes**

1. National Polio Eradication Programme
2. National Leprosy Eradication Programme
3. National Yaws Eradication Programme

➢ **Disease Control Programmes**
    National Antimalaria Programme
    National Filaria Control Programme
    National TB Elimination Programme
    National AIDS Control Programme
    National STD Control Programme
    National Diarrhoeal Diseases Control Programme
    National ARI Control Programme
    Integrated Disease Surveillance Programme

➢ **National Nutrition Programmes**
    Vitamin A Prophylaxis Programme
    National Nutritional Anemia Control Programme
    Iodine Deficiency Disorders Control Programme
    Supplementary Nutrition Programme
    Balwadi Nutrition Programme
    Integrated Child Development Services
    School Mid–day Meal Programme

➢ **National Programmes for Mother & Child Health**
    RCH
    National Health Mission - NRHM, NUHM
    Vande Mataram Programme
    UIP
    RBSK

➢ **National Family Welfare Programme**

➢ **National Programmes for Non-Communicable Diseases**
National Programme to Control Blindness (NPCB)
National Programme for Prevention & Control of Cancer, Diabetes, Cardiovascular
Diseases and Stroke
National Mental Health Programme

➢ **National Water Supply & Sanitation Programme**

National Family Welfare Programme

Milestones of National Family Welfare Programme

1951:

India was the first country in the world to launch a Family Planning Programme.
Clinic based approach.

1961-66:

Extension education approach.
Expansion of services facilities and spread of message on small family norm.
3rd Plan - Dept of Family Planning created in the Ministry of Health
Adopted a Target Oriented Approach.
Lippes Loop introduced and massive effort to promote IUCD and condoms.

1969-74:

4th Plan.
All India Hospital Post-Partum Programme.
MTP Act 1971.

1974-79:

5th Plan.
Campaign for male sterilisations
Renaming Family Planning to Family Welfare Programme.
1978 Primary Health Care, Community Participation, Child Marriage Restraint Act.

1980-85:

6th Plan.
1983 - National Health Policy, strengthening MCH and Family Welfare.

1985-90:

7th Plan.
Inclusion of various programmes under MCH-UIP, ORT.

1992-97:

8th Plan.

1992 - Child Survival and Safe Motherhood Program

1994 - International Conference on Population & Development, Cairo

1996- Target Free Approach

1997-2002:

9th Plan.

Reproductive and Child Health (RCH) Programme.

2000 - National Population Policy

2002 - National Health Policy

2002-07:

10th Plan.

2005 - RCH II, National Rural Health Mission (NRHM)

2007-12:

11th Plan. NRHM

2012-17:

12th Plan. NRHM

Social Marketing Scheme

Social marketing is a process of bringing about a social change towards health and health behaviour pattern.

It is to generate demand for Health Care Services from those who need health interventions but are presently not seeking the same.

It is an application of marketing principle for welfare of public eg. Social Marketing Programme for condoms and oral pills.

Operational Research (OR)

OR is the application of quantitative methods to the solution of management problems.

Important areas of OR:

- Male involvement and issues affecting male behaviour and attitude
- Behavioural and operational barriers to women accessing contraceptive services
- How can effective linkages be built among field workers from different departments
- Mechanisms to involve women in planning/monitoring health services
- Identification and dissemination of best practices in the area of contraceptive services

Reproductive and Child Health (RCH) Programme

Definition

People have the ability to reproduce and regulate their fertility

Women are able to go through pregnancy and childbirth safely

The outcome of pregnancies is successful in terms of maternal and infant survival and well-being

Couples are able to have sexual relations free of fear of pregnancy and contracting disease. RCH Programme addresses women's health across their lifecycle.

RCH Package

Family Planning	Child Survival & Safe Motherhood
Client Approach to Health Care	RTI/STD/AIDS Prevention & Management

RCH I

Interventions in all Districts

Child Survival Interventions - Immunization, Vit A, ORT, ARI, Diarrhoea, PEM Management and Prevention

Safe Motherhood Interventions - Antenatal check-up, TT, Anemia Control Programme, safe delivery

Family Planning - Target Free Approach
Safe Abortion Facilities at PHCs

Capacity Building - High quality training
Information Education Communication
RCH Package specially designed for urban slums and tribal areas

District sub-projects
RTI/STD clinics at District Hospitals
Community Participation through Panchayats, women's groups and NGOs
Adolescent Health and Reproductive hygiene

Interventions in Selected States/Districts

Screening and treatment of RTI/STD
Essential Obstetric care by providing Public Health Nurse/Staff and drugs at PHC

Additional ANM at sub-centres

Sub-centre improvement of delivery services and emergency care by providing equipment kits, IUD insertions and ANM kits

Transport facilities for referrals through Panchayat

RCH I

- Early registration of pregnancy (within 12-16 weeks)
- Minimum of 3 Ante-natal check-ups by ANM/Medical Officer
- Promotion of Institutional delivery and provision of safe delivery at home
- Provision of post-natal care

RCH II (2004-2009)

Objectives:

- Improve access to skilled care and emergency obstetric care
- Improve coverage and quality of antenatal care
- Increase coverage of postpartum care

Components of RCH

1. Population Stabilisation
2. Maternal Health (Essential Obstetric Care)
3. Reproductive Tract & Sexually Transmitted Infections control the programme
4. Newborn and Child Health through IMNCI including Diarrhoeal Disease Control Programme, ARI Control Programme, Breast feeding, Baby Friendly Hospital Initiative, Behaviour Change Communication
5. Prevention and Control of Anemia
6. Prevention and Control of Vit A Deficiency
7. Universal Immunization Programme
8. Polio Eradication - Pulse Polio Programme
9. Adolescent Health
10. Behaviour Change Communication
11. Community Participation
12. Public Private Mix
13. Procurement and Logistics
14. Monitoring, Evaluation and Health Management Information System

Strategies

(a) Increasing the number of facilities (PHCs/CHCs/FRUs) offering safe delivery and Emergency Obstetric Care (EmOC)

(b) Operationalising CHCs and 50% PHCs to provide 24 hours safe delivery and EmOC by 2010
(c) Operationalising Comprehensive EmOC at 2000 FRUs by 2010
(d) Ensuring access to safe blood at all District Hospitals and FRUs
(e) Training of MOs in Anaesthesia for EmOC
(f) Training of MBBS MOs in Caesarian Section
(g) Providing EmOC services to BPL families at recognised private facilities

First Referral Units (FRUs)

Specialists - Obstetricians, Pediatricians, Physicians, Surgeons

Services:

Vacuum Extraction, Anaesthesia administration, Caesarian Section, Blood transfusion, Manual removal of Placenta, Suction Curettage for incomplete abortion, Insertion of IUCD, Sterilisation operations (Vasectomy and Tubectomy)

Vande Mataram Scheme

Government launched a scheme to involve private sector in safe motherhood/FP activities. OBG specialist will volunteer to provide free Outpatient Care Services (Ante-natal and family planning) to pregnant women on a fixed day each month.
Government will provide the specialist a kit consisting of IFA tablets, TT Injections, condoms, OCPs, IUCDs for free distribution.

Reproductive Tract Infection & Sexually Transmitted Infections

Objectives

➢ Promote recognition and referral for those with suspected RTI/STI
➢ Strengthen services for diagnosis and treatment of RTI/STI at PHCs, CHCs, FRUs and District Hospitals
➢ Strengthen linkages with NACO activities

Strategies

(a) *Community Level*
Train ANMs to provide presumptive treatment to cases and their partners for common RTI/STI
Train AWW and Link Workers to identify and refer cases of RTI/STI
Promote community awareness regarding RTI/STI for prevention, early diagnosis and treatment

(b)   Facility Level
- Operationalise services for diagnosis and treatment at all FRUs, CHCs, and 50% of PHCs
- Provide first line drugs at PHCs
- Revise essential drug list
- Strengthen labs and post technicians
- Train MOs and LHVs

Integrated Management of Neonatal and Childhood Illness (IMNCI)

IMNCI is the Indian adaptation of WHO-UNICEF Integrated Management of Childhood Illness (IMCI).

IMNCI encompasses a range of interventions to prevent and manage the 5 major childhood illnesses - ARI, Diarrhoea, Measles, Malaria, Malnutrition and the major causes of Neonatal Mortality (Prematurity, Sepsis).

IMNCI also teaches about nutrition on breastfeeding, complementary feeding and micronutrients.

It focuses on preventive, promotive and curative aspects, a holistic outlook to the program.

Major Components

1. Strengthening skills of health care workers
2. Strengthening health care infrastructure
3. Involvement of community

Strategy

o Evidence based interventions
o Approach integrated with RCH program
o Equity-driven implementation and monitoring
o Rational mix of community and facility-based interventions
o Decentralised priority setting at state and district levels
o Participation of private sector

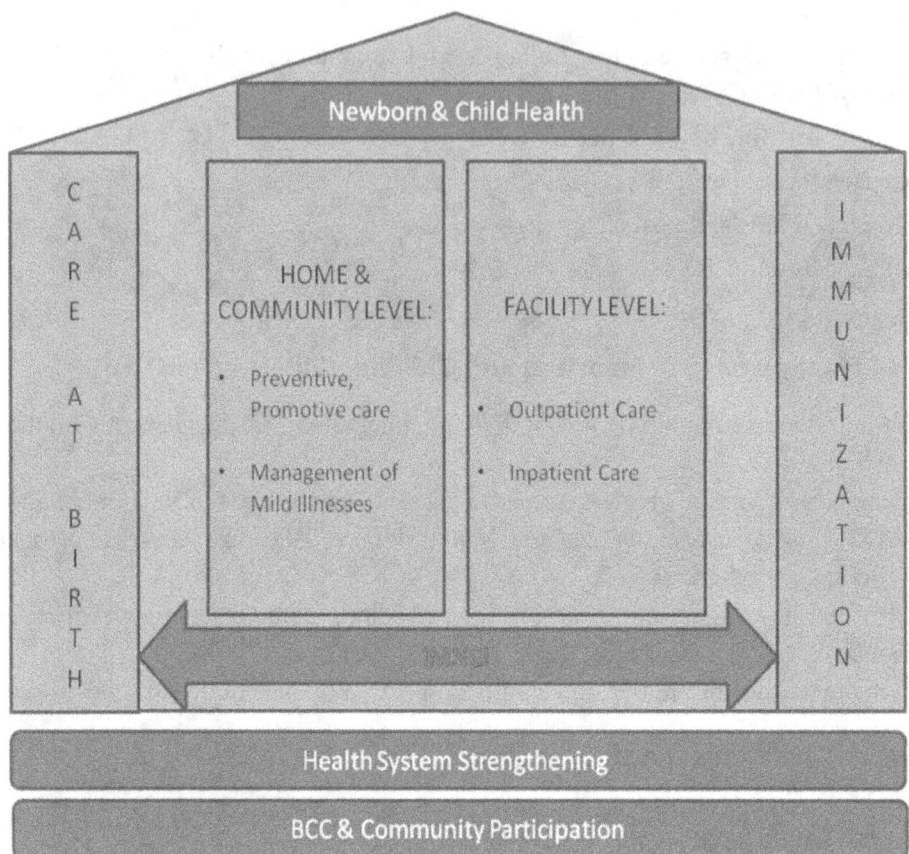

For all sick children age up to 5 years who are brought to a first-level health facility

ASSESS THE CHILD: Check for danger signs (or possible bacterial infection). Ask about main symptoms. If a main symptom is reported, assess further. Check nutrition and immunization status. Check for other problems.

CLASSIFY the child's illnesses: Use a colour-coded triage system to classify the child's main symptoms and his or her nutrition or feeding status.

IF **URGENT REFERRAL** is needed and possible	IF **NO** URGENT REFERRAL is needed and possible
IDENTIFY URGENT PRE-REFERRAL TREATMENT(S) needed for the child's classifications	**IDENTIFY TREATMENT** needed for the child's classifications: Identify specific medical treatments and/or advice.
TREAT THE CHILD: Give urgent pre-referral treatment(s) needed.	**TREAT THE CHILD:** Give the first dose of oral drugs in the clinic and/or advise the child's caretaker. Teach the caretaker how to give oral drugs and how to treat local infections at home. If needed, give immunizations.
REFER THE CHILD: Explain to the child's caretaker the need for referral. Calm the caretaker's fears and help resolve any problems. Write a referral note. Give instructions and supplies needed to care for the child on the way to the hospital.	**COUNSEL THE MOTHER:** Assess the child's feeding, including breastfeeding practices, and solve feeding problems, if present. Advise about feeding and fluids during illness and about when to return to a health facility. Counsel the mother about her own health.

FOLLOW-UP care: Give follow-up care when the child returns to the clinic and, if necessary, reassess the child for new problems.

IMNCI Plus

Package of IMNCI plus Immunization, Care at Birth and Behavior Change Communication (BCC).

Objectives

Implement by 2010 a comprehensive Newborn and Child Health Package at all Sub-centres through ANMs, PHCs through MOs, nurse and LHVs and in FRUs through MOs and nurses.

Implement by 2010 a comprehensive Newborn and Child Health Package at the household level in 250 districts through AWWs.

Sick Newborn Care

Sick newborn care units opened in CHCs, FRUs, District Hospitals and equipped with skilled manpower.

Home-based Newborn Care

Home-based newborn care based on Gadchirolli Model. ASHAs and ANMs are trained on newborn care.

Diarrheal Disease

Diarrhoeal Diseases Control Programme

- 1980-81: National Cholera Control Programme
- 1986–87: Oral Rehydration Therapy Programme started
- 1997: RCH Programme, incorporates Diarrhoeal Diseases Control Programme with stress on Rational Management of Diarrhoea with
    i.   Increased intake of Home Available Fluids (HAF)
    ii. Continued feeding, and
    iii. When to take child to Doctor/health facility

ORS is promoted & supplied as part of Sub-centre kits and in Anganwadi Centres

Definition

Diarrhoea is the passage of loose/watery stools more than 3 times per day
Acute Diarrhea may last up to 14 days.
Persistent Diarrhea > 14 days.

Dysentery is blood and mucus in stools.
Complications of Diarrhea

(a) Death due to Dehydration

(b) Malnutrition

Classification of Dehydration

		A	B	C
LOOK	Condition * Eyes Tears Tongue, mouth Thirst *	Well, alert Normal Present Moist Drinks normally, not thirsty	Restless, irritable Sunken Absent Dry Thirsty, drinks eagerly	Lethargic, unconscious, floppy Very sunken, dry Absent Very dry Drinks poorly or not able to drink
FEEL	*Turgor (Skin pinch)	Goes back quickly	Goes back slowly	Goes back very slowly
DECIDE	Degree of Dehydration	No signs of Dehydration	Has 2 or more signs including one key * sign Some Dehydration	Has 2 or more signs including one key sign * Severe Dehydration
Observation in Diarrhoeal Episodes		90%	9%	1%
Treatment Plan		Plan A Home Available Fluids (HAF)	Plan B Oral Rehydration Salt Solution (ORS)	Plan C Intravenous Fluid Therapy

TREATMENT PLAN A
TREAT DIARRHOEA AT HOME

> ### USE THIS PLAN TO TEACH THE MOTHER TO:
>
> *   Continue to treat at home her child's current episode of Diarrhoea
> *   Give early treatment for future episodes of Diarrhoea

EXPLAIN THE THREE RULES FOR TREATING DIARRHOEA AT HOME:

1. GIVE THE CHILD MORE FLUIDS THAN USUAL TO PREVENT DEHYDRATION:
    • Use recommended home fluids.

These include ORS solution, food-based fluids (Such as soup, rice water, yoghurt drinks) and plain water.

Use ORS solution for children described in the box below (Note if the child is < 6 months old & is not yet taking solid food, give ORS solution or water rather than a food-based fluid).

    • Give as much of these fluids as the child will take. Use the amounts shown below for ORS as a guide.
    • Continue giving these fluids until the Diarrhea stops.

2. GIVE THE CHILD PLENTY OF FOOD TO PREVENT MALNUTRITION
    • Continue to breast-feed frequently.
    • If the child is not breast-fed give the usual milk.
    • If the child is 6-months or older or already taking solid food give cereal or another starchy food mixed, if possible, with pulses, vegetables and meat or fish.
      Add 1 or 2 teaspoonfuls of vegetable oil to each serving.
      Give fresh fruit juice or mashed Banana to provide Potassium.
      Give freshly prepared foods. Cook and mash or grind food well.
      Encourage the child to eat: Offer food at least 6 times a day.
      Give the same foods after Diarrhea stops and give an extra meal each day for two weeks.

3. TAKE THE CHILD TO THE HEALTH WORKER IF THE CHILD DOES NOT GET BETTER IN 2 DAYS OR DEVELOPS ANY OF THE FOLLOWING:

Many watery stools	Marked thirst	Fever
Repeated vomiting	Eating or drinking poorly	Blood in the stool

IF THE CHILD WILL BE GIVEN ORS SOLUTION AT HOME, SHOW THE MOTHER HOW MUCH ORS TO GIVE AFTER EACH LOOSE STOOL AND GIVE HER ENOUGH PACKETS FOR 2 DAYS

Age	Amount of ORS to give after each loose stool
< 2 years	50-100 ml
2 -10 years	100-200 ml
≥10 years	As much as wanted

TREATMENT PLAN B

TO TREAT DEHYDRATION

APPROXIMATE AMOUNT OF ORS SOLUTION TO GIVE IN FIRST 4 HOURS

Age: *	< 4 mths	4–11 mths	12–23 mths	2–4 yrs	5–14 yrs	≥ 15 yrs
Weight:	<5 kg	5-7.9 kg	8–10.9 kg	11–15.9 kg	16–29.9 kg	≥30 kg
In ml	200-400	400–600	600-800	800-1200	1200-2200	2200-4000

* Use the patient's age only when you do not know weight. Approximate amount of ORS (in ml) can also be calculated; patient's weight (in kg) X 75

• If the child wants more ORS than shown, give more

• Encourage mother to continue breast-feeding

• Infants <6-months who are not breast-fed, also give 100-200 ml clean water during this period.

OBSERVE THE CHILD CAREFULLY AND HELP THE MOTHER GIVE ORS SOLUTION

• Show her how much solution to give the child.

• Show her how to give it, a teaspoonful every 1-2 minutes for a child under 2 years, frequent sips from a cup for an older child.

• Check from time to time to see if there are problems.

• If the child vomits, wait 10 minutes and then continue giving ORS, but more slowly, for example, a spoonful every 2-3 minutes.

• If the child's eyelids become puffy, stop ORS and give plain water or breast milk. Give ORS according to Plan A when the puffiness has gone.

AFTER 4 HOURS, RE-ASSESS THE CHILD USING THE ASSESSMENT CHART. THEN SELECT PLAN A, B, OR C TO CONTINUE TREATMENT

• If there are no signs of Dehydration, shift to Plan A. When Dehydration has been corrected, the child usually passes urine and may also be tired and fall asleep.

• If signs indicating some Dehydration is still present, repeat Plan B, but start offering food, milk and juice as described in Plan A.

• If signs indicating Severe Dehydration has appeared, shift to Plan C.

IF THE MOTHER MUST LEAVE BEFORE COMPLETING TREATMENT PLAN B:

• Show her how much ORS to give to finish the 4-hour treatment at home.

• Give her enough ORS packets to complete Rehydration and for 2 more days as shown in Plan A.

• Show her how to prepare ORS solution.

• Explain to her the three rules in Plan A for treating her child at home:

- To give ORS or other fluids until Diarrhea stops

- To feed the child

- To bring the child back to the health worker, if necessary.

TREATMENT PLAN C

TO TREAT SEVERE DEHYDRATION QUICKLY

START HERE

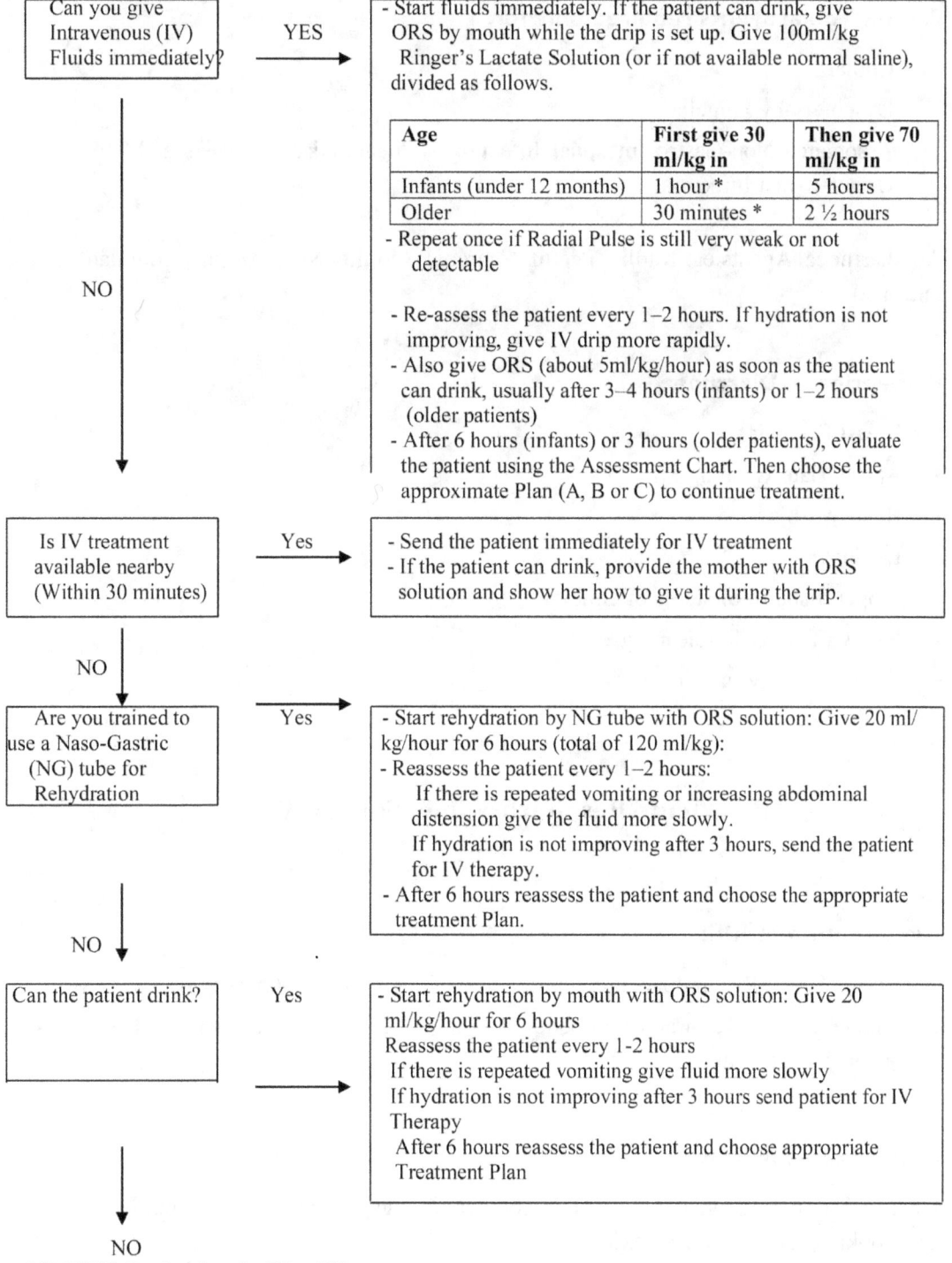

| Can you give Intravenous (IV) Fluids immediately? | YES → | - Start fluids immediately. If the patient can drink, give ORS by mouth while the drip is set up. Give 100ml/kg Ringer's Lactate Solution (or if not available normal saline), divided as follows. |

Age	First give 30 ml/kg in	Then give 70 ml/kg in
Infants (under 12 months)	1 hour *	5 hours
Older	30 minutes *	2 ½ hours

- Repeat once if Radial Pulse is still very weak or not detectable

- Re-assess the patient every 1–2 hours. If hydration is not improving, give IV drip more rapidly.
- Also give ORS (about 5ml/kg/hour) as soon as the patient can drink, usually after 3–4 hours (infants) or 1–2 hours (older patients)
- After 6 hours (infants) or 3 hours (older patients), evaluate the patient using the Assessment Chart. Then choose the approximate Plan (A, B or C) to continue treatment.

NO ↓

| Is IV treatment available nearby (Within 30 minutes) | Yes → | - Send the patient immediately for IV treatment
- If the patient can drink, provide the mother with ORS solution and show her how to give it during the trip. |

NO ↓

| Are you trained to use a Naso-Gastric (NG) tube for Rehydration | Yes → | - Start rehydration by NG tube with ORS solution: Give 20 ml/kg/hour for 6 hours (total of 120 ml/kg):
- Reassess the patient every 1–2 hours:
  If there is repeated vomiting or increasing abdominal distension give the fluid more slowly.
  If hydration is not improving after 3 hours, send the patient for IV therapy.
- After 6 hours reassess the patient and choose the appropriate treatment Plan. |

NO ↓

| Can the patient drink? | Yes → | - Start rehydration by mouth with ORS solution: Give 20 ml/kg/hour for 6 hours
Reassess the patient every 1-2 hours
If there is repeated vomiting give fluid more slowly
If hydration is not improving after 3 hours send patient for IV Therapy
After 6 hours reassess the patient and choose appropriate Treatment Plan |

NO ↓

NO
URGENT: Send patient for IV or NG treatment

Drug Therapy in Diarrhoea

Antimicrobial drugs not required in majority of Acute Diarrhoea as they are caused by viruses or E Coli that act by elaborating Enterotoxins.

Antimicrobial agents required only for:

1. Cholera
2. Dysentery by Shigella
3. Associated Non-Gastro Intestinal Infection – Pneumonia, Septicaemia, Meningitis, Urinary Tract Infection.

Antidiarrhoeal Agents eg. Kaolin, Pectin, Charcoal, Motility Suppressants, Stimulants not indicated.

Prevention of Diarrhoea

- Breast Feeding
- Appropriate Weaning Practices
- Hand Washing
- Latrines
- Proper disposal of stools of children
- Plenty of water for cleaning
- Measles, Rotavirus Vaccination

Acute Respiratory Infections (ARI)

Classification of ARI:

1. Acute Upper Respiratory Infection (AURI) - Common cold, Pharyngitis, Otitis Media
2. Acute Lower Respiratory Infection (ALRI) - Epiglottitis, Laryngitis, Bronchitis, Bronchiolitis, Pneumonia

Risk Factors for ALRI

Lack of breast feeding, URTI/LRTI in mother/siblings, inappropriate immunization for age, cooking fuel, passive smoking

Classification of Illness

Age of child	Very Severe Disease	Severe Pneumonia	Pneumonia	No Pneumonia
< 2 months	(Any 1 or 2 signs) Stopped feeding well Convulsions Abnormally sleepy Difficult to wake Stridor in calm infants Wheezing in calm infants Fever (38^0 C) or low body temp (35.5^0 C)	Fast breathing ≥ 60/min Severe chest indrawing	-	No fast breathing No severe chest indrawing
Treatment	Give 1st dose antibiotic Refer to hospital	Refer urgently to hospital for treatment Keep baby warm Breast feed newborn	-	Home care
2 months – 5 years	All the above Not able to drink Severe undernutrition	Chest indrawing	No chest indrawing Fast breathing ≥ 50/min (2m – 12m) ≥ 40/min (12m – 5yrs)	No chest indrawing No fast breathing
	Refer urgently to hospital Give 1 dose antibiotic Treat fever Treat wheezing	Refer urgently to hospital Give 1 dose antibiotic Treat fever Treat wheezing	Advise home care Give antibiotics for 5 days Treat fever Treat wheezing	Home care Treat fever

Home Care in ARI

Fever – Paracetamol

Continue feeding

Adequate fluids

Cough treatment – Home remedies – (Honey, ginger, tulsi, hot water)

Saline drops for running & blocked nose.

Discourage use of antimicrobials, cough syrups containing Ephedrine, Codeine, Atropine, Alcohol, Medicated Nasal/Ear drops.

Prevention of ARI

- Breast Feeding
- Appropriate Complementary Feeding
- Immunization
- Passive smoking prevention
- LPG instead of firewood

Universal Immunization Programme (UIP)

Definition

Immunization – A cost-effective intervention for disease prevention.
IMR has come down from 104/1000 Live Births in 1984 to 42/1000 Live Births in 2014.
Vaccine preventable diseases were the major cause of Morbidity, Mortality and lifelong physical and mental disabilities prior to the Immunization Programmes.

Aim:

To improve access to sustainable Immunization Services.
Overall Immunization coverage amongst 12-23 months is 77.3%.
Coverage of routine Immunization is being enhanced with a focus on underserved communities.

The output of UIP is measured in terms of:

(a) Antigen Coverage and
(b) Dropout Rates

Antigen Coverage Rates are a measure of access to Immunization services.
Dropout Rates indicate the service utilisation.

Most Common Constraints of UIP:

Non-uniform coverage, poor implementation, poor monitoring, high dropout rates, over reporting, poor injection safety, lack of reorientation of staff, cold chain replacement plan not made, staff vacancies not filled, poor surveillance of VPDs, poor vaccine logistics, poor maintenance of equipment.

Under RCH II- 6 Goals

1. Districts will provide efficient and safe Immunization Services to all infants and pregnant women
2. Contribute to Global Polio Eradication, Measles Mortality Reduction and Neonatal Tetanus Elimination

3. Sufficient and sustainable funding with established adequate, accountable and efficient fund flows
4. Sustain demand and reduce social barriers to access Immunization Services
5. Accelerated introduction of licensed new vaccines against diseases with significant Mortality and Morbidity eg. MMR, JE, Hepatitis B
6. Accurate, complete and timely data on Vaccine Preventable Diseases (VPDs), Adverse Events Following Immunizations (AEFIs), Antigen Coverage and Dropout Rates by district.

Rashtriya Bal Swasthya Karyakram (RBSK)

This programme was launched in Feb 2013

In NRHM, significant advance has been made to decrease Mortality.
However, there is a need to improve survival by early detection and management of following conditions from birth to 18 years:
It is estimated that 270 million children from birth to 18 years will be benefited by the Programme.

4Ds
Defects at birth
Deficiencies
Diseases
Development delays and disability

At birth - Screening by MOs, Staff nurses, ANMs
After 48 hours to 6 weeks – Screening by ASHAs at home
Within 6 weeks to 6 years - Outreach screening by Mobile Health Teams at Anganwadi Centres
From 6 to 18 years – Screening of children to be done at school

Treatment/Intervention at zero cost to the family

Health Conditions to be Screened:

Defects at Birth

Neural Tube Defects, Down's Syndrome, Cleft Lip and Palate, Talipes, Hip Dislocation, Congenital Cataract, Congenital Deafness, Congenital Heart Disease, Retinopathy of Prematurity

Deficiencies

Anemia, Vit A deficiency (Bitot's Spots), Vit D deficiency (Rickets), Severe Acute Malnutrition, Goitre

Diseases of Childhood

Skin conditions (Scabies, Fungal infection, Eczema), Otitis Media, Rheumatic Heart Disease, Reactive Airway Disease, Dental conditions, Convulsive disorders

Developmental Delays and Disabilities

Vision impairment, hearing impairment, Neuromotor impairment, Motor delay, Cognitive delay, Language delay, Behavior disorder (Autism), Learning disorder, Attention Deficit Hyperactive Disorder, Congenital Hypothyroidism, Sickle Cell Anemia, Beta Thalassemia.

Mechanism of Screening

Child screening at 2 Levels:

1. Community level
2. Facility level

Community Level

Screening to be done by Mobile Health teams at Anganwadi Centres, Govt/Govt Aided schools

Facility Level

To be done at PHCs, CHCs, DHs by MOs, Nurses, ANMs

Mobile Health Teams

The team consists of_4 members - 2 Doctors (one male, one female), 1 ANM/Staff nurse, 1 Pharmacist

Referrals to DEIC (District Early Intervention Centre)

Team of Pediatrician, MO, Staff nurses, Paramedics provide services.
Referrals to Tertiary Care Facilities.
Funds are provided by NHM for management.

Polio Eradication Programme

In 1988, the World Health Assembly passed a resolution to eradicate Polio by 2000.
Only 2 countries are still endemic for Polio - Pakistan, Afghanistan

India - No case has been reported since 13 Jan 2011.

1995 - National Immunization Days - Pulse Polio Immunization (PPI) initiated.
"Pulse" means sudden, simultaneous, mass administration of OPV on a single day to all children between 0-5 years irrespective of their previous vaccination status.

Immunization replaces the wild virus with vaccine virus thereby eradicates harmful virus in the community.

Even a single case is treated as an outbreak and prevention measures are initiated within 48 hours of notification of the case.

Basic Strategies to Eradicate Polio

➢ Routine Immunization - Immunize all infants with Trivalent OPV
➢ National Immunization Days (Pulse Polio Immunization Programme, Subnational Immunization Days) - Additional doses of OPV given 4-6 weeks apart to children < 5 years.
➢ Surveillance of Acute Flaccid Paralysis (AFP) & Outbreak Response
➢ Conduct Extensive house to house Immunizations - Mopping up campaigns
Mopping up conducted when surveillance shows evidence of the Polio Virus Transmission in an area.

Certification of Polio Eradication

Feb 2014 - India was certified Polio Free by WHO.

Single Programme-based strategy of Public Health should not be conducted whereas multipronged strategy should be instituted
Vaccination, water and sanitation, nutrition, socio-economic development, urban development, family welfare.

Integrated Child Development Services (ICDS) Scheme

The ICDS Scheme was launched on 2nd Oct 1975 by the Ministry of Social Welfare.

The Beneficiaries are:

1. Children below 6 years
2. Pregnant and lactating women
3. Women between 15-45 years
4. Adolescent girls

12th 5-year Plan
Restructured ICDS is a critical component of the 12th Plan strategy for Child Development.

Objectives

- To improve the nutritional and health status of preschool children between 0-6 years.
- To lay the foundation for proper Psychological Development
- To reduce Mortality, Morbidity, Malnutrition and school dropout rate
- To achieve effective coordination of policy and implementation among various departments to promote child development
- To enhance capability of the mother to look after the normal health and nutritional needs of the child through Nutrition and Health Education.

Organisation

Anganwadi - A courtyard play centre located within the village/slum area.
It covers a population of 1000.
Manpower - 1 Anganwadi Worker, 1 Helper

Mukhya Sevika

Supervises work of 20, 25, 17 Anganwadi workers in urban, rural and tribal projects.
Visits the Anganwadi once/month.
Coordinates with LHV in nutritional and health activities.

Child Development Project Officer (CDPO)

1 CDPO, 1 Assistant CDPO
Covers one community development block with a population of 80,000-120,000.
CDPO supervises, guides, coordinates the work of ICDS project, supervises 4-5 Mukhya Sevikas.

Services

Supplementary Nutrition, Immunization, Health Check-up, Treatment of minor illnesses, Referral services, Nutrition and Health Education, Non-Formal Education to 3-5-year-old children, Convergence of other supportive services ie. Safe water, Sanitation, Functional literacy for adult women, provide Supplementary Nutrition and Nutrition & Health Education to Adolescent girls of 11-18 years.

Role of Health Department

Health check-ups, Handling referrals from Anganwadis, Immunization, Health and Nutrition education, Continuing education of ICDS staff, Monitoring of health component of ICDS.

Indicators for Analysis

(a) Monthly Basis
- Enrolment efficiency at Anganwadi Centres (AWCs)
- Weighment efficiency
- Rate of moderate or severe malnutrition
- Projects and AWCs – Operational vs Sanctioned

(b) Annual Basis
Monthly basis indicators plus

- % children fully immunized
- % AWCs that provide supplementary nutrition 300 days/year
- % AWCs housed in own building vs rented
- % operational AWC vs AWC with toilet facility &/or drinking water facility
- % children who left AWC and enrolled at primary schools
- % children under various degrees of malnutrition
- % children with low birth weight
- % children breastfed with Colostrum and exclusively breastfed for 6 months
- Average No. of AWCs visited by the Supervisor in a year/month

Challenges

In spite of big infrastructure, the nutritional status of women and children is almost the same as in the previous years.

Reasons

Inadequate coverage of children, irregularities of food deliveries, poor quality of food which is not accepted by majority of children, poor nutrition education to mothers, inadequate training of Anganwadi workers, poor supervision, poor coordination and linkage with health workers, lack of community ownership and participation.

Poshan Abhiyan

This was launched on 18 Dec 2017. It was launched in 36 States/UTs

Goals

Improvement in the Nutritional Status of 0-6 years children, adolescent girls, pregnant and lactating women.

Objectives & Targets

1. Prevent and reduce stunting in children of 0-6 years by   6%
2. Prevent and reduce undernutrition and underweight in 0-6 years children by 6%

3. Reduce and prevent Anemia (6-59 months) by   9%
4. Reduce and prevent Anemia (15-49 years) by   9%
5. Reduce low birth weight by   6%

Implementation through various programs:

ICDS
Pradhan Mantri Matri Vandana Yojana
Schemes for Adolescent Girls
Janani Suraksha Yojana
National Health Mission
Swachh Bharat Mission
Rajiv Gandhi Scheme for Empowerment of Adolescent Girls

Balwadi Nutrition Programme

The Balwadi Nutrition Programme was started in 1970.
Its aim was to provide Nutritional Supplementation.

Beneficiaries

Children between 3-6 years in rural areas

Diet

Children – 300 Kcals; 10g proteins per child per day

Ministry

Ministry of Social Welfare

Special Nutrition Programme

The Programme was started in 1970 to provide Nutritional Supplementation

Beneficiaries
Children < 6 years
Pregnant women   In urban slums, tribal areas, backward rural areas
Lactating mothers

Diet
Children - 300 kcals; 10g proteins/child/day
Adults – 500 kcals, 25g protein/day   For 300 days a year

Ministry

Ministry of Social Welfare

Vit A Prophylaxis Programme

The Programme was started in 1970

One of the components of NPCB (National Programme for Control of Blindness) is to administer massive dose of Vit A to preschool children on a 6-monthly basis.

Vit A 1-lakh at 9 months (with Measles), 2-lakh at 1½ years (with DPT OPV Booster), 2-lakh from 2 to 5 years every six months.

Ministry

Ministry of Health and Family Welfare

Applied Nutrition Programme

The Programme was started in 1960

Objectives:

1. To make people conscious of Nutritional Needs
2. To increase production & consumption of nutritious foods
3. To provide Supplementary Nutrition to vulnerable groups through locally produced foods

Specific Activities

(a) Supplementary feeding
(b) Non-formal preschool education
(c) Nutrition education
(d) Poultry farming
(e) Beehive keeping
(f) Providing better seeds and seedlings
(g) Raising kitchen gardens

Beneficiaries

Children between 2-6 years
Pregnant women
Lactating mothers

Funding

UNICEF

National Nutritional Anemia Prophylaxis Programme

Anemia is a serious concern in children as it can affect Cognitive Performance, Behavioural and Motor development, Language development, Scholastic achievement and increased Morbidity from infectious diseases.

Hb levels are classified into 3 categories:
Mild - 10-10.9 gm/dl
Moderate - 8-8.9 gm/dl
Severe < 8 gm/dl

Prevalence of anemia in adults:
58% in pregnant and lactating women
56% in women 15-49 years
24% in adult males

Ministry of Health & Family Welfare Guidelines:

Short Term Measures

- Infant 6-12 months should also be included in the Programme
- Children 6-60 months should be given 1-ml (20mg Elemental Iron+100 mcg Folic acid) daily for 100 days.
- School children 6-10 years should be included in the Programme and provided 30 mg Iron + 250 mcg Folic Acid per child for 100 days annually.
- Adolescents 10-19 years will be supplemented at same doses and duration as adults.
- Pregnant and lactating women to be given 100 mg Elemental Iron + 500 mcg Folic Acid for 100 days.
- Double fortification of salt

Intermediate Measures

Food Fortification - Cereals, milk, sugar, salt with iron.

Long Term Measures

Nutrition Education to improve dietary intake of Iron rich food and food which helps in the absorption of Iron.

12 by 12 Initiative for Anemia Control

2007 – Launched at AIIMS to ensure every child should have Hb 12 g by age 12.

National Iron Plus Initiative

12th 5-year Plan - Aim to decrease Anemia in girls and women by 50%.

Strategy

- 6-59 months by weekly 20mg Elemental Iron + 100 mcg Folic Acid
- 1-5th Grade (6-10 years) – Weekly 45mg Elemental Iron + 400 mcg Folic Acid
- Adolescents (10-19 years) weekly 100 mg Elemental Iron + 500 mcg Folic Acid
- Women in reproductive age, pregnant and lactating women - Weekly 100 mg Elemental Iron + 500 mcg Folic Acid

National Iodine Deficiency Disorders (IDD) Control Programme

1962 - National Goitre Control Programme
1986 - National IDD Control Programme

Goal

To reduce prevalence of IDD to < 10% by 2012 AD

Objectives

1. Surveys to assess the magnitude of IDD
2. Supply Iodized salt
3. Re-survey after 5 years to assess the prevalence of IDD and impact of Iodated salt
4. Laboratory monitoring of Iodated salt and Urinary Iodine Excretion
5. Health education and publicity

Components

1. Iodized Salt
   Effective, economical method for Prophylaxis.
   PFA Act - Not < 30 ppm at production point, 15 ppm at consumer level
   Iodized Oil Inj. IM
   Iodized Oil oral or Sodium Iodate tablet

2. Monitoring Iodine
   Laboratories for
   i. Iodine excretion determination
   ii. Determination of Iodine in water, soil, food
   iii. Determination of Iodine in salt

3. Manpower Training
   Health workers to be trained on IDD Programme, legal enforcement, public education.

4. Mass Communication
   IEC on IDD, Iodized salt

Mid-day Meal Programme

Neither a child who is hungry nor a child who is ill can be expected to learn.
150 million children are present in 800,000 schools in India.

1961 – Mid-day Meal Scheme launched.

Aims:

- Improve school attendance
- Reduce dropouts
- Beneficial impact on children's nutrition in primary classes
- Impart Health and Nutrition education to children, parents, community
  Each child should receive 300 kcals and 8-12 g protein per day

Principles

- Meals should be a supplement and not substitute to home food
- Should supply at least one-third energy and half protein requirement
- Low cost
- Easily prepared in schools
- Locally available foods
- Menu frequently changed to avoid monotony

Recommendations

-Beneficiaries - Children in classes 1-8

-Meals should contain good quality vegetables, dark green leafy vegetables

-Meals should be hygienically prepared

-Urban areas - Centralised kitchen, meal prepared, transported, served hygienically (done in Chennai, Hyderabad, ISKON group in Bangalore)

-Rural areas – Self-help groups and Panchayats should be involved

-Every state should have a separate fund for effective implementation of the scheme

12th 5-year Plan

-Convergence of Millenium Development Goals with School Health Programme

-Management Information System for monitoring the scheme

The Programme is good for improving nutrition of underprivileged society. Sustainability requires political will, community participation, monitoring and evaluation and quality of services.

Adolescent Girls' Schemes

(a) Kishori Shakthi Yojana

Target - Girls 11-18 years
Addresses self-development, nutrition, health, literacy, numerical skills, vocational skills
Implemented through ICDS

(b) Nutrition Programme for Adolescent Girls

Target 11-18 years
Services - Undernourished girls – 6 kg free food/month

National Tuberculosis Elimination Program (NTEP)

RNTCP has been renamed NTEP in 2020

Objectives

1. To achieve Cure Rate of 85%
2. To detect 70% of cases

Revised Strategy

*   Augmentation of organisational support at Central and State levels for meaningful coordination
*   Increased budget outlay
*   Use of Sputum Testing as primary method of diagnosis
*   Standardised treatment regimens
*   Augmentation of peripheral level supervision through creation of subdistrict supervisory unit
*   Ensuring a regular uninterrupted supply of drugs up to the most peripheral level
*   Emphasis on training, IEC, Operational Research and NGO involvement in the Programme

Interventions

(a) Strengthening of TB cells at Central and State levels
(b) Strengthening Training Institutions for TB at Central and State levels
(c) Gradual implementation of revised strategy for TB control
(d) Strengthening National TB Control Programme in remaining Short Course Chemotherapy Districts as transitional step to adopting RNTCP
(e) Providing uninterrupted supply of antiTB drugs

Components of DOTS (Directly Observed Treatment Supervised)

-Case detection with the help of microscope
-Regular and uninterrupted supply of drugs
-Direct observation while patient is getting treatment
-Systematic evaluation and monitoring
-Political and administrative commitment to ensure financial support and sustainability

Diagnosis of TB

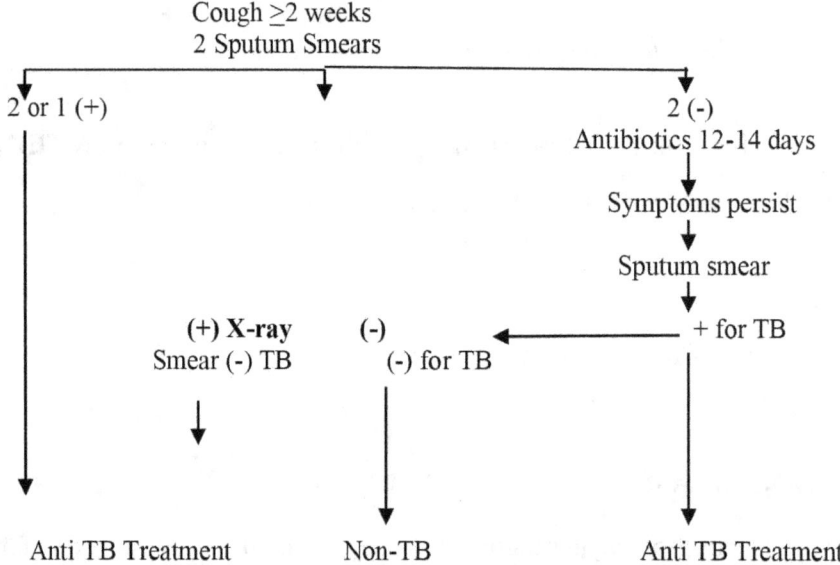

Category		Type of Patient	Regimens (mths)	Duration (mths)
CAT I New cases		New Sputum Smear (+) Seriously Ill Smear (-) Seriously Ill Extrapulmonary Sputum (-) Extrapulmonary not Seriously Ill	$2(HRZE)_3 + 4(HR)_3$	6
CAT II Re-treatment cases		Sputum (+) relapse Sputum (+) failure Sputum (+) treatment after default		8
MDR TB				

Public Private Partnership (PPP)

Aim is to provide standardised treatment to all TB patients
GOI developed guidelines for NGOs and private sector for TB Control

Advocacy, Communication and Social Mobilisation

IEC Strategy
Detailed planning, communication channels, monitoring
States and Districts to develop Specific Communication Plans
Special communication initiatives for special groups and hard to reach population eg Tribals

At Individual Level

IEC to understand disease, compliance to medicines, social stigmas, disposal of Sputum

At Community Level

Health education - Informs, motivates and helps people adopt and maintain healthy practices and lifestyles

School Awareness Programme

Awareness Programmes on TB, early detection and DOTS Treatment, myths, stigmas in schools and colleges.

Collaboration of NTEP Activities within NRHM and NUHM

NTEP incorporated with NRHM and NUHM

Prevention

Chemoprophylaxis - Children < 5 years INH 5mg/kg x 6 months
Screening and if symptomatic a full course of AntiTB Treatment
BCG Vaccination

Global Plan to Stop TB

Vision – A TB-free world.

Mission

 i.   Ensure every TB patient has access to effective diagnosis, treatment & cure
 ii. To stop transmission of TB
 iii. To reduce inequitable social & economic toll of TB
 iv. To develop & implement new preventive, diagnostic & therapeutic tools & strategies to stop TB

Targets

By 2005
To be sustained/exceeded by 2015
70% diagnosed & at least 85% cured

By 2015
Global burden of TB (Prevalence and deaths) reduced by 50% from 1990 levels

By 2050
TB eliminated as a global public health problem

Strategy- 6 components

1. To pursue high quality DOTS expansion & enhancement
2. Address TB/HIV, MDR-TB and other challenges
3. Contribute to Health System Strengthening
4. Engage all care givers
5. Empower people with TB and communities
6. Enable and promote Research

New Initiatives

1. *NIKSHAY*
   TB Surveillance using case-based, web-based IT system
   TB patient details, registration, diagnosis, DOT provider, HIV status, follow-up, contact tracing, outcomes
   Referral, transfer

Private Health Facility Registration & TB Notification

SMS alerts to patients
Automated periodic reports

2. *TB Notification*
   It is mandatory for Health Care Providers to notify all TB cases to authorities

3. *Ban on TB Serology*
   Serological Tests should not be used for diagnosing Pulmonary/Extrapulmonary TB

4. *Direct Benefit Transfer Schemes*
   To deliver benefits to TB patients and providers

Newer Initiatives

1. Daily Regimen for Pediatric TB
2. Daily Regimen for All forms of TB
3. Pilots for Universal Access to TB Cases
4. Universal Drug Susceptibility Testing (DST)
5. Shorter Regimen & Bedaquiline
6. Campaign Mode - Active Case Finding

Management of Drug Resistant TB

National Expert Technical Working Group developed National Policies
State PMDT Committee develops plan of action for implementation

District DR-TB Centre

For initiation and management of uncomplicated DR-TB patients eg RR-TB;
H-mono/poly DR-TB

Nodal DR-TB Centre

Patients with resistance to second line drugs

TB-HIV Coordination

ICTC - Integrated Counseling & Testing Centres

National Strategic Plan (2017-2025) for TB Elimination

Outcome Expected:

80% reduction in TB Incidence
90% reduction in TB Mortality
0% having Catastrophic Expenditure due to TB

National Leprosy Eradication Programme

Objectives

(a) Elimination of Leprosy (Prevalence <1 case/10,000 population in all districts)
(b) Strengthen disability prevention & medical rehabilitation of patients affected by Leprosy
(c) Reduction in level of stigma associated with Leprosy

Strategies

i. Integrated Leprosy Services through general health care system - Early diagnosis and treatment
ii. Capacity building
iii. Intensified IEC
iv. Prevention of disability and medical rehabilitation
v. Intensified monitoring and supervision

Case Detection and Management

States to have innovative plans:
(a) To improve access to services
(b) To involve women including Leprosy affected persons in case detection

(c) To organise skin camps

(d) To undertake contact survey

(e) To increase awareness through ANM, AWW, ASHA

Major Initiatives

1. Focus on New Case Detection Rate

2. Treatment Completion Rate

3. Disability prevention and medical rehabilitation
    - Dressing materials, medicines, ulcer kits
    - Microcellular footwear
    - Rs 5,000 for Leprosy patient undergoing Reconstructive Surgery
    - Rs 5,000 per Reconstructive Surgery

4. ASHAs to bring Leprosy suspects for diagnosis, treatment and follow-up

Cash incentives on diagnosis - Rs 250

Completion of treatment, Paucibacillary Leprosy - Rs 400

Multibacillary Leprosy - Rs 600

Early case before deformity - Rs 250

New case with deformity of hands, feet, eyes - Rs 200

Dosage (Adult PB)	Dosage (Child PB 10-14 years)
Monthly treatment: Day 1 - Rifampicin 600 mg - Dapsone 100 mg Daily Treatment: Days 2-28 - Dapsone 100 mg Duration of Treatment: - 6 Blister Packs to be taken monthly within a maximum period of 9 months	Monthly treatment: Day 1 - Rifampicin 450 mg - Dapsone 50 mg Daily Treatment: Days 2-28 - Dapsone 50 mg Duration of Treatment: 6 Blister Packs to be taken monthly within a maximum period of 9 months

Dosage (Adult MB)	Dosage (Child PB 10-14 years)
Monthly treatment: Day 1 - Rifampicin 600 mg - Clofazimine 300 mg - Dapsone 100 mg Daily Treatment: Days 2-28 - Clofazimine 50 mg - Dapsone 100 mg Duration of Treatment: - 12 Blister Packs to be taken monthly within 18 months	Monthly treatment: Day 1 - Rifampicin 450 mg - Clofazimine 150 mg - Dapsone 50 mg Daily Treatment: Days 2-28 - Clofazimine 50 mg every other day - Dapsone 50 mg daily Duration of Treatment: - 12 Blister Packs to be taken monthly within 18 months

Lepra Reactions

Reversal Reaction or Type-1 Reaction	ENL Reaction Erythema Nodosum Leprosum or Type-2 Reaction
Clinical Features: Skin lesions become reddish, swollen, peripheral nerves painful, tender, swollen Signs of Nerve Damage - Loss of sensation, muscle weakness Fever, malaise Hands and feet may be swollen Rarely new skin lesions may appear Treatment: Diagnosis and treatment is urgent because of risk of permanent damage to Peripheral Nerve Trunks If mild - (a) Rest (b) Analgesics If severe (Nerve involvement) Above + Corticosteroids	Tender reddish skin nodules, fever, joint pains, malaise, occasionally painful swollen nerves, eye involvement sometimes Mild- Bed rest Analgesics - Paracetamol/Aspirin If severe-

Prednisolone   40mg OD x 2 wks
                  30mg OD for wks 3 and 4
                  20mg OD for wks 5 and 6
                  15mg OD for wks 7 and 8
                  10mg OD for wks 9 and 10
                  5mg OD for wks 11 and 12
	Prednisolone
	Immobilization of Affected Nerve
	
	Note: During reactions continue MDT along with Antireaction Treatment

Surveillance

(a) PB Leprosy - Clinically examined once a year for 2 years after completion of treatment.
(b) MB Leprosy - Clinically examined once a year for 5 years

Immunoprophylaxis

BCG Vaccine gives some protection against Leprosy

Chemoprophylaxis

Dapsone/Acedapsone for 3 years or till index case becomes negative.

Deformities

Hand & Feet

Grade 0 - No anaesthesia, no visible deformity
Grade I - Anaesthesia but no visible deformity
Grade II - Visible deformity present

Eyes

Grade 0 - No eye problem

Grade I - Eye problem but vision not affected

Grade II - Severe visual impairment, Lagophthalmos, Iridocyclitis, Corneal Opacity

Face

Mask face, Leonine Facies, Lagophthalmos, loss of eyebrows, eyelashes, Corneal Ulcers, Opacities, Perforated Nose, Depressed Nose, ear deformities (Nodules on ear, Elongated Lobules)

Hands

Claw Hand, Wrist Drop, ulcers, Absorption of Digits, Hollowing of Interosseous Spaces, swollen hand

Feet

Claw Toes, Foot Drop, Inversion of Foot, Plantar Ulcers, Absorption of Toes, Collapsed Foot, swollen foot, Callosities

Others

Gynaecomastia, Perforation of Palate

Prevention of Deformities

(a)   Care of Palms and Soles - Heal wounds, ulcers, skin cracks

(b)   Prevent Injuries - Protective gloves, footwear

(c)   Prevent joint stiffness in paralytic deformities by physiotherapy

(d)   Protect eyes

Rehabilitation

The physical, mental restoration of treated patients to normal activity so that they may be able to resume their place in the home, society and industry.

Medical, surgical, social, educational and vocational rehabilitation.

Health Education

Regarding the disease, regular treatment, regular follow-ups, remove wrong beliefs, superstitions

Social Support

Department of Social Welfare - Assistance for travel to and from clinic, food grains, clothes, job,

abolishing social evil of beggary

Non-Government Organizations

Hind Kusht Nivaran Sangh
Gandhi Memorial Leprosy Foundation, Sevagram, Wardha
Damien Foundation

Reasons Leprosy Eradication not possible

1. Extra-human Reservoirs
2. Modes of transmission disputed
3. Incubation period long and variable
4. Subclinical cases and inability to detect them
5. Disease Manifestations - Complicated Spectrum
6. Failure of Cell Mediated Immunity in Lepromatous Cases
7. Bacterial resistance and persistence in human body
8. Absence of Vaccine
9. Social and cultural taboos resulting in concealment of disease

National Vector Borne Disease Control Programme (NVBDC)

- NVBDC Program is for the prevention and control of major Vector Borne Diseases of public health importance namely Malaria, Filaria, Japanese Encephalitis, Kala Azar, Dengue and Chikungunya.
- This program comes under National Rural Health Mission (NRHM).
- Integrated vector control methods are used - Environmental management, chemical, biological methods.
- Proper Solid Waste Disposal and improved water storage practices.

Vision

Well informed and self-sustained healthy India free from Vector Borne Diseases with equitable access to quality health care.

Mission

Integrated and accelerated action towards reducing Mortality on account of Malaria, Dengue, JE by half and elimination of Kala Azar by 2010 and elimination of Filariasis by 2015.

Millenium Development Goal 6 - Combat HIV/AIDS, Malaria and other diseases

Target 6 - Halt and begin to reverse incidence of Malaria and other major diseases

Objectives

Reduce Malaria Morbidity and Mortality by 50% by 2012

Targets

- Annual Blood Examination Rate (ABER) over 10%
- Annual Parasite Incidence (API) $\leq$ 1.3
- 25% Reduction in Morbidity and Mortality due to Malaria by 2010 & 50% by 2012

Indicators

- % of Blood Smears examined from population during the year
- No. of laboratory confirmed Malaria cases per 1000 population (API)
- No. of Malaria deaths per 100,000 population

Strategies

(a) Against the Parasite
(b) Against the Vector

1. ***Disease Management***
   - Early Case Detection and Treatment
   - Strengthening Referral Services
   - Epidemic preparedness and Rapid Response

2. ***Improve Efficiency and Quality of Services***
   Primary Level
   - ASHA under NRHM, AWW under ICDS and NGOs trained to serve Fever Treatment Depots
   - PHCs and CHCs equipped to provide In-Patient Treatment for PF cases
   - Lab Surveillance from private sector enhanced

   Secondary Level
   - Training of Medical Officers, Lab Technicians and Community Volunteers of Public and Private sector
   - District Level Hospitals equipped with Ventilators and appropriate Lab Services
   - Medical Audit to measure effectiveness of Program

   Tertiary Level
   - Medical College Hospitals to manage all referral cases
   - Undertake Operational Research on effectiveness of Rapid Diagnostic Kits, efficacy of Combi-pack
   - Renal Diagnosis for management of severe Malaria cases

3. ***Legislative Measures***
   Enforcement of Civic Bylaws and Building Bylaws

4. **Involvement of NGOs/Private Sector/Community/Local Self-Government**

5. **Quality Assurance on Laboratory Diagnosis**

6. **Long Lasting Insecticide Treated Bed-nets (LLIN)**

7. **Environmental Management**
    Burrow Pits, river bed pools cleared; land leveling and filling to eliminate depression areas; seepage control; piped or covered canals and drains; weed control

    Wells, tube wells and hand pumps should have platform sloping towards periphery which should lead to drainage system or soakage pit.

    Wells and overhead tanks to be covered.

8. **Monitoring and Evaluation**
    NAMMIS - National Anti-malaria Management Information System for Data Analysis from Sentinel Sites, Field reviews/visits by personnel from State/District Level and ICMR Institute.

9. **Collaboration with National Institute of Malaria Research (NIMAR) and Medical Colleges**

10. **Intersectoral Collaboration**
    PPP - Public Private Partnership, Agriculture, Social Welfare, Education, Railway, Armed Forces

11. **Behaviour Change Communication**
12. **Research**
    Drug Resistance in Parasite & Insecticide Resistance in Vector.

H/O Malaria Control in India
1946 - Bhore Committee Report
1953 - National Malaria Control Program
1958 - National Malaria Eradication Program
1971 - Urban Malaria Scheme
1977 - Modified Plan of Operation (MPO)
1995 - Malaria Action Program (MAP)
1997 - Enhanced Malaria Control Program (EMCP)
1999 - National Anti-Malaria Program (NAMP)
2002 - National Health Policy
2004 - National Vector Borne Disease Control Program
2005 - Intensified Malaria Control Project & National Rural Health Mission

Bhore Committee (1946)

Recommended a countrywide program to control Malaria.

1953 - National Malaria Control Program

Objectives:

- To bring down Malaria Transmission to a level where it would cease to be a public health problem
- Thereafter, maintenance by each state

Strategies:

- Residual Insecticide spraying of human dwellings and cattle sheds
- Malaria control teams to monitor program
- Anti-malarial drugs

Good results obtained.

1958 - National Malaria Eradication Program

Objective:

To eradicate Malaria in 7-9 years.

Programme was divided into

- o Preparatory Phase
- o Attack Phase
- o Consolidation Phase &
- o Maintenance Phase

Preparatory Phase

This phase of collection of preliminary data was omitted because it was done during NMCP.

Attack Phase

DDT spraying done twice a year in Endemic areas.
Objective of DDT spraying was to intercept transmission ie. To kill the mosquitoes after they had picked up Malarial Parasites but before they become infective to man.

Active Surveillance
Malaria field worker visits each of the 2000 houses (10,000 population) allotted to him once a fortnight and enquires whether anyone is suffering from fever or had suffered from it since his previous visit or if any guest or visitor with fever had stayed with them.
If yes, he takes a thick and thin blood smear from him & sends slide to the PHC.

He administers presumptive treatment, Chloroquine 600mg.

If blood report is positive, he returns & gives radical treatment – Chloroquine 600 mg stat & primaquine 15mg Day 1 – Day 5.

Passive surveillance
Medical Officers of hospitals & dispensaries and Private Practitioners should obtain blood smears from every Febrile Case & hand over the slides to surveillance worker when he comes
(Once in 15 days).
In large hospitals the worker sits in the OPD & obtains smears from every febrile case & administers presumptive treatment.

Consolidation Phase

Surveillance done to detect persons infected with Malarial Parasites during mopping up operation of the consolidation phase & treated so as to wipe out residual Foci of infection.

Maintenance Phase

This is the last phase of NMEP.
If despite active & passive surveillance no case of malaria is detected for 3 years, maintenance phase commences.
In this phase strict vigil is kept in order to detect cases of malaria.
If a case is detected immediate Focal Insecticidal Spray is done, epidemiological investigations conducted & all positive cases radically treated.

Factors Responsible for Resurgence of Malaria (OAT)

1. *Operational Failure*
    Starting project without idea of epidemiological factors & trends
    Inadequate Surveillance & Case Detection
    Inadequate coverage of Insecticidal Spray during house-to-house
    Undue reliance on PHCs which are ill equipped & ill prepared for the task
    Several staff left the job due to better opportunities & salaries
    Premature take off into consolidation & maintenance phase

2. *Administrative Failure*
    Inadequate Insecticides
    Inadequate Anti-malarial Drugs
    Insufficient Trained Staff
    Difficulty in recruitment of labourers for spraying
    Improper budget allocation for purchasing insecticides,

Spraying equipment
Rising Cost of Operation
Laxity of government & staff
Improper lab facilities & transport

3. *Technical Failure*

Resistance of mosquitoes to DDT
Resistance of Plasmodia to Chloroquine

1971 - Urban Malaria Scheme

Anti-larval measures in Urban Malaria Scheme.

1977 - Modified Plan of Operation (MPO)

Objectives:

- Elimination of Malarial Deaths
- Reduction of Malaria Morbidity
- Maintenance of gains achieved by Reducing Transmission

Strategy

Areas divided on basis of API.

API ≥ 2

1. Insecticide Spray
2. Entomological Study
3. Malaria Surveillance
4. Treatment of cases
5. Efforts intensified in rural areas with SIDA Assistance (Swedish International Development Agency)
6. Decentralisation of Laboratory Services to PHC level
7. Establishment of Drug Distribution Centres (DDCs)/Fever Treatment Depots (FTDs)

API < 2

1. Focal Spray of DDT/BHC/Malathion if case of PF occurred
2. Surveillance – Active & Passive
3. Treatment of cases
4. Epidemiological Investigation of Malaria cases

1995 - Malaria Action Program (MAP)

Expert committee identified problem areas: Tribal areas, Epidemic Prone areas (North-Western plains, Indo-Ganjetic plain, Project areas, Triple Insecticide Resistant areas, Urban areas

Strategies:

1. Case Detection and Treatment
2. Surveillance
3. IEC
4. MPW trained to identify and refer severe cases to PHC

1997 - Enhanced Malaria Control Project (EMCP)

Objectives:

- Effective control of Malaria to decrease Morbidity
- Prevention of deaths
- Consolidation of gains achieved so far

Strategies:

1. Early Case Detection and treatment
2. Vector Control by Indoor Residual Spray in rural and Antilarval Measures in urban areas
3. Health education and community participation

Number of PF cases decreased from 0.7 million to 0.4 million

1999 - National Anti-Malaria Program (NAMP)

NMEP renamed National Anti-Malaria Program.
Later this program became part of National Vector Borne Disease Control Program coming under National Rural Health Mission in 2005.

2002 - National Health Policy

Goal:

Reduction in Mortality due to Malaria and other vector borne diseases by 50% by 2010 and Morbidity Control.

2004 - National Vector Borne Disease Control Program (NVBDCP)

Malaria included in the program.

2005 - National Rural Health Mission (NRHM)

NVBDCP is included in NRHM.

Goal in MDG 6:

Combating HIV/AIDS, Malaria and other diseases.

Target:

Halting and beginning to Reverse Incidence of Malaria and other major diseases.

Intensified Malaria Control Project

This was launched in 2005 with assistance from Global Fund AIDS, TB, Malaria in North-East states, Orissa, Jharkhand and West Bengal.

Objectives:

(a) To increase access to Rapid Diagnosis and Treatment
(b) To reduce Malaria Transmission through Risk Reduction by use of Insecticide treated Bed-nets and Larvivorous Fish
(c) To enhance awareness about Malaria Control, and
(d) To promote community, NGO and private sector participation

Strategies:

- Early Case Detection and Prompt Treatment through Active and Passive Surveillance
- Antilarval Measures through Larvicides
- Minor Engineering Methods eg Source Reduction, Channelisation, De-weeding
- Biological Control using Larvivorous Fish
- IEC Campaigns for community awareness and their involvement

Treatment of Uncomplicated Malaria:

All fever cases investigated by Rapid Diagnostic Test.
P Vivax treated with Chloroquine for 3 days and Primaquine for 14 days.
P Falciparum treated with ACT – Artesunate 3 days + Sulphadoxine - Pyremethamine 1 day. Pregnant women should be treated with Quinine in 1st Trimester; ACT in 2nd and 3rd Trimesters.

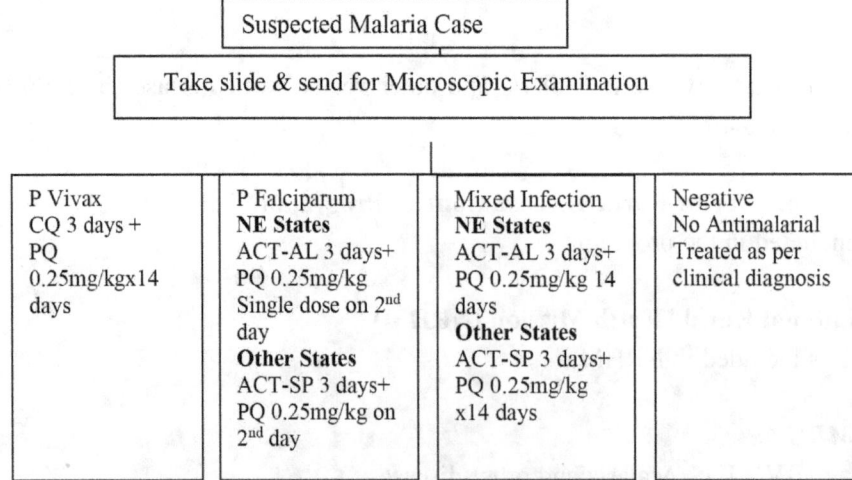

Insecticide Treated Bed-nets Program

Deltamethrin impregnated mosquito nets should be used

Community Participation

Promote Community Participation through NGOs, local self-governments.

Computerised MIS

Web-based Management Information System from National to District level.
This will facilitate Early Detection of Epidemics and Control.

Intersectoral Convergence

Public Private Partnerships involving NGOs, Community-based organisations, Non-Health sector departments (Education, railways, tribal welfare, CRPF, BSF, Armed Forces), Corporate Sector.

Behavior Change Communication

BCC targeting caretakers, care providers, political/opinion leaders/planners/resource givers/media for prevention and control of Vector Borne Diseases.
Early case detection, reporting, complete treatment, drug compliance, referral of severe cases, home based morbidity management, outbreak preparedness, integrated vector management.

Capacity Building

Training of Medical College Faculty and Private Practitioners on Vector Borne Diseases and Control.

Operation Research

Operation Research conducted in collaboration with State Program Managers, ICMR.

Remote Sensing

Tool for surveillance of habitats, densities of vector species and prediction of incidence of diseases.
Remote Sensing is likely to become a Rapid Epidemiological Tool for surveillance of Vector Borne Diseases and Malaria in particular.
Geographical Information System (GIS), statistical analysis, knowledge of ecology of mosquito, remote sensing will play a key role in Macro-stratification of vast Malarious areas for prioritising the control measures in a cost-effective way.

Roll Back Malaria

1998 - Roll Back Malaria – A global partnership by WHO, UNDP, UNICEF, World Bank.

Aim:

Halve the world's Malaria burden by 2010

Strategies:

- Prompt access to Effective Treatment
- Prevention and Management of Malaria in pregnancy
- Improving prevention and response to Malaria epidemics
- Promotion of Insecticide Treated Bed-nets and improved Vector Control
- Encourage Research for New Drugs, Insecticides, Malaria Vaccines
- Strengthening Health System
- Capacity Building
- Involvement of private and other sectors

Malaria Vaccine

They are under trial.

Types:

(a) *Merozoite Vaccine*
Asexual Blood Stage Vaccine.
Prepared from Polypeptides of Merozoites (Blood Stages) of Pl Falciparum.
They prevent the RBCs alone from being infected.

(b) *Sporozoite Vaccine*
Prepared from Antigens of Sporozoites.
Prevent both Liver cells and RBCs from being infected.

(c) *Gamete Vaccines*
Prepared from Gametes.
Mosquito picks up antibodies when it bites vaccinee thereby preventing development in the mosquito.
But vaccinee is not prevented from getting infected.

(d) *A synthetic cocktail vaccine*
Pf S 66 for Pl Falciparum is a Peptide-Alum combination.
It is 30% effective.

(e) *Transmission blocking vaccine*
Pf S 25 - Under trial.

2016-2030 - National Framework for Malaria Elimination

Goal:

Elimination of Malaria by 2030
Maintain Malaria-free status where Malaria Transmission has been interrupted & prevent reintroduction of Malaria

Classification of States/UTs for Malaria Elimination in India

CATEGORY	DEFINITION
0 - Prevention of re-establishment phase	States/UTs with 0 Indigenous cases of Malaria (none)
1 - Elimination phase	States/UTs with API <1 in all districts (15 states)
2- Pre-elimination phase	States/UTs with API <1 in some districts with API >1 (11 states)
3. Intensified Control Phase	States/UTs with API > 1 (10 states)

District as a Unit of Planning and Implementation

Each district should stratify PHCs and SCs into 5 Strata:

1. 0 cases
2. API > 0 to < 1
3. API 1 to < 2
4. API 2 to < 5
5. API > 5

Broad Strategies

- Early Diagnosis & Treatment
- Case-based Surveillance & Rapid Response
- Integrated Vector Management - Indoor Residual Spraying (IRS), Long Lasting Insecticidal Nets (LLIN), Larval Source Management (LSM)
- Epidemiological preparedness & early response
- Monitoring & Evaluation
- Advocacy, Coordination, Partnership
- BCC & Community Mobilisation
- Program Planning & Management

Category 3 (Intensified Control Phase States/UTs API >1)

- Massive scaling up of Management and Preventive approaches
- Screening all fever cases
- Classification of areas based on Malarial Epidemiology and Tailored Interventions

- Intersectoral Coordination
- One-stop Centres/Mobile Clinics on fixed days in tribal/conflict areas
- Referral of severe cases
- Strengthening District and Sub-district hospitals
- IEC

Category 2 (Pre-elimination Phase States/UTs API<1 but some districts API>1)

Malaria Elimination Interventions, Elimination Surveillance Systems and Initiating Elimination Phase activities in districts with API < 1 per 1000 population

Category 1 (Elimination Phase States/UTs/All districts API <1)

- All efforts interrupting transmission wherever Active Foci of Malaria
- Mandatory Notification - Government and private hospitals
- Case-based Surveillance
- Investigation and Classification of all Foci
- Effective Vector Control measures
- Early Detection and Treatment of cases
- State and National level database
- Mobile and Migrant Populations - Interventions for Effective Screening, Management and Prevention
- Epidemic forecasting and Response System
- Quality assurance of medicines, Diagnostics
- National level reference lab for quality checking and training
- Surveillance of special groups, migrant populations, populations in industrial areas

Category 0

- Detect any reintroduced case of Malaria
- Notify
- Determine causes
- Rapid Curative and Preventive Measures
- Prevent re-introduction and re-establishment of Malaria Transmission
- Maintain Malaria-free status

Filaria Control

1955 - National Filaria Control Program launched.

Goal:

Eliminate Lymphatic Filariasis by 2015

Objectives:

- Reduction of problem
- Control in urban areas through recurrent Antilarval & Antiparasitic measures

Strategy

1. Vector Control

Anti-mosquito, Anti-larval measures
DDT 1-2 rounds residual insecticide spray 1g/sq m in endemic areas

Temephos (Antilarval) in water storage tanks every week & MLO (Mineral Larvicidal Oil) on water surface

Biological Control through Larvivorous Fishes

Environmental Engineering through source reduction and water management

2. Antiparasitic Measure

Diagnosis & Treatment of Microfilaria carriers and cases
Di Ethyl Carbamazine (DEC) 6mg/kg orally x 12 days (Bancroftian Filariasis) in divided doses (100 mg TDS)
Brugian Filariasis 3-6mg/kg

Mass Treatment - Every member of community treated
DEC Medicated Salt: 1-4g DEC/kg common salt (Lakshadweep & Pondicherry)

National Filaria Day once a year for 5 years.

3. Behavior Change Communication

IEC for community awareness and to change behavior for healthy practices

4. Capacity Building

For home-based management of Lymphoedema and Hydrocelectomy at CHCs and hospitals.

Implemented through:
206 Filaria Control Units,
199 Filaria Clinics,
27 Survey Units

Japanese Encephalitis

In India, Japanese Encephalitis is prevalent in the states of Andhra Pradesh, Karnataka, Tamil Nadu, Kerala, Maharashtra, Bihar, West Bengal, Assam, Manipur, Uttar Pradesh, Haryana

Prevention & Control

Strategy

- Strengthening surveillance activities through Sentinel Centres in Tertiary Health Care institutions
- Early diagnosis and proper case management at PHCs, CHCs and hospitals
- Behavior Change Communication to promote early case reporting, personal protection, isolation of amplifier host
- Integrated Vector Control Measures - Fogging, space spraying in animal dwelling, Antilarval operations, Larvivorous fishes, personal protection
- Capacity Building - Training of medical and nursing staff
- Vaccination of high-risk population - Children aged 1-15 years

JE Vaccination

Mouse Brain derived inactivated JE Vaccine SC 3doses 0.5-1ml day 0, 7, 30.
Booster to be given every 3 years.
Vaccination should be done in the Inter-epidemic period for 1-15 years population.
JE vaccination done as part of UIP in 11 Endemic districts of 4 states - UP, Assam, W Bengal, Karnataka

Kala Azar Control

Strategy for Control

- Integrated vector control
- Enhanced case detection and treatment including introduction of rK39 Rapid Diagnostic Kits and Oral Miltefosine
- Communication for behavior change and intersectoral coordination
- Capacity building
- Monitoring, Supervision and Evaluation
- Operational Research

Integrated Vector Control

Sandfly Control

i. DDT 2 rounds - Spraying in human dwellings, animal shelters and all resting places upto 6ft from floor level in Feb-Mar and May-June.
ii. BHC where there is resistance to DDT

Enhanced Case Detection and Complete Treatment

rK39 Rapid Diagnostic Kits and ELISA used.
IM or IV Sodium Antimony Stibogluconate 20mg/kg body weight x 20 days.
IV Pentamidine Isethionate 3mg/kg x 10 days
Oral Miltefosine, Paramomycin or Amphotericin B 1mg/kg x 20 days.

Communication for Behavior Change & Intersectoral Coordination

- Avoid sleeping on the floor.
- Use Bed-nets.
- Cleaning human dwellings and animal shelters.
- Cracks, crevices to be closed by cement.

Capacity Building

All staff trained on early detection and treatment.

Monitoring, Supervision, Evaluation

This is vital to the program.
Linked with Malaria and other VBD control.

Operational Research

- Integrated Vector Management Strategies
- Health seeking behavior of different community groups
- Community behavior towards use of Insecticide Treated Bed-nets
- Drug compliance studies and drug response monitoring
- Satellite based health mapping for Kala Azar

Dengue Fever

Strategy:

1. Surveillance for disease and vector through Sentinel Centres in Tertiary Health Care institutions
2. Early and prompt case management
3. Vector (Aedes Aegypti) control through source reduction, personal protection, Behavior Change Communication campaign for community participation and social mobilisation
4. Intersectoral Coordination for mosquito breeding, source reduction, personal protection and early reporting of cases
5. Capacity Building - Training of Health Staff

Vector Surveillance

Larval Surveys

- House Index (HI) - % of houses infected with Larvae and/or Pupae

$$HI = \frac{\text{No. of houses infected}}{\text{No. of houses inspected}} \times 100$$

- Container Index (CI) - % of water holding containers infected with Larvae and/or Pupae

$$CI = \frac{\text{No. of positive containers}}{\text{No. of containers inspected}} \times 100$$

- Breteau Index (BI) - No. of positive containers per 100 houses inspected

$$BI = \frac{\text{No. of positive containers}}{\text{No. of houses inspected}} \times 100$$

- Pupae Index (PI) - No. of Pupae per 100 houses

$$PI = \frac{\text{No. of Pupae}}{\text{No. of houses inspected}} \times 100$$

Adult Surveys

- Landing/biting collection
  Landing/biting counts per man hour

- Resting collection
  No. of adult mosquitoes per house, or
  No. of adult mosquitoes per man hour of human effort

- Oviposition Traps
  Ovitraps are devices used to detect presence of Aedes Aegypti where population density is low.

Control

No separate budget for Dengue.
IEC for preventing and controlling all Vector Borne Diseases under National Vector Borne Disease Control Program.

Vector Management

(a) Environmental Management

- Environmental Modification - Improved water supply, mosquito proofing
- Environmental Manipulation - Removal of Breeding Sites
- Changes in human habitations - Mosquito proofing of houses with screens or doors/windows

(b) **Personal Protection**
Protective clothing, repellents, mosquito coils, Pyrethrum space spray

(c) **Biological Control**
Larvivorous Fish - In large water bodies and large water containers
Bacillus Thuringiensis - Endotoxin producing Bacteria

(d) **Chemical Control**
Larvicides - Temephos 1ppm (1mg/lit of water)
Adulticides - Pyrethrum, Malathion

Legislative Measures

1. **Model Civic Bylaws**
Fines/punishment should be implemented if breeding is detected
trictly enforced in Mumbai, Chandigarh, Delhi Municipal Corporations

2. **Building Construction Regulation Act**
Building bylaws should be made for appropriate overhead/underground tanks, mosquito proofing buildings, designs of sunshades, porticos for not allowing stagnation of water.

3. **Environmental Health Act**
Bylaws for proper disposal or storage of junk, discarded tins, old tyres.

Health Education for Community Mobilisation & Intersectoral Coordination

- Involvement of households, community for Aedes Mosquito Control.
- Behavior Change Communication campaign is crucial.
- Community must be assured that this is a preventable disease and empowered with knowledge about mode of transmission, vector control options, treatment facilities available.

Chikungunya Fever

Derived from the word "Kungunyala" of the Makonde language of South-eastern Tanzania & Northern Mozambique, and means "to dry up or become contorted".

The disease resembles Dengue Fever and is characterised by Severe Persistent Joint Pain (Arthritis), fever and rash.

Socio-economic Impact

Poor people are mainly affected.
Productivity at work declines, income decreases, farmers cannot do agriculture, school children cannot attend school.

Treatment

No specific treatment.

Supportive Therapy - NSAID, rest.

Aspirin to be avoided.

Infected persons should be isolated from mosquitoes to avoid transmission of infection to other people.

Prevention

- No vaccine
- No disease specific drugs
- Prevention mainly by avoiding mosquito bite and eliminating mosquito breeding sites
- Prevention of mosquito bites by long sleeved shirts and long pants, mosquito repellents, screening, bed-nets
- Controlling breeding of Aedes by Source Reduction, use of Larvicides (Temephos), Adulticides (Pyrethrum Spray), Biological Control (Larvivorous Fish).

National AIDS Control Program

1987 - National AIDS Control Programme launched.

Ministry of Health & Family Welfare set up the National AIDS Control Organisation (NACO) to implement the Programme.

1992-1999 - NACP I

Objectives:

To control spread of HIV Infection

To decrease Morbidity, Mortality

Activities:

- Expansion of infrastructure of blood banks, separation of blood components
- Infrastructure for treatment of STDs increased in District Hospitals, Medical Colleges
- Sentinel Surveillance System for HIV was initiated
- NGOs involved in prevention interventions, focus on awareness generation
- State AIDS Cells established

1999-2006 - NACP II

New Initiatives Undertaken

Targeted Interventions (TI) for High-Risk Groups (HRG) - Commercial Sex Workers (CSW), Men who have Sex with Men (MSM), Injecting Drug Users (IDU) and Bridge populations (Truckers and Migrants)

Services:

Behaviour Change Communication (BCC), STD Management, Condom Promotion

School AIDS Education Programme - To build up life skills of adolescents

IEC - Awareness programmes about HIV/AIDS, promote safe behaviours, condom promotion

2007-12 - NACP III

2012-17 - NACP IV

Goal:

To halt and reverse the epidemic in India

Objectives:

Reduce Incidence Rate by 60% in first year of Programme in high prevalence states and by 40% in vulnerable states

Strategies:

HIV Surveillance Centres
Identification and screening of High-Risk Groups
Guidelines for Management of Cases and follow up
Guidelines for blood bank, blood product manufacturers, blood donors, dialysis units
Information Education and Communication (IEC)
Research - Indigenous vaccine development, Microbicides
Control of STDs
Capacity Building
Condom Promotion

Services:

1. **Prevention Services**
   Targeted Interventions for High-Risk Groups
   Needle-Syringe Exchange Programme and Opioid Substitution Therapy for IDUs
   Prevention interventions for migrant population at source, transit and destination
   Linkwork Scheme for HRGs and vulnerable populations in rural areas
   Prevention and Control of STDs/RTIs
   Blood Safety
   HIV Counselling and Testing
   Prevention of Parent-To-Child Transmission

School AIDS Education Programme
. Family Health Awareness Campaign (FHAC)
. National AIDS Telephone Helpline

2. *Care, Support and Treatment Services*
   Lab Services for CD4 testing and other investigations
   Free 1st line and 2nd line ART through ART Centres, Link ART Centres, Centres of Excellence (CoE) and ART Plus Centres
   Pediatric ART for children
   Early Infant Diagnosis for HIV exposed infants and children < 18 months
   Nutritional and Psychosocial support through Care and Support Centres (CSC)
   HIV/TB Coordination (Cross-referral, detection and treatment of co-infections)
   Treatment of Opportunistic Infections
   Drop-in-Centres for People Living with HIV (PLHIV) networks
   Post Exposure Prophylaxis (PEP) for Health Care Workers

Red Ribbon Express

On 1st Dec 2007 it began its journey from Delhi and traversed 27,000 km throughout the country.

It spread IEC on HIV/AIDS, promoted safe behavioural practices, measures to prevent epidemic, reduce stigma and discrimination against People Living with HIV/AIDS (PLHA).

STD Control Programme

1946 - STD Control Programme launched
It is now linked to the National AIDS Control Programme

Strategies:

(a) Management of STDs through Syndromic Approach through general health service
(b) Treatment of RTIs/STDs under RCH and now NRHM Programme
    STD Clinics in District/Block/First Referral Units/Medical Colleges
(c) Training of Medical, Paramedical workers
(d) Counselling Services
(e) Condom Promotion

Integrated Disease Surveillance Project

2004 – The Integrated Disease Surveillance Project was launched.

Objective:

1. To detect early warning signals of impending outbreak and help initiate effective response in a timely manner
2. To provide essential data and monitor progress of On-going Disease Control Programmes

Components of Surveillance Activity:

- Collection of Data
- Compilation of Data
- Analysis & Interpretation
- Follow-up Action
- Feedback

Syndromes Under Surveillance

1. Fever
   - < 7 days duration without localising signs
   - With rash
   - With altered sensorium/convulsions
   - Bleeding from skin or mucous membrane
   - Fever > 7 days with or without localising signs
2. Cough > 2 weeks duration
3. Acute Flaccid Paralysis
4. Diarrhoea
5. Jaundice
6. Unusual events causing death/hospitalisation

Diseases Under Surveillance:

Malaria, Typhoid, Cholera, Japanese Encephalitis, Dengue, Measles, TB, Polio, Hepatitis, Leptospirosis, Yellow Fever, Anthrax, Plague, Emerging Epidemics, Road Traffic Accidents

National Programme for Prevention & Control of Cancer, Diabetes, Cardiovascular Diseases & Stroke (NPCDCS)

NPCDCS was launched in 2008.

Objectives:

1. Prevent and Control NCDs through behavior and lifestyle changes
2. Provide early diagnosis and management of NCDs
3. Capacity Building at various levels of health care for Prevention, Diagnosis and Treatment of NCDs
4. Train Manpower - Doctors, Nurses, Paramedics
5. Establish Palliative and Rehabilitative Care

NCD Clinics at CHCs & District Hospitals

Behaviour Change Communication:

- Healthy Balanced diet
- Physical Activity
- Decrease/Maintenance of BMI < 23
- Avoidance of Tobacco
- Avoidance of Alcohol
- Stress Management

Activities at Sub-centre & PHC

1. Health promotion for behavior and lifestyle change through camps, interpersonal communication, posters, banners
2. Screening of people > 30 years for BP, Diabetes
3. Referral of suspects to higher facilities for diagnosis and management

Activities at Community Health Centre

- NCD Clinic
- OPD & In-patient Services
- Referral of complicated cases to District Hospital

Activities at District Hospital

- NCD Clinic
- Screen persons > 30 years for Diabetes, Hypertension, Cardiovascular Disease
- Referrals from CHC - Investigation and Treatment
- Home-based Palliative Care
- Promotion of healthy lifestyle through Health Education and Counseling to patients and attendants

Urban Health Check-up Scheme

1. To screen urban slum population for Diabetes and High BP
2. To create database for prevalence of Diabetes and High BP in urban slums
3. To sensitise the urban slum population on healthy lifestyle

Cancer Component under NPCDCS

Objectives

(a) Primary Prevention by Health Education
(b) Secondary Prevention by Early Detection of Common Cancers eg. Cervix, Breast, Mouth and tobacco related cancers by Screening and self-examination
(c) Tertiary Prevention by strengthening existing institutions of Comprehensive Therapy including Palliative Care.

Schemes under Revised Programme

1. *Regional Cancer Centre Scheme*
   Regional Cancer Centres strengthened as Referral Centres and Rs 3 crore funding given.

2. *Oncology Wing Development Scheme*
   Central assistance Rs 3 crore given per institution for purchase of equipment eg. Cobalt unit.

3. *District Cancer Control Programme*
   District projects on prevention, health education, early detection and pain relief where funding of Rs 22 lakh per district has been provided.

4. *NGO Scheme*
   For IEC and early detection of cancer Rs 5 lakh given.

5. *IEC Activities at Central Level*
   To give publicity to Antitobacco legislation for discouraging consumption of Cigarettes and other Tobacco-related products and creating awareness among masses about the ill effects of Tobacco and Tobacco-related products.

6. *Research and Training*
   Training programmes, monitoring and research activities will be organised at Central Level.

Tobacco control legislation

"The Cigarettes and other Tobacco Products Act 2003 (COTPA) states:

(a) Prohibition of Smoking in Public Places
(b) Prohibition of direct and indirect advertisement of Cigarette and other products
(c) Prohibition of sale of Cigarette and other Tobacco products to a person below 18 years.
(d) Prohibition of sale of Tobacco products near educational institutions
(e) Mandatory depiction of statutory warnings on Tobacco packs.
(f) Mandatory depiction of Tar and Nicotine contents along with maximum permissible limits on Tobacco packs.

National Programme for Control of Blindness and Visual Impairment

Vision 2020 - The Right to Sight

The Right to Sight, a global initiative to eliminate avoidable blindness by the year 2020. It was launched by WHO in 1999.

Objective

To assist member countries to develop sustainable systems to eliminate avoidable blindness from Cataract, Refractive Error, Xerophthalmia, Trachoma etc by 2020.

Strategies

(a) Target diseases are Cataract, Refractive Errors, Childhood Blindness, Corneal Blindness, Glaucoma, Diabetic Retinopathy
(b) Human Resource Development
(c) Infrastructure and Technology Development at various levels of health system

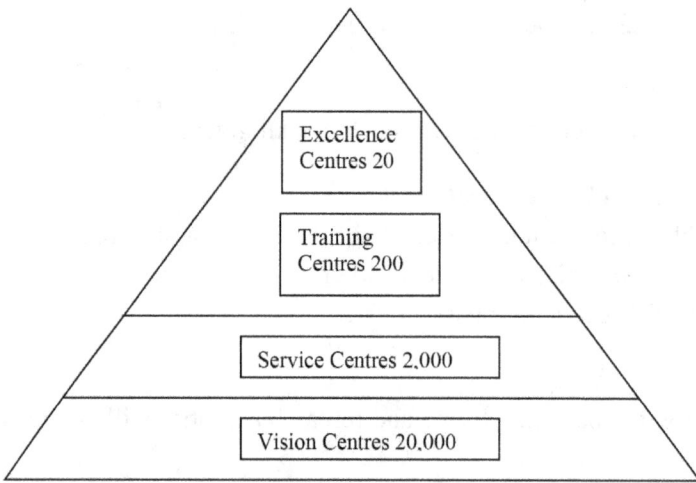

Proposed Structure for Vision 2020 - The Right to Sight

1976 - NPCB launched

100% Centrally Sponsored Programme and incorporates the earlier Trachoma Control Programme.

Strategies:

1. Strengthening Service Delivery
2. Developing Human Resources for Eye Care
3. Promoting Outreach Activities and Public Awareness
4. Developing Institutional Capacity
5. To Establish Eye Care Facilities for every 5 lakh persons

Revised Strategies:

1. To make NPCB more comprehensive by strengthening services for other causes of blindness eg. Corneal blindness, refractive errors in school children, improving follow-up services of cataract operated patients, glaucoma treatment.

2. To shift from eye camp approach to fixed facility surgical approach; from conventional surgery to IOL.
3. To expand the World Bank project to District level eg. Construction of Operation Theatres, Eye Wards.
4. To strengthen Voluntary Organisations' participation in the programme and improve performance of Govt Medical Colleges, District Hospitals, CHCs, PHCs
5. To enhance coverage of eye care services in tribal and underserved areas through identification of blind patients, preparation of village-wise Blind Registers and preference to Bilateral Blind Patients for Cataract Surgery.

Infrastructure Development

- National Institute of Ophthalmology - Dr Rajendra Prasad Centre for Ophthalmic Science in AIIMS, New Delhi.
- 10 Regional Institutes of Ophthalmology for manpower development, research and referral services.
- Strengthening PHCs
- Paramedical Ophthalmic Assistants trained and posted in PHCs
- Central Mobile Units
- Strengthening District Hospitals
- District Mobile Units
- DBCS - District Blindness Control Societies
- Upgrading Departments of Ophthalmology in Medical Colleges
- Eye Banks

National Guinea Worm Eradication Programme

1984 - Launched with Technical Assistance from WHO
1996 - Onwards zero cases
2000 - International Commission for Certification of Dracunculiasis Eradication recommended India be certified free of Dracunculiasis Transmission

Activities Continuing as per Recommendations of above Committee:

i. Health Education of school children & women in rural areas
ii. Rumour Registration & Rumour Investigation
iii. Guinea Worm Disease on list of notifiable disease & surveillance continued
iv. Supervision of hand pumps, drinking water; provision of additional units where necessary.

National Mental Health Programme

1982 – National Mental Health Programme (NMHP) was launched

Aims:

- Prevention & Treatment of Mental and Neurological Disorders and their associated disabilities
- Use of Mental Health Technology to improve general health services
- Application of mental health principles in total national development to improve quality of life

Objectives:

1. To ensure availability and accessibility of minimal mental health care for all in the foreseeable future particularly to the most vulnerable and underprivileged sections of population
2. To encourage application of mental health knowledge in general health care and in social development
3. To promote community participation in the mental health services development and to stimulate efforts towards self-help in the community

Strategies:

- Integrating mental health with primary health care through the National Mental Health Programme
- Provision of Tertiary Care institutions for treatment of mental disorders
- Eradicating stigmatisation of mentally ill patients and protecting their rights through Regulatory Institutions like the Central Mental Health Authority and State Mental Health Authority
- District Mental Health Programme
- Life Skills Education in Schools

WHO's 10 Life Skills:

1. Problem Solving
2. Decision Making
3. Critical Thinking
4. Creative Thinking
5. Communication Skills
6. Self-Awareness
7. Empathy
8. Interpersonal Relationship
9. Management of Stress
10. Management of Emotions

District Mental Health Programme Components:

1. Training for all workers at the state institutes
2. Early detection and treatment, mental health camps

3. Health education of public to increase awareness and reduce stigma
4. Data collection, analysis for future planning of services
5. Upgrading department of Psychiatry in medical colleges
6. Research

National Water Supply & Sanitation Programme

The National Water Supply and Sanitation Programme was initiated in 1954.

Objective:

Providing safe water supply and adequate drainage facilities for the entire urban and rural population

1972 - Accelerated Rural Water Supply Programme
Central Government supports the State Governments to identify problem villages and gives assistance.

Problem Village

A village where no source of safe water is available within a distance of 1.6 km, or
Where water is available at a depth of > 15 metres, or
Where water source has excess salinity, Iron, Fluorides and other toxic elements, or
Where water is exposed to the risk of Cholera.

Minimum Needs Programme

1974-78 – The Minimum Needs Programme was introduced in the 5th Five Year Plan.

Objectives:

To provide basic minimum needs and thereby improve living standards

Components:

1. Rural Health
2. Rural Water Supply
3. Rural Electrification
4. Elementary Education
5. Adult Education
6. Nutrition
7. Environmental improvement of Urban Slums
8. Houses for landless labourers

20 Point Programme

1975 – The 20-Point Programme was initiated.

1986 – It was revised.

Objectives:

Eradication of poverty, raising productivity, reducing inequalities, removing social and economic disparities, improving quality of life

8 of the 20 points are related to health:

Point 1	Attack on Rural Poverty
Point 7	Clean Drinking Water
Point 8	Health for All
Point 9	Two Child Norm
Point 10	Education
Point 14	Housing
Point 15	Improvement of Slums
Point 17	Protection of Environment

India Demographic Profile

Total Population	1.4 billion
CBR	20.0
CDR	6.0
Annual Growth Rate	1.2%
Life expectancy at birth Male	67.3
Female	69.6
Adult Literacy Rate	74%
Male	82
Female	65
Sex Ratio	899
Population <15 yrs	25.9%
Population >60 yrs	9.0%
Age at marriage female	22.3yrs
Total Fertility Rate	1.8
Child Mortality Rate	36
IMR	32
Neonatal Mortality Rate	23
Early Neonatal Mortality Rate	18
Late Neonatal Mortality Rate	5

Post-neonatal Mortality Rate	9
Perinatal Mortality Rate	22
Annual per capita GNP (Rs)	126,521
No. of Medical Colleges	542
Sub-centres	151,684
PHCs	24,448
CHCs	5,187
Health Expenditure as % of GDP	1.1

MCH Goals & Current Level of Achievement

Indicator	Current Level	Target in NPP 2000 (2010)
A) FP Indicators		
Crude Birth Rate	21.6	21
Total Fertility Rate	2.4	2.1
Net Reproduction Rate	1.08	1.0
Couple Protection Rate %	55.0	Meet all needs
B) Mortality Indicators	178	<100
Maternal Mortality Ratio (per 100,000)	42	<30
Infant Mortality (per 1000)	31	-
Neonatal Mortality (per 1000)	52	-
Child Mortality Rate (0-4 yrs)	56	
Under 5 Mortality (per 1000)		
C) Services (% Coverage)	77	100
Infants (Fully Immunized)	74	100
Measles	72	100
DPT3	70	100
Polio3	87	100
BCG	70	100
Hepatitis B3	87	100
Pregnant Women TT	74	100
Antenatal Care at least once	37	100
At least 4x	47	10
Institutional Deliveries	52	
Deliveries by Trained Personnel	22.3	
IFA Tab x 100 days (%)	36.4	
PNC within 2 days (%)		
D) Prevalence of Low Birth Weight Babies (%)	28	

List of Public Health Interventions Provided by Government

- Antenatal care, Intranatal care, Postnatal care
- HIV Testing, Counseling, ART
- Skilled Birth Attendance and Emergency Obstetric Care
- Immunization of mother and child
- Home-based Newborn Care
- Promotion of exclusive breast feeding till 6 months
- Community-based care for sick children
- Referral of sick children to higher levels of care
- Regular treatment of Intestinal Worms in children and reproductive age women
- Iron and Folic Acid Supplements
- Universal use of Iodized Salt
- Vit A Supplementation for 9-59 months children
- Family Planning and Contraceptives, Safe Abortion Services
- Malaria Prophylaxis, LLINs, Rapid Diagnostic Kits, Treatment
- Diarrhoea Management, ORS
- TB Treatment including MDR-TB
- Leprosy Treatment
- Hepatitis B Vaccine for high-risk groups
- Health Education services
- School Health Check-up, Immunization, Treatment
- Adolescent Reproductive and Sexual Health
- Patient Transport 108

BIBLIOGRAPHY

1. Park K. Park's Textbook of Preventive and Social Medicine, 26th Ed, 2021, M/s Banarsidas Bhanot Publishers

2. Mahajan BK, Gupta MC. Textbook of Preventive and Social Medicine, 3rd Ed. 2003, Jaypee Brothers Medical Publishers (P) Ltd.

3. Shridhar Rao B. Principles of Community Medicine, 4th Ed. 2005, AITBS Publishers and Distributors

4. Prabhakara GN. Short Textbook of Preventive and Social Medicine, 2003, Jaypee Brothers Medical Publishers (P) Ltd.

5. Kulkarni AP, Bardide JP. Textbook of Community Medicine 2nd Edition, 2002, Vora Medical Publications

6. J Kishore. National Health Policies and Programs of India 11th Ed. Century Publications, 2014.

7. Mangala Subramanian. Handbook of Community Medicine 2012. Jaypee Brothers Medical Publishers (P) Ltd

8. http://www.mohfw.nic.in

9. http://www.nrhm.gov.in

www.ingramcontent.com/pod-product-compliance
Lightning Source LLC
Chambersburg PA
CBHW081102170526
45165CB00008B/2293

* 9 7 8 1 6 3 6 4 0 6 3 0 5 *